Just Health
Inequality in Illness, Care and Prevention

Edited by

Charles Waddell PhD
Senior Lecturer in Anthropology,
The University of Western Australia

Alan R. Petersen PhD
Lecturer in Sociology,
Murdoch University, Western Australia

CHURCHILL LIVINGSTONE
MELBOURNE EDINBURGH LONDON MADRID NEW YORK AND TOKYO 1994

CHURCHILL LIVINGSTONE
Medical Division of Longman Group UK Limited

Distributed in Australia by Longman Cheshire Pty Limited,
Longman House, Kings Gardens, 95 Coventry Street, South
Melbourne 3205, and by associated companies, branches and
representatives throughout the world.

© Longman Group UK Limited 1994

First published 1994

ISBN 0-443-04953-X

National Library of Australia Cataloguing in Publication Data

Just health: inequality in illness, care and prevention.

ISBN 0 443 04953 X.

1. Social medicine - Australia.   2. Health services accessibility -
Australia.   3. Right to health care - Australia.   4. Medicine,
Preventive - Australia.   I. Waddell, Charles.   II. Peterson, Alan
R.

362.10420994

Produced by Churchill Livingstone in Melbourne

Printed in Malaysia

Just Health

Acknowledgements

We thank the contributors to *Just Health*, together with the people at Churchill Livingstone, particularly Judy Waters, for their co-operation and support with the hunting, gathering and producing of this book. We also thank colleagues in our respective departments for their support during this endeavour. Finally, thanks to Ros and Greg for promoting our health and caring for our illnesses during the venture.

C.W.
A.R.P.

For Churchill Livingstone:
Publisher: Judy Waters
Co-ordinating Editor: Maja Ingrassia
Copy Editor: John Macdonald
Desktop Preparation: Sandra Tolra
Typesetting: Danny Chan
Indexing: Master Indexing
Production Control: Peter Hylands
Design: Churchill Livingstone

Contents

PART 3

Inequalities in prevention

Introduction 315

Contributors

Dorothy H. Broom PhD
Senior Research Fellow, National Centre for Epidemiology and Population Health, Australian National University, Canberra

Colette J. Browning MSc MAPsS
Lecturer in Behavioural Health Sciences, La Trobe University, Melbourne

Elizabeth Cameron-Traub PhD
Professor and Dean of Nursing, University of Technology, Sydney

Rosemary Cant MEd(WA) PhD (Newcastle)
Senior Lecturer in Health Sciences, University of Sydney

Murray Couch BA(Hons) LTh
Senior Project Officer, South Australian Occupational Health and Safety Commission

Jeanne Daly PhD
Research Fellow, La Trobe University, Melbourne

Ann E. Daniel PhD
Associate Professor, School of Sociology, The University of New South Wales, Sydney

John Duff BAHons MSc (London)
Associate Professor of Sociology, Edith Cowan University, WA

Liz Eckermann PhD
Lecturer in Sociology of Health and Illness, School of Social Inquiry, Deakin University, Geelong

Victoria M. Grace PhD
Lecturer in Feminist Studies, University of Canterbury, Christchurch NZ

Dennis Gray PhD
Senior Research Fellow, National Centre for Research into Prevention of Drug Abuse, Curtin University of Technology, Perth WA

Lindsey Harrison PhD
Lecturer in Public Health and Nutrition, University of Wollongong

Lynne Hunt BA DipEd MSc
Lecturer in Health Studies, Edith Cowan University, WA

Helen Keleher RN BA MA
Senior Lecturer in Health Studies, La Trobe University, Bendigo

Allan Kellehear PhD
Senior Lecturer in Sociology, La Trobe University, Melbourne

Hal Kendig PhD FASSA
Director, Lincoln Gerontology Centre, La Trobe University, Melbourne

Varoe Legge BA(Hons) MA PhD
Senior Lecturer in Sociology, University of Sydney

Martha MacIntyre PhD
Senior Lecturer in Anthropology, University of Melbourne

Lenore Manderson BA(Asian Studies) PhD
Professor of Tropical Health, University of Queensland Medical School

Dennis McIntyre Dip Teach (NCAE) BA(Hons)(Newcastle)
Associate Lecturer in Health Sciences, University of Sydney

Julie Mulvany BA(Hons) Dip Ed PhD
Senior Lecturer in Sociology, Swinburne University, Melbourne

Jake M. Najman PhD
Associate Professor of Anthropology and Sociology, Social and Preventive
Medicine, University of Queensland

Arthur O'Neill PhD
Teaching Fellow in Administrative, Higher and Adult Education Studies,
La Trobe University, Melbourne

Alan F. Patterson BDS, GDHSM
Director, Westmead School of Dental Therapy, Sydney

Alan R. Petersen PhD
Lecturer in Sociology, Murdoch University, WA

Janice C. Reid BSc MA (Hawai) MA (Stan.) PhD
Pro-Vice Chancellor (Academic), Queensland University of Technology

Margie Ripper PhD
Lecturer in Women's Studies, University of Adelaide

Michael W. Ross MHPEd MPH PhD
Professor of Public Health, University of Texas

Sherry Saggers PhD
Lecturer in Aboriginal and Intercultural Studies,
Edith Cowan University, WA

Leonie M. Short BA MHP
Senior Lecturer in Health Management, University of New England, Armidale NSW

Stephanie D. Short PhD
Senior Lecturer in Health Services Management, University of New South Wales

Karen Teshuva MPH
Research Fellow, Lincoln Gerontology Centre, La Trobe University, Melbourne

Gavin Turrell BA (M qual.)
PhD Candidate in Anthropology and Sociology, University of Queensland

Charles Waddell PhD
Senior Lecturer in Anthropology, The University of Western Australia

Mary T. Westbrook BA(Hons) MA(Hons) PhD
Associate Professor in Psychology, University of Sydney

John S. Western Ph D
Professor of Anthropology and Sociology, University of Queensland

Kevin White BA DipSocSci PhD
Lecturer in Sociology and Social Work, Victoria University of Wellington

Rob White PhD
Senior Lecturer in Criminology, University of Melbourne

Evan Willis PhD
Senior Lecturer in Sociology, La Trobe University, Melbourne

Prologue

The personification of sickness and death as lawless ones, ones who strike at random without regard to a person's rank, place or situation, has long been regarded as a folk myth-conception. The poor and Aboriginal or Maori people get sick most frequently and are far more likely to die prematurely than are others in Australia and New Zealand.

A parallel misconception, still widely held, is that because of their inevitability, sickness and death are primarily biological in nature. However, biological reasons do not explain the disproportional incidence of morbidity (sickness) and mortality (death) among the poor and Aboriginal or Maori people. Social reasons do.

Inequalities in illness. The rich/poor and Aboriginal/Maori/European disparities in sickness and death can be explained by the way we live with each other, the value decisions our governments, churches and businesses make in their day-to-day political and economic activities, and the priorities health officials set as they go about their duties. Sickness and death are not lawless ones, nor are they solely distributed according to biological laws. Rather the disproportional incidence of morbidity and mortality among the poor and aboriginal people is tied into the very socially unjust fabrics of Australian and New Zealand societies.

Inequalities in care. Furthermore, health resources—money, equipment and personnel—are not always distributed in the most effective manner: not enough goes to health care services other than medical care. Much more can and must be done for the 'Cinderellas' of our country—the growing number of elderly and people with chronic, terminal and mental illnesses and physical disabilities.

Inequalities in prevention. Also, what does kill us today is often referred to as 'lifestyle diseases' such as cancers and heart diseases. Not only must a greater proportion of the health budget be spent on health promotions like the Quit Smoking, Safe Sex, Fat and Alcohol Abuse campaigns that attempt to get people to adopt healthier ways of living but these programmes need to be better directed to reach those people most at risk.

The term 'lifestyle diseases' frequently conjures up the notion that people who smoke, drink excessively or are sexually promiscuous or engage in homosexual acts are solely responsible for whatever poor health they may suffer: this is the 'blame the victim' mentality. It is difficult to dismiss this notion since there frequently is an element of truth in it. Nevertheless, by and large, wealthier people live healthier lifestyles than do poorer people. Is this because wealthier people have stronger social and moral characters than do poor people or because health education reaches them better and the motivations and opportunities to adopt healthier lifestyles are more available to them? (A quick look at the characters under investigation by any current Royal Commission makes the answer obvious to all.)

Thus, lifestyle diseases are not the sole responsibility of the individual but enter the political and economic arenas of Australia and New Zealand. Politicians and business people are aware of their obligation not to seek gain by allowing harmful products to reach the consumer; indeed, increasingly they are becoming sensitive to their responsibility of promoting healthy products to ensure a healthy population.

Finally, many ill people are not treated justly by us in our everyday lives. How often do we avoid physically or mentally ill people or the elderly or dying as though they are totally alien to us?

In short, health, illness and death and the way we treat these things, are not just biological phenomena but social phenomena tied into the way we live with each other. Since health, illness and death, their care and possible prevention, are much more social than biological, a healthy life is the responsibility not only of health professionals but of all members of society. It is here in the social environment where inequalities in illness, its care and prevention largely take place and it is here where just health will be achieved. For to care for the sick and dying and do nearly nothing about those things that cause some groups of Australians or New Zealanders to get sick more often and live far fewer years than others is obscene; to feed and shelter the poor and not query the politics and economics of poverty in either country is myopic; and to run readily accessible private hospitals for the rich and leave the poor queuing for public hospitals, and not ask governments, medical associations and churches why, is irresponsible. It is only by addressing these social issues that we will improve the health of all the people of Australia and New Zealand. Towards that end *Just Health* is dedicated.

Just Health is divided into three parts: Inequalities in illness; Inequalities in care; Inequalities in prevention. However, as will become obvious as you read through the book, these divisions are largely heuristic; illness, its care and prevention are highly interrelated. A short introduction proceeds each part which serves not only to introduce the respective chapters but to put them into the larger anthro-sociological literature on health. An Epilogue further explaining how this book came about concludes *Just Health*. Its purpose, however, is not just explanation but to inspire you to engage in our anthro-sociological enterprise.

PART 1

Inequalities in illness

Introduction

Students frequently first learn about the social nature of illness by courses of study along the lines of Thomas McKeown's fascinating book, *The Origins of Human Disease*. Firstly, they learn that most diseases, except for those at or soon after fertilization, result from unhealthy ways of life and can be prevented if those ways are changed. The basics noted, the students move on to understanding the deleterious influences of human ways of life. Here, the standard fare is discussion on deficiences of resources, of which food is most important, and of natural and human-made hazards. After duly noting that health depends primarily on removal of the long standing deficiencies and hazards, students are ready for grappling with specific situations.

The menu will vary considerably at this point in the course's polemics, but for anthropologists it typically includes hunters and gatherers: here, the students learn that non-communicable diseases were rare and morbidity and premature mortality were due largely to environmental hazards and to food deficiency leading to starvation or malnutrition and infection. For early agriculturalists students again learn that non-communicable diseases were rare, but that as size and density of stationary populations increased so too did unhygienic conditions, inadvertently giving rise to infectious diseases as the predominant cause of morbidity and premature death. Sociologists, on the other hand, may typically note that with industrialization, food supply and hygienic conditions increased but that the human way of life became far removed from that under which humans evolved; as a result, non-communicable diseases such as cancers and strokes, displaced infections as the common causes of disease and premature death.

At the end of the course nearly everyone involved is usually pleased except the esoteric creationist to whom none would listen, the biological determinist who entered the course by mistake and, of course, the students who received bad grades. The doctor-bashers are pleased with the course because it seemingly shows (in an apparently sophisticated manner) the irrelevance of medicine to improving human health; the more tender hearted are pleased because it shows the relevance (and possible employment potential) of social scientists in helping to remove environmental deficiencies and hazards; and the lecturer is satisfied because it is always a delight to query if disease is really an escapable reality of human life. If examples of the social aetiology of

3

disease have been judiciously selected, and the discussion has been lively, it may go entirely unnoticed that something crucial has been left out, that somehow the essence of human health has been discarded with the anthro-sociological bathwater.

To see that this is the case, that the critical essence of human health has not been achieved in the described course, one needs only to reflect upon the situations and dispositions of the many intelligent and perceptive people who, even without disease, visit the doctor. There's the long suffering woman, an expert on childhood diseases, routinely visiting her GP for stress as though it was some biological entity. There's an accomplished business-man, deeply schooled in efficiency, acting as though his GP can cure his obesity, alcoholism and inactivity. And it is not impossible to find astute anthropologists and sociologists, who would never dream of asserting fact from deconstructed text, faithfully cluttering up doctors' waiting rooms without the slightest shred of evidence to support their hope of magic tablets to fix their aches, pains and cramps.

For the few who concern themselves with this phenomenon, there is no lack of social and psychological theories which purport to explain these medical junkies. We may airily dismiss fraudulent use of GPs as socialist by-products of the medicare system or as ideological whitewash to cope with economic recession.

On the other hand, not all so-called fraudulent use of GPs is causally dependent upon weaknesses in the national health system nor upon feelings of stress in a recession. GP junkies are simply too diverse to be explained by any single theory, if that theory is to be defended on empirical rather than metaphysical ground.

For the purposes of this book, a major criticism of both the polemics outlined above and the theories just mentioned is that both operate on the false assumption that being healthy is centrally a matter of avoiding disease. Thus, to be unhealthy is to have a disease; having a disease is the proper reason to see a doctor. This analysis is neat and concise, yields measure of morbidity and mortality for epidemiologists, and has the widespread support of medical officialdom.

Of course it is often true that unhealthy people have a disease but there are several reasons for rejecting this fact as the fundamental difference between the healthy and unhealthy, let alone the essence of health. One is that prior to 1950, no one died of what is called cystic fibrosis; after cystic fibrosis was defined, hundreds of people did. If diseases are socially constructed through scientific discourse, then it seems possible that healthy infants may not be distinguishable by a disease from unhealthy infants.

A second reason for refusing to divide the healthy from the unhealthy by disease is that this position leaves the stance of some very ill people both unexplained and inexplicable. There is the case of the chronic fatigue sufferer, who feels unhealthy but has no diagnosed disease. If a person may be ill without any clearly defined disease, then it seems possible that this person may be unhealthy despite medical science's disease ontology.

Another case is the mature, well educated and psychologically sound person who may have a disease but feels healthy. Cancers and the human immunodeficiency virus (HIV) may appear dormant in a person for years without causing unhealthy symptoms or being clinically detected. It may be true that having these diseases may cause premature death, but this consideration does not obviate the distinction between having a disease and feeling unhealthy.

All these cases show that the reason for being ill remains mysterious as long as we continue to assume that its essence is having a disease. A more productive approach, and the crucial missing link in the opening course outline, begins with regarding health and non-health as social entities, with central emphasis on the notion that they are socially constructed — in our heads and in our bodies. Disease is surely involved, but the heart of the matter lies deeper, in each individual's sense of personal identity and worth; in each individual's fundamental perspective on the world of his or her experience and in the value priorities each individual establishes by living and making choices from day to day. And these individual things do not happen in isolation, as the readings in this section show; rather they come from society and culture and from one's particular location within this milieu. Lenore Manderson and Janice Reid present a number of vignettes to illustrate the complex interactions of culture and immigrant health. Jake Najman focuses on the effects that one's location in the class structure has on health. Rob White, Dennis McIntyre and Murray Couch each focus on the relationship between occupation and health. Social class has become such an important determinant of health that elaborate conceptual and empirical strategies have been devised with which to measure it as Gavin Turrell, John Western and Jake Najman illustrate. Margie Ripper's chapter shows the health inequalities women experience due to gender biases in medical explanations of illness. Finally, Dennis Gray and Sherry Saggers discuss structural and cultural factors effecting the health of Aboriginal people.

Besides illustrating the social aetiology and inequality of illness, these readings easily lead into Parts 2 and 3 of this book: Inequalities in care and in prevention.

REFERENCE

McKeown T 1988 The origins of human disease. Blackwell, Oxford

1. What's culture got to do with it?

Lenore Manderson   Janice C. Reid

This chapter draws on research undertaken with immigrant Australians over the past decade. It is written drawing upon a number of case studies and vignettes to illustrate the complex interactions of culture and health.[1] Sometimes, as we show, the interaction or influence of culture on health is highly significant: in influencing food choice, cooking style, and diet, for instance, it is for many people a major protective factor against ischaemic heart disease. On the other hand, the importance of culture is often overstated, and at times it is unclear whether the incidence of infection or development of disease, or quality of treatment, is due to or determined by sex, class, race, ethnicity or other factors.

The cultural production of illness

In the discussion which follows, focusing on the ways in which culture influences health, we use Linton's (1940) definition of culture: 'the sum total of knowledge, attitudes, and habitual behaviour patterns shared and transmitted by members of a particular society' (in Keesing 1981:68). More recent anthropological definitions are similar to this, and include the material base and economic activities of a particular group of people as well as their values, ideas, and institutions. All of these are learned and shared.

Kleinman, in his writings on the cultural construction and clinical manifestations of suffering, distinguishes between illness and disease. *Illness* is defined as the 'human experience of symptoms and suffering' including the physical dimensions (e.g. having a headache, feeling nauseous) and the social and behavioural consequences (e.g. taking drugs, not being able to work). *Disease*, in contrast, is the physiological (or psychological) pathology—'an alteration in biological structure or functioning' (Kleinman 1988:3–6). The experiences of health and illness, understandings of the aetiology of disease, and the diagnosis, treatment and expected outcome (prognosis) of ill health, are all culturally shaped.[2] But to understand the epidemiology of a disease, we need to take into account both the biological and social risk factors of infection, pathology, or disability. Heart disease is a good example of this. The risk of developing heart disease is influenced by family history (genetic predisposition), diet, exercise, stress (including individual responses), and perhaps personality type, together with culturally based appreciations of the significance of heart disease (for example, as a treatable condition, death sentence or chronic illness), and different views about appropriate treatment and responses to rehabilitation (e.g. Kleinman 1988).

Anthropologists maintain that the natural world, including bodily dysfunction, is known, understood, interpreted and mediated by culture. Thus peoples from different cultures may have very different perceptions of a particular disease, its cause or appropriate treatment, and may cluster together and give different weight to various signs and symptoms of illness, and give different significance to afflictions in different parts of the body.[3]

Prior experience of an illness, personally or within the wider community, may lead to different assessments and subsequent action, including with respect to the care of the sick person and the treatment of any underlying pathology. Measles, for instance, was regarded in Australia in the 1950s and 1960s as 'normal', and young children would be intentionally exposed to ensure that they 'caught it while they're young'.[4] Immunization and greater familiarity with the sequelae of measles in Australia has lead to a greater concern to prevent infection (through immunization). In other societies, measles still causes high mortality and women justifiably regard it as a serious illness which results in high mortality of infants and small children (Aaby 1990). Conversely the dramatic reduction in the incidence of such diseases as diphtheria and poliomyelitis in the last 30–40 years in Australia has meant that fewer adults have seen their effects and this has led to some young parents failing to have children immunized—and also to a belief among some that immunization holds greater risks than the disease itself.

Culture-specific syndromes

The so-called 'culture-bound' or 'culture-specific' syndromes are the most dramatic examples of the cultural elaboration of bodily dysfunctions and feelings of ill health. The aetiology, symptoms and management of particular named illnesses appear to be unique to particular cultures or settings (Rubel 1977, Pow 1977), although such health problems may exist in other settings (e.g. following migration), since individuals carry with them their culturally based beliefs, ideas and understandings. A variety of health problems have been described as culture-bound syndromes; in western cultures these include obesity, anorexia nervosa and bulimia (Rittenbaugh 1982, Prince 1983).

Susto is the prototypical example of a culture-bound syndrome. *Susto*, 'soul loss' or 'magical fright', occurs throughout Latin America and is characterized by disturbed or restless sleep patterns, loss of appetite, listlessness, loss of interest in personal appearance and attention to personal hygiene, and feelings of depression. Its treatment, undertaken usually by a *curandero*, involves diagnostic and curing sessions that are aimed to remove illness and encourage the soul to return to the body (Rubel 1977, Helman

1984: 158–160). In Latin America, *susto* is found among both Indian and non-Indian communities, but it occurs also among Hispanic Americans in the United States. In Australia, too, immigrants from Latin America may suffer from *susto*, but generally must manage their symptoms without the help of culturally appropriate healers (Allotey 1992).

However, *susto* and similar illnesses of 'loss of soul' or 'fright' might in other contexts be described as instances of depression or anxiety, and there is considerable debate about the accuracy of describing any illness as 'culture-bound'. In many instances their discrete existence ceases as we learn more about them and are able to establish the underlying biological basis or physical pathology that results in certain behaviours or signs (Hahn 1985, Landy 1985). In other cases the underlying disorder (e.g. depression) may occur cross-culturally, although the expression of the disorder and social responses to it are culturally patterned. Folk understandings of the cause of the illness will be concordant with a general understanding of bodily function, health and illness.

Folk interpretations

Culture-specific syndromes provide a striking example of the way in which culture patterns illness. Folk interpretations of the signs and symptoms of illness are universal, though they are less readily recognized and interpreted when they occur within a familiar cultural framework. Medical information is always filtered through existing knowledge and beliefs, whether in urban western settings ('feed a cold, starve a fever') or in rural Vietnam ('a woman should not eat 'hot' foods postpartum'). Action is taken on the basis of the understandings formed at the intersection of professional and lay knowledge and experience. People may understand hypertension, for example, as 'too much tension' or stress, or high blood pressure as 'too much blood' (Snow 1976, Kleinman 1988: 132–134). Commonsense understandings are derived from the diagnostic terminology, sometimes leading to confusion and misunderstanding (for example, the difference between hypertension and 'hyper-tension'), or they are derived from the explanations offered by health professionals to patients of particular dysfunctions or pathology. For example:

Nurse: Your baby's got jaundice and he's got to go under the lights.
Mother: Why?
Nurse: Because he has immature kidneys and there's a high level of bilirubin; sunshine washes it out but the lights speed it up. I'll take him now.
Mother: No. I don't understand. Sunshine doesn't *wash*. Explain it to me properly.
Nurse: I can't explain it to you any more simply (Manderson, 1984).

In a multicultural society such as Australia, where individuals may recognize and respond to perceived ill health in a variety of ways and as a consequence of very different understandings of the 'normal' and the pathological, the possibilities for misunderstanding are manifold. Cross-cultural interactions between health professionals and their clients often highlight the problems of communication, with both parties making certain assumptions about the other's perceptions and interpretation of symptoms within their own cultural or professional frame of reference. Good and Good (1981), for instance, describe the case of a Mexican-American woman who rang the hospital for emergency assistance terrified that her baby was going to die because its fontanel appeared to be depressed—a sign of a traditional Mexican illness category *caida de la mollera* or 'fallen fontanel'. Notwithstanding an explanation by the resident on duty when the mother brought the baby to Emergency that there were no signs of impending brain damage, the mother continued to believe that her baby was in danger.

Whilst cultural practices, beliefs, values and institutions are important components of the experience of illness, these in turn are shaped by wider social, political, institutional and economic factors. The incidence of *susto*, for example, may itself be a reflection of personal and social factors, such as stress and anxiety related to migration, family breakdown, unemployment, or poverty. See, for example, the case of Celia, a Mexican-American school-girl from a broken family, diagnosed by a traditional healer as having *susto* after she developed gastrointestinal symptoms and refused to go to school (Stafford 1978).

Seeking the appropriate healer

Where people hold to an understanding of illness that differs from that of the health professionals they consult, then they may consult not only western medical practitioners but practitioners of other therapeutic traditions. The case of Dr Wong (Tang 1990) illustrates this. Dr Wong suffered from lower back pain diagnosed as being due to ligament and soft tissue damage to his spine. Rest did not resolve the pain. Subsequently over a period of eighteen months he had physiotherapy, manipulation, traction, facet joint injecting and epidural injections, without improvement, further inconclusive diagnostic tests, then referral to a psychologist. Wong's condition deteriorated.

> This led him in turn to traditional Chinese medicine. After a few consultations, he took up *Qigong*. In addition, he underwent a course of acupuncture, massage, moxibustion and herbal medicine...(and) was diagnosed as having suffered from *'yang* deficiency through a blockage of *qi'*. He was told that while undergoing Chinese medical treatment he should initially rest in bed for at least 100 days (Tang 1990: 27).

The presence of traditional or alternative therapists, or access to remedies other than pharmaceuticals (e.g. herbs, tonics and other mixtures to be ingested, inhaled or applied topically), enable people to self-medicate or present to the most appropriate practitioner on the basis of their own cultural readings or diagnosis of signs and symptoms of illness. There is a good deal of ethnographic evidence that where there is choice in health care options, people will seek relief for symptoms pragmatically, using treatments which are efficacious from both traditional and western medical systems. Their own models of illness, however, may remain unchallenged by those of the other culture—thus, they may continue to believe that an illness is due to 'evil eye', sorcery or supernatural forces whilst utilizing a range of different treatments (see Landy 1977, Section XIV).

Whose culture?

Within Australia, suppositions about the role of culture in health and illness behaviour take place—sometimes tacitly—in the context of discussions of the health of immigrant Australians (Bottomley & de Lepervanche 1990: 66–68, cf. Eisenbruch & Handelman 1990, Eisenbruch 1991). In contrast the health and illness behaviour of Anglo-Australians is presumed to be culture-free. Their health beliefs, actions, and outcomes are seen as determined 'scientifically' and objectively, in keeping with the theory and practice of biomedicine.[5] People who, by virtue of their name, first language, country of birth, race, or ethnic identity are regarded as different are therefore presumed to present distinctive problems, needs and challenges in terms of their access to and use of health services and their compliance with treatments and interventions. In ethnic health policies and programs, these cultural and personal variables are often collapsed to issues of language or more broadly to communication. Issues of access to, and use of, health services are often considered able to be resolved through the provision of translated information, interpreter services, and training for various health workers in cross-cultural communication.

Recognition of the heterogeneity of immigrant Australia and the distinctive social, cultural and linguistic background of clients of health services is critical in health care encounters. However, much of the literature and discussion by health professionals and policy makers about migrant health has given greater attention to cultural difference than to other factors that may also be significant in understanding patterns of sickness such as social isolation, poverty, age, gender or immigrant status. Broader political and economic considerations influence both health services and our knowledge of particular groups. For example, researchers have tended to work with those peoples most recently arrived, who for reasons of language or ethnic background may be considered most different from Anglo-Australian society (e.g. not speaking English as a first language, not being Christian, and so on); and their 'differences' might be relevant to the Australian government with respect to service provision, social adjustment, integration within the community, and health and illness (Garrett & Lin 1990, Lin & Pearse 1990). On this basis, the most recent immigrant community has tended to be the one whose health and other social welfare, educational and economic problems are under scrutiny—Italian and Greek migrants in the 1950s, for example; the Turkish community in the late 1960s and early 1970s; Vietnamese in the 1980s—with shifts of subject community reflecting shifts in the source countries of Australian migrants. Earlier immigrant communities will become the subject of new topics of research—for example, 'the care of the ethnic aged' as large numbers of these earlier groups retire and age (McCallum & Lerba 1989, McCallum 1990, Thomas not dated)—whilst other topics of research again focus on the perceived health needs of the most recent arrivals.[6]

Defining the community

It is important to note the way in which different groups of immigrants have been presented and their health priorities identified in health policies and in academic or professional publications. Research into the Turkish community, for example, has been largely concerned with return migration and occupational mobility, not with access to health services, although there is no prima facie evidence to suggest that Eastern Turkish peasant migrants without knowledge of English are better served by Australian health services than say, Lao refugees. Similarly, mental health amongst the Indochinese refugee community has received rather more attention than the Lebanese immigrant community, for example, although again without reason to suggest that war, trauma or fear were experienced less by many in the latter community. Whilst some recent work highlights the commonality of the experiences of torture and trauma, common health needs, and common responses to conventional health services (Reid & Strong 1987, Allotey 1992), the literature on mental health often emphasizes instead cultural aspects without regard to such issues as lack of community support, social isolation and poverty (e.g. Eisenbruch 1991).

Much of the work to date has made light of differences within groups, dissolving cultural specificity under general terms (e.g. Southern Europeans, Indochinese), and has concentrated on particular health issues whilst others are disregarded. Only recently have researchers begun to distinguish within groups, to write not of Indochinese but of Hmong, Lao, Khmer, Vietnamese-Chinese, and Vietnamese, and to distinguish between urban and rural dwellers, peasant farmers and professionals. Such ethnic, class and geographic differences are themselves a short-hand for major differences in native and second languages, cultural practice, belief systems, familiarity with, access to, and use of health services, educational levels, income and prior and present class position. These factors are all relevant to how people think of illness and health, and what they do—in terms of diagnosis, treatment advice and medication—when they are sick.

Expectations of difference

Writers on migrant health have tended to characterize people in terms of certain behavioural traits (Martin 1978:162), resulting in neglect of the complex sets of factors that influence individual's histories, current social and economic circumstances, their health status, and their access to and use of various health services. Scholarly and popular writings about Indochinese communities, for example, have been influenced by the concern of health professionals with mental health problems following dislocation through war and trauma, and a genuine concern by government to ease the difficulties of immigration and settlement.[7] Certain cultural differences among Vietnamese, Lao and Cambodian immigrants may affect health behaviour, of course, but expectations of differences tend to derive from various dated ethnographies based on fieldwork undertaken many years ago in the country of origin (Manderson 1990) and these have led professionals, bureaucrats and students of the immigrant experience to presume that there would be problems of adaptation to Australian institutions and social organisations. Obvious areas of difference in behaviour and understanding, resulting in conflict within the health care system, reinforce these expectations, although such conflicts need to be and are easily resolved (Manderson & Mathews 1985, Hopper 1992). The following is an example of this:

Inner city maternity hospital wards in the early 1980s were concerned with the refusal of Vietnamese women postpartum to eat fruit and vegetables, and their reluctance to get up and move around. On enquiry it was found that their reluctance was influenced by humoral medical theory, according to which women postpartum were in a state of extreme 'cold' and should therefore only eat 'hot' food which would restore the humoral balance to a state of equilibrium. Failure to do so might result in ill health at a later date. Similarly, women's reluctance to move about related to fear of being exposed to draughts and 'catching cold', again because of vulnerability due to humoral imbalance. Hospital dietitians when apprised of this were able to modify meals to provide a range of nutritional foods that the women would eat, that both met their needs and the dietitians' own notions of a 'balanced diet', and hospital staff were able to adjust their expectations of women's activities after giving birth (for background information, see Manderson & Mathews 1981, Mathews & Manderson 1981).

Often, the stereotypes of immigrants used to explain their health problems are simply ahistorical. Locke (1985: 1332–6), for example, asserts that Vietnamese women are 'accorded low status in society', that their status and home life are threatened by their participation in the paid work force in Australia, and that they are distrustful of Western medicine, hospitals and surgery and so are reluctant to seek medical attention even in potentially life threatening circumstances. Along the same lines, Boman and Edwards (1984) write of Vietnamese distrust of Western medicine, reluctance to accept hospitalization, and class-consciousness, the women again isolated and subjugated to men. In these representations, the observers often present culture as fixed and resistant to change, taking normative statements as reflections of practice, and presuming that the population is homogenous. Writings such as these say to us, 'This is what all Vietnamese are like'.

Such accounts associate culture or ethnic background, different medical traditions, and the presence of alternative medical systems with poor use of Australian health services, whilst underestimating the immediate causes of various patterns of use and failing to take account of the fact that most immigrants, from Vietnam and elsewhere, are quite familiar with hospital based medicine and biomedical care. The 'class conscious' Vietnamese working as unskilled labourers upon migration to Australia include qualified doctors and allied health workers. Their low utilization of Australian health services or failure to comply with suggested medical treatment may not relate to unfamiliarity with western biomedicine, but to a limited understanding of the health system in Australia. Language difficulties also affect access to health services: Chak et al (1984), for example, in their study of Indochinese families using hospital medical services in Brisbane, suggested that only 21% were able to communicate satisfactorily without assistance from an interpreter.

Immigrants may also experience discrimination and depersonalization in some health interventions, which would discourage their future use. The first contact many refugees have with the Australian health care system is compulsory screening immediately after arrival, for diseases of public health significance such as tuberculosis, STDs and malaria. This is not an experience which would necessarily leave a positive impression. Reid et al (1986: 271) comment that 'we frequently heard, from observers and visitors the view that it (the screening program) is like a cattleyard or a sausage factory with people entering at one end, being processed and extruded at the other'.

When culture makes a difference

Our understandings of immigrants are largely politically and socially constructed, built upon presumptions of what a particular people are like rather than on empirical data of the experience and behaviours of those people. We need to take account far more of the ways in which health status is influenced by social and economic as well as cultural factors. Employment (or its absence), occupation and industry, income, education, residential patterns, age and gender may all influence the incidence of disease, injury or disability, and access to and use of health services (see also Lewins 1984:30). The experience of medical and rehabilitative services of an elderly Anglo-Australian woman pensioner may in the most important ways be indistinguishable from that of an elderly Polish woman suffering the same injury.

This is not to deny the importance of culture, nor the need for health professionals to understand the ways in which culture might affect health outcomes. At all points along the line, from the point of transmission of infection, development of symptoms or sustaining an injury, and throughout the course of the illness, culture is a variable. Patterns of diet and exercise, attitudes to our bodies, our ability to recognize and react to signs of sickness, our choice of healers, our willingness to follow treatment advice, and the resources and supports that are available and that may promote or retard speedy recovery, are all influenced by culture as well as social, economic and political factors.

Food habits, diet and disease

Culture can be an important risk factor or determinant of disease, or conversely, it may be protective (Webb & Manderson 1990:161–170). For example, although diet is certainly influenced by the availability of food in the market place and by family income and expenditure patterns, cultural background is a major influence on food choice and eating behaviour, including food preferences and food avoidances, cooking styles, menu composition, variety in diet and the nutritional balance of meals. These in turn affect individual risk of developing certain diseases such as diabetes, some cancers, and cardiovascular disease (Webb & Manderson 1990).

Considerable change occurs following migration. Although the rates of ischaemic heart disease and diseases of the circulatory system tend to be lower among most immigrants from non-English speaking backgrounds than among Anglo-Australians, shifts towards Australian eating patterns and behaviour (sedentary lifestyle, smoking and so on) have occurred and all increase the risk of hypertension and heart disease (Powles & Gifford 1990). Middle-class Anglo-Australians have changed their diet away from fatty foods and refined sugar in response to health education, leading to a decline in the death rate from ischaemic heart disease. But over the same time period, the rate of ischaemic heart disease among immigrants, for example among southern European men (Wise et al 1990), has increased, and this appears to relate to the fact that most immigrants, regardless of country of origin, increase their consumption of meats, sugar, butter and other high fat dairy products following migration, while decreasing their consumption of cereals, vegetables, and sometimes also fish and fruit (Webb & Manderson 1990).

Powles and colleagues, for example, document the nature of dietary change following migration within one community (Greek) and their work provides further evidence of protective aspects of a 'traditional' diet (Powles et al 1988, Powles 1990). This study compared food consumption of immigrant and non-immigrant siblings. Non-immigrants consumed twice the amount of vegetables, fruit and alcoholic beverages, but only half the amount of meat of immigrants; in particular non-immigrants ate more leafy vegetables, cheese, eggs and olive oil whilst their immigrant siblings ate more margarine, more milk and ice-cream, and more meat (chicken, lamb and beef).

The behaviour here is not 'cultural' in terms of culture of origin, but is one of a shift of culture and the availability and costs of different foodstuffs, with dietary modification so that food consumption patterns are nearer to those of most Anglo-Australians. In addition, however, socioeconomic factors (i.e. being poor) may affect food habits, purchases and consumption patterns. Poor people, regardless of ethnicity or place of birth, tend to eat cheaper, more fatty foods and refined sugar (Health Targets and Implementation Committee 1988).

Traditional diets are not always advantageous. The case of Mr L.A.

(Hoskins 1990), a 67-year-old Portuguese man, illustrates the way in which cultural practices—including diet, smoking and drinking—may be implicated in the development and management of diabetes.

Mr L.A. had developed non-insulin dependent diabetes six years earlier, but his condition had deteriorated and he now required insulin therapy. He was still smoking 30 cigarettes a day, drinking up to 2 litres of wine per day, and eating a traditional diet high in salt and fat. As Hoskins notes, the difficulties that faced the health worker advising Mr L.A. included the fact that he and his compatriots would not regard the amount of alcohol consumed to be excessive, were unaware of the risks of smoking, and would reject a new diet that required major changes to a cooking style that represented important cultural links. In addition, Hoskins points out that Mr L.A. and many others would perceive the need for insulin therapy as a 'death sentence', had a poor understanding of the chronic nature of diabetes, and would be reluctant to discuss other related health issues such as the development of impotence (Hoskins 1990: 41–42).

Kinship and perceptions of women

Adherence to a traditional diet is often protective. But other 'traditional' or 'cultural' factors may not be so beneficial. A recent article by de Costa (1988), for example, draws attention to the high perinatal mortality rate and high incidence of birth abnormalities among Lebanese women. She describes Lebanese women as isolated by language and limited social and medical interaction, ground down by frequent pregnancies, and at risk from repeated caesarean sections. The paper significantly links birth abnormalities to cultural practice: that of marriages to close relatives such as cousins. Other discussions of the health of Lebanese women draw attention to their high crude birth rate and fertility rate (Yusuf 1986) which is implicated in the high rate of birth complications such as anaemia and antepartum haemorrhage (de Costa 1988).

In addition, health care providers speak of women's poor attendance and late presentation at clinics and their reluctance to allow internal examinations, as well as less specific, supposedly cultural values and beliefs, affecting behaviour during pregnancy and birth (Hickey et al 1991:2). However, these comments need to be read against other more positive portrayals of women's lives. Hickey et al (1991), for example, note the support that many Lebanese women say they enjoy from husbands and relatives during pregnancy and postpartum. Their study does not substantiate assertions that women do not present for medical care when pregnant, although women in this study did delay presentation at the public antenatal clinic. The explanations offered for this are instructive:

Do you think it's important to see a doctor when you're pregnant? (Yes) Why?
To be certain that I'm pregnant and to be sure everything is OK. It's very important, if something happens, all of a sudden happens, the doctors won't have any of the details (if you don't come). Tests will be done, I have a sister-in-law, she was five months pregnant, and she had a stillbirth. She didn't think she had to

go to a doctor for her pregnancy. Even when you're pregnant just two months, you have to go. It's safer. You'll feel more comfortable, you'll know what's happening. My sister-in-law, she had a hard lesson to learn. She learned the hard way (Hickey et al 1991:17).

But women's reluctance to attend antenatal sessions reveals how culture and class coincide in clinical settings, and underline a commonality in the experience of public patients whether they be Anglo-Australian, Lebanese, or other:

> I choose to go see a private doctor because...when I used to go and see the doctor in the clinic...they give you an appointment to go and see a doctor. So we go there thinking we will be examined by only one doctor. So they'll ask you to lie down on the bed, so they (put in) the speculum when they examine you internally, and one doctor goes and one comes, and the sisters and the student doctors. And if you say I'm in pain or I don't want these things, they'll say, well you don't have a say because you're coming here as a clinic patient (Hickey et al 1991:18).

In general, the women interviewed in this study were motivated primarily to ensure the best possible outcome of pregnancy. Similarly, a report on the health status of Vietnamese women in Brisbane indicated that women made reasonable use of antenatal and child health services, although their knowledge of services appeared to be limited, and they were reluctant to present with certain health problems which they regarded as embarrassing (e.g. vaginal infections and haemorrhoids) (Tran 1991). For these women, lack of mobility, lack of family encouragement, and domestic and work obligations all affected their access to services and potential participation in health courses. Suppositions are made frequently of women from various immigrant communities, about their relative (and sometimes simply presumed) lack of mobility, their lack of economic independence, and their subordination, but discussions of the status of women have often been insensitive and ill-informed, focusing on sensational cases (such as female circumcision) or emphasizing their isolation. Community reluctance to be identified with practices subject to disapprobation by the wider community has lead also to a silencing of other health problems and issues, such as that of domestic violence, no less common a problem among immigrant communities than the Australian-born population (see e.g. Hetzel 1990).

Encounters in the clinic

The impact of culture on health is perhaps most marked in health care settings, the point at which interaction between peoples from different cultural (and social) backgrounds occurs. Experiences with health services, as well as the conditions of daily life that provide the context of health and illness, vary considerably according to a range of factors, including ethnicity and culture. Misunderstandings and difficulties in communication, and lack of knowledge of the range of health services, may result in the under-utilization of clinical services, although in some circumstances immigrant groups are said to over- rather than under-utilize services. Figures from the 1983 Australian Health Survey (Australian Bureau of Statistics 1984), for instance, indicate that both men and women of all ages from non-English speaking backgrounds are less likely to take 'health-related action', but this covers any health action, including self-medication (vitamins, other supplements, prescribed and over-the-counter pharmaceuticals) and, presumably, resort to alternative practitioners. Persons from non-English speaking backgrounds are in fact more likely to consult with a doctor: this might reflect either higher utilization of professionals or higher morbidity rates in the population.

In clinical encounters, both the importance and, paradoxically, the irrelevance of culture are highlighted. The following case study illustrates this point:

Clara, a young woman who had recently arrived in Australia from El Salvador, found she was expecting a child to her boyfriend, who had been unable to follow her to Australia. Clara had emigrated with her sister and brother-in-law, but had left their home to take up a position as a housekeeper after the brother-in-law had become abusive. When she went into labour she was admitted to a large public maternity hospital and the baby was born uneventfully. She shared a public ward with several other immigrant women, a common experience in this hospital which had a catchment population in which 60% were overseas-born of non-English speaking background, or the children of overseas-born. Within a day Clara complained to nursing staff of discomfort, nausea and feeling unwell. Her complaints were disregarded and no examination was made. She complained the following day, and an examination revealed a severely prolapsed cervix. She was told that nothing could be done, and that it would improve slowly. The following day, again, she complained of feeling ill and she was feverish. On the fourth day her sister, who was medically trained, visited her, and complained to nurses that she could 'smell' an infection. At this point the researcher (Australian-born) became involved too, and complained to the medical director of the hospital; investigation revealed a puerperal infection and a course of antibiotics was commenced (Reid 1989).

This case illustrates the difficulty of invoking culture to explain the vagaries of the quality of health care. While Clara was an immigrant and while staff may have been predisposed to ignore her complaints because she was not an articulate middle-class Anglo-Australian, it is equally true that she was a public patient in a large teaching hospital and prejudice was just as likely to be based on class as ethnicity. The hospital staff did not learn until the situation was serious that Clara's sister was a medical graduate and that the researcher was a university professor, and these two social facts, as much as the signs and symptoms of illness, finally prompted action.

Our fieldnotes from a variety of research projects provide corroborative evidence of the powerlessness of most patients in hospitals, regardless of language or cultural background, although it is also true that staff tend to ignore or 'speak over' patients from non-English speaking backgrounds because they presume (often falsely) that English is not understood. Further, regardless of ethnicity, women perceive that they are disadvantaged and poorly treated in clinical settings. Discussions concerning presentation to hospitals and compliance by women from non-English speaking backgrounds draw attention to women's subordination to men and their 'modesty' as a barrier to health care. However, such suppositions fail to take account of the fact that this 'modesty'—a reluctance to be examined by male doctors—is shared by many women, regardless of ethnicity, who are dissatisfied with the health services provided to them, feel that they are denied information, treated summarily, and do not have an adequate choice of care, including the choice of female rather than male doctors (Australia, Department of Community Services and Health 1989).

Error and ignorance

The difficulty in establishing the relative role played by ethnicity and class is evident also in the following example, where an immigrant mother faces both a social worker and a doctor. In this case, professional support is compromised as a consequence of unfamiliarity with a racial characteristic:

An Afghani woman living in Sydney, already a mother of a 14 month old child, gave birth to twins by caesarean section. Her husband was overseas, so home help was arranged to assist her on return home with the babies. Six weeks after her return home, one of the twins was admitted to hospital with a respiratory tract infection. Monitoring of the family after the discharge of the sick infant indicated that breast feeding had failed, that the infants were being bottle fed, and that the older child was jealous and difficult to manage. At this point, the social worker called in, unexpectedly, with a doctor, to take all three babies into custody on the grounds of child abuse and to 'give the mother a rest'. The evidence of abuse were 'bruises' on the babies—Mongolian spots (Rudolph 1987: 838) that are character-istic discoloration on the lower back of most Asian infants. Neither the Australian doctor nor social worker had seen these bluish marks before, did not know that they were a racial feature and that they faded, and were unwilling to listen to or accept the mother's explanation of their significance (Manderson 1989).

This extract suggests the need for the Australian professional health commu-nity to be better informed in order to deliver health care to people of backgrounds different from their own. But again the lives of this woman and her children were influenced by individual circumstance (a poor single mother with three children under the age of 15 months) as well as cultural factors. Apart from the misinterpretation of the markings, there is little to suggest that an Australian-born woman in the same circumstances would have fared better. On the basis of the fieldnotes, too, we cannot assume that the social worker was influenced by the woman's ethnic background, although the literature in general highlights the way in which racism predetermines professional/ client encounters and interventions, as well as determining the social, economic and physical environments that are the preconditions of their poor health (Bottomley & de Lepervanche 1990).

'Over-reading' culture

Interactions in health settings draw attention to the differences between health professionals and patients of other cultures in interpreting illnesses and in responding to pain, disability and care. Differences in perceptions and the articulation of pain are an interesting example of this. Each culture has its own 'language of distress' or means by which the experience of pain or discomfort are communicated to others, and the form of this pain behaviour, as well as response to it, are culturally determined (Helman 1984:99, Parsons & Wakeley 1991, Wolff & Langley 1977). In clinical settings where such cultural differences are not well understood, this has led to considerable misunderstanding of individual patient behaviour and response. For example, health professionals have assumed different levels of pain tolerance based on whether the patient did or did not verbalize reaction to pain. In maternity hospitals, in the past much more so than today, nurses would compare the vocal or non-vocal responses of different immigrant women in labour, with the behaviour of Anglo-Australian women (presumed to be 'normal' and normative). They assumed that Southern European women were 'exaggerating' labour pain (and did not recognize vocalization as a means of pain management, for instance), or that Indochinese women who were relatively quiet 'don't feel pain like we do' (and ignored non-vocalized expressions of pain) (Manderson 1981).

In cross-cultural contexts, culture is often presumed to be the major or determining factor in the encounter. The case of Tessa Martin (Parsons 1990, Parsons & Najman, 1990) illustrates how culture can be inappropriately presumed to be important in the aetiology and management of sickness, in Tessa's case a suspected brain tumour that finally led to her death.

Tessa Martin was the daughter of a working-class Maori family. After a period of several months characterized by prolonged sleeping and social withdrawal, she was admitted to a Brisbane hospital for medical tests. A dispute developed between doctors and Tessa's family over appropriate therapy and care. The family, represented in the press as believing that their daughter was 'under an evil spell', were concerned at the lack of information that they were given regarding the child's care, discontinued her sedation because she seemed 'like a zombie', and refused permission for the administration of an 'experimental drug' without a clear diagnosis and reason for the course of action. Failure to return Tessa to medical care led to a court case which placed her in temporary custody. She died within two months, without any abnormality or pathology being detected.

Conflict between the child's parents, extended family and community, the doctors and the police was precipitated by the failure of the consulting physician to meet with and negotiate treatment with the child's family, exacerbated by media reportage which construed the family as culturally deviant, believing in evil spells and black magic, and magnified by police action (reports of child abuse, and forcible removal of the child which was broadcast around Australia on the evening news). The case highlights not so much the cultural basis of the child's illness or her care—there is no evidence of this—but presumptions of cultural difference which resulted in 'mis-communication and conflict, therapeutic mismanagement, non-compliance, and dissatisfaction of both clients and health professionals' (Parsons 1990:148).

Compliance and response

The Tessa Martin case highlights the ways individuals understand, interpret and comply with or reject advice. Misunderstanding, disagreement, differing interpretations or personal circumstances result not only in people refusing to comply, but also in rejecting medical recommendations or altering prescribed treatment regimes or doses of medicine. Consider this example:

Nguyen is a 40-year-old man who participated in a community health screening in Cabramatta...His local general practitioner (an Anglo-Australian) had prescribed medication to control his blood pressure, but Mr Nguyen did not comply with the doctor's instructions, because 'that amount of medication could kill a buffalo, so I took only half the amount...' He was counselled to reduce his fat and salt intake, to give up smoking, and to exercise more. At these suggestions he smiles and nods politely...(and says) 'When you feel depressed or lonely, a cigarette is your closest friend. If only I had my whole family here, it would be easier to give up smoking and to eat properly' (Humphrey & Nguyen 1990:45).

Nguyen's reference to buffalo might be regarded as cultural but his non-compliance is not especially so: that is, he does not question the diagnosis or treatment, only the dosage, and the only apparent cultural component is when he considers consulting an alternative practitioner rather than a general practitioner regarding his poor sleep and appetite. On the other hand, many Australian-born people also consult herbalists, naturopaths, and other alternative practitioners for a range of health problems, including chronic disease and disability as well as less precisely defined states of 'illness' (Bates & Linder-Pelz 1987: 100-103). What is significant in this case is the fact that Nguyen has moderately raised blood pressure and blood cholesterol, that he is lonely and smokes, and that his diet has moved from a conventional Vietnamese diet that is high in complex carbohydrates and fibre, a phenomenon already discussed (Webb & Manderson 1990).

Conclusion

When we speak of culture in the context of health and health equity, we often use the term to cover a variety of issues that are affected by immigration or by language. This chapter addresses the need for us to be precise about the way culture affects the incidence, diagnosis and treatment of ill health. This is not to argue against closer examination of the effects of cultural background on health, but rather the need to be sensitive also to other cultural, social and economic factors that influence health status and health behaviour. The Australian Government, through the Better Health Commission, identified newly arrived immigrant people from non-English speaking backgrounds as having special needs (Australia, Better Health Commission 1986:145–6). This draws attention to continuing disparity among Australians with respect to health status and access to health care. Access to health care may be related, as we have indicated, to unfamiliarity with the Australian health care system, to lack of fluency in English, to discrimination, direct or indirect, in health-care settings, to fear of health services (an issue particularly salient for torture and trauma survivors), or to lack of money. While cultural factors affect risk of disease, other factors colour both the health status and health-seeking behaviour of new immigrants: the occupational health risks to those who are employed in unskilled and semi-skilled capacity, for example (Casey & Yaman 1982, Lin & Pearse 1990, Watson 1985); or the difficulties and deprivations faced by people with low income who reside in poorer areas of the cities (e.g. Coughlan 1989). Being old and being female also influence access to and use of health care services, ability to pay for treatments, and the care provided. Working class Australians are all subject to inequitable health risks and health services.

Over the past two decades, there have been many calls by concerned ethnic communities, health professionals, policy makers, and academics (such as anthropologists) to give greater recognition to the health needs and experiences of immigrants in health service planning and delivery. This has lead to a range of culturally appropriate programs—health care interpreter services, torture and trauma rehabilitation services, ethnic health promotion programs, ethnospecific midwifery clinics and post-birth services, 'clustering' of the elderly according to country and language of origin in nursing homes, and so on. There is no doubt that a recognition of culturally specific needs, beliefs and practices in health care delivery has, in places, enhanced the accessibility and experience of care for people of non-English speaking backgrounds. Paradoxically, however, it has also reified 'culture' (including language) as the pre-eminent variable in health behaviour and access to services. As a result, other factors are at times overshadowed: being a woman in a public obstetric ward under the care of mainly male medical staff, being too poor and isolated to sustain a healthy lifestyle, being old, frail and alone, or alternatively, being prosperous, professional and well informed about health care options. Issues of dignity, choice and quality of care are the outcome of a 'mosaic' of factors (McCallum 1990) of which culture is but one.

NOTES

1.   In particular, we draw on a number of case studies published in the Instructor's manual to *The Health of Immigrant Australia* (Reid & Trompf 1990).
2.   Much of the work of medical anthropologists is built on an understanding that illness and disease are culturally constructed; see for example Paul (1955), Landy (1977), Foster and Anderson (1978), Kleinman (1980), and Helman (1984).
3.   This influences patterns of presentation for care, and is reflected in cases of somatization, where pain in a particular site is a reflection of a psychological, mental or

emotional problem. For example, the cultural significance of the stomach (*hara*) in Japan as a site of emotion, as well as the high frequency of stomach cancer, leads to greater emphasis on stomach related problems than, say headache (Ohnuki-Tierney 1984); elsewhere pain or perceived pathology in the head or the heart may be regarded as more serious than gut problems.

4. There was advantage to this strategy: the severity of measles infection depends on intensity of exposure to the virus, and children infected outside the home tend to have lighter infections and so be less sick than those infected by siblings in the home (Aaby 1988).

5. In this context, biomedicine is regarded as if 'outside of culture' whilst in contrast, humoral medical theories, Chinese medicine, and other medical theories and practices are considered 'cultural'.

6. In 1990-1991, one quarter of all immigrants to Australia were from Europe and the United Kingdom, but the majority of settler arrivals to Australia were from Asia, in particular from Hong Kong, Vietnam, the Philippines, India, China, Taiwan, Malaysia and Singapore. The other major area, contributing 9% of new settler arrivals, was Oceania, primarily New Zealand.

7. In this respect, in fact these communities face the same kinds of problems as other refugees, see especially Reid and Strong (1987) and Allotey (1992).

REFERENCES

Aaby P 1988 Malnutrition and overcrowding-exposure in severe measles infection: a review of community studies. Reviews of Infectious Diseases 10:478-491

Aaby P 1990 Social and behavioural factors affecting transmission and severity of measles infection. In: Caldwell J et al (eds) What we know about health transition: the cultural, social and behavioural determinants of health. The Health Transition Centre, National Centre for Epidemiology and Population Health, Canberra

Allotey P A 1992 Perceived health status: health needs and utilisation of health services among Latin American refugee women in Perth. Unpublished thesis, University of Western Australia, Perth

Australia, Better Health Commission 1986 Looking forward to better health, Vol 3. AGPS, Canberra

Australian Bureau of Statistics 1984 Australian health survey 1983. ABS, Canberra

Australia, Department of Community Services and Health 1989 National women's health policy: advancing women's health in Australia. AGPS, Canberra

Bates E, Linder-Pelz S 1987 Health care issues. Allen & Unwin, Sydney

Boman B, Edwards M 1984 The Indochinese refugee: an overview. Australia and New Zealand Journal of Psychiatry 18:40-52

Bottomley G, de Lepervanche M 1990 The social context of immigrant health and illness. In: Reid J, Trompf P (eds) The health of immigrant Australia. Harcourt Brace Jovanovich, Sydney

Casey H, Yaman N 1982 Slow down the line: occupational health hazards amongst South American and Turkish workers in Flemington. Flemington Community Health Centre, Melbourne

Chak S, Nixon J, Dugdale A 1984 Primary health care for Indochinese children in Australia. Australian Paediatric Journal 2:57-58

Coughlan J 1989 The spatial distribution and concentration of Australia's three Indochinese-born communities: 1976-1986. Centre for the Study of Australia-Asian Relations, Griffith University, Nathan

de Costa C 1988 Pregnancy outcomes in Lebanese-born women in western Sydney. Medical Journal of Australia 149:457-459

Eisenbruch M 1991 The post-traumatic stress disorder to cultural bereavement: diagnosis of Southeast Asian refugees. Social Science and Medicine 33 (6):673-680

Eisenbruch M, Handelman L 1990 Cultural consultation for cancer: Astrocytoma in a Cambodian adolescent. Social Science and Medicine 31 (12):1295-1299

Foster G M, Anderson B G 1978 Medical anthropology. Wiley, New York

Garrett P, Lin V 1990 Ethnic health policy and service development. In: Reid J, Trompf P (eds) The health of immigrant Australia. Harcourt Brace Jovanovich, Sydney

Good B J, Good M-J D 1981 The meaning of symptoms: a cultural hermeneutic model for clinical practice. In: Eisenberg L, Kleinman A (eds) The relevance of social science for medicine. D.Reidel, Dordrecht

Hahn R A 1985 Culture-bound syndromes unbound. Social Science and Medicine 21 (2):165-172

Health Targets and Implementation Committee 1988 Health for all Australians: report to Australian health minister's advisory council. AGPS, Canberra

Helman C 1984 Culture, health and illness. John Wright, London

Hetzel S 1990 Maria: a battered wife, case 8. In: Reid J, Trompf P (eds) Instructor's manual for The health of immigrant Australia. Harcourt Brace Jovanovich, Sydney

Hickey K, Trompf P, Reid J 1991 Antenatal care for Muslim Lebanese women: a pilot study of utilisation, health beliefs and practices, women's health studies. Discussion papers and research reports no. 4. Cumberland College of Health Sciences, The University of Sydney, Sydney

Hopper U 1992 Developments in migrant health services for pregnancy. Migration Action, April:28-32

Hoskins P 1990 Cross-cultural issues in diabetic care, case 20. In: Reid J, Trompf P (eds) Instructor's manual for The health of immigrant Australia. Harcourt Brace Jovanovich, Sydney

Humphrey B, Nguyen N 1990 Cardiovascular health issues for Vietnamese immigrants, case 22. In: Reid J Trompf P (eds) Instructor's manual for The health of immigrant Australia. Harcourt Brace Jovanovich, Sydney

Keesing R M 1981 Cultural anthropology: a contemporary perspective. Holt, Rinehart & Winston, New York

Kleinman A 1980 Patients and healers in the context of culture. University of California Press, Berkeley

Kleinman A 1988 The illness narratives: suffering, healing and the human condition. Basic Books, New York

Landy D (ed) 1977 Culture, disease and healing: studies in medical anthropology. Macmillan, New York

Landy D 1985 Pibloktoq (hysteria) and Inuit nutrition: possible implications of hypervitaminosis A. Social Science and Medicine 21 (2):173-186

Lewins F 1984 The significance of factors influencing early Vietnamese settlement in Australia. Journal of Intercultural Studies 5 (2):29-50

Lin V, Pearse W 1990 A workforce at risk. In: Reid J, Trompf P (eds) The health of immigrant Australia. Harcourt Brace Jovanovich, Sydney

Linton R 1940 Acculturation. In: Linton R (ed) Acculturation in seven American Indian tribes. Peter Smith, Gloucester, Mass.

Locke M 1985 Risk factors impinging on Vietnamese women of childbearing age in Australia. Australian Family Physician 14 (12):1332-1336

McCallum J 1990 The mosaic of ethnicity and health in later life. In: Reid J, Trompf P (eds) The health of immigrant Australia. Harcourt Brace Jovanovich, Sydney

McCallum J, Lerba C 1989 Crosscultural differences in health and mobility in the 'old' old in Australia. Advances in Behavioural Medicine 6:483-505

Manderson L 1981 Fieldnotes

Manderson L 1984 Fieldnotes

Manderson L 1989 Fieldnotes

Manderson L 1990 Indochinese health: creating cultural fictions. In: Nguyen Xuan Thi, Cahill D, Bertelli L (eds) Australia and Indo-Chinese health issues. Australian Association of Vietnamese Studies, Melbourne

Manderson L, Mathews M 1981 Vietnamese attitudes towards maternal and infant health. Medical Journal of Australia 1 (2):69-72

Manderson L, Mathews M 1985 Care and conflict: Vietnamese medical beliefs and the Australian health care system. In: Burnley I, McCall G, Encel S (eds) Immigration and ethnic studies. Longman Cheshire, Melbourne

Martin J 1978 The migrant presence: Australian responses 1947-77. Allen & Unwin, Sydney

Mathews M, Manderson L 1981 Vietnamese behavioural and dietary precautions during confinement. Ecology of Food and Nutrition 11:9-16

Ohnuki-Tierney E 1984 Illness and culture in contemporary Japan: an anthropological view. Cambridge University Press, Cambridge

Parsons C 1990 Cross-cultural issues in health care. In: Reid J, Trompf P (eds) The health of immigrant Australia. Harcourt Brace Jovanovich, Sydney

Parsons C, Najman J 1990 Reading culture into health care: generating lego-ethical dilemmas, case 15. In: Reid J, Trompf P (eds) Instructor's manual for The health of immigrant Australia. Harcourt Brace Jovanovich, Sydney

Parsons C D F, Wakeley P 1991a. Idioms of distress: somatic responses to distress in everyday life. Culture, Medicine and Psychiatry 15:111-132

Paul B D (ed) (1955) Health, culture and community. Sage, New York

Pow Meng Yap 1977 The culture-bound reactive syndromes. In: Landy D (ed) Culture, disease and healing. Macmillan, New York

Powles J W 1990 Best of both worlds: attempting to explain the persisting low mortality of Greek migrants to Australia. In: Caldwell J et al (eds), What we know about Health transition: the cultural, social and behavioural determinants of health. The Health Transition Centre, National Centre for Epidemiology and Population Health, Canberra

Powles J, Ktenas D, Sutherland C, Hage B 1988 Food habits in southern European migrants: a case study of migrants from the Greek island of Levkada. In: Truswell A S, Wahlqvist M L (eds) Food habits in Australia. Rene Gordon, Melbourne

Powles J, Gifford S 1990 How healthy are Australia's immigrants? In: Reid J, Trompf P (eds) The health of immigrant Australia. Harcourt Brace Jovanovich, Sydney

Prince R H 1983 Is anorexia nervosa a culture-bound syndrome? Transcultural Psychiatric Research Review 20:299-300

Reid J, Strong T 1987 Torture and trauma: the health care needs of refugee victims in New South Wales. Cumberland College of Health Sciences, Sydney

Reid J, Trompf P (eds) (1990) The health of immigrant Australia. Harcourt Brace Jovanovich, Sydney

Reid J C 1989 Fieldnotes

Reid J C, Goldstein G B, Keo L 1986 Refugee medical screening in NSW: refugee welfare versus public risk? Community Health Studies X(3):265-274

Rittenbaugh C 1982 Obesity as a culture-bound syndrome. Culture, Medicine and Psychiatry 6:347-361

Rubel A 1977 The epidemiology of a folk illness: *susto* in Hispanic America. In: Landy D (ed) Culture, disease and healing. Macmillan, New York

Rudolph A 1987 Paediatrics. Prentice Hall, Norwalk, Conn.

Snow L F 1976 'High blood' is not high blood pressure. Urban Health 5:54-55

Stafford A M 1978 The application of clinical anthropology to medical practice: case study of recurrent abdominal pain in a pre-adolescent Mexican-American female. In: Bauwens E E (ed) The anthropology of health. C V Mosby, St Louis

Tang K C 1990 Evaluating alternative therapies. In: Reid J, Trompf P (eds) Instructor's manual for The health of immigrant Australia. Harcourt Brace Jovanovich, Sydney

Thomas T (n.d.) Vietnamese elderly women in Australia: health issues. Mimeograph, Department of Psychology, Royal Melbourne Institute of Technology, Melbourne

Tran Le Trinh 1991. Report on health status of Vietnamese women living in Brisbane. Mimeograph, The Women's Health Centre, Brisbane

Watson J 1985 A case of status degradation: or how insult is added to injury. In: Manderson L (ed) Australian ways. Allen & Unwin, Sydney

Webb K, Manderson L 1990 Food habits and their influence on health. In: Reid J, Trompf P (eds) The health of immigrant Australia. Harcourt Brace Jovanovich, Sydney

Wise M, Bekiaris J, Gleeson S 1990 The 'good heart, good life' heart disease prevention project, case 19. In: Reid J, Trompf P (eds) Instructor's manual for The health of immigrant Australia. Harcourt Brace Jovanovich, Sydney

Wolff B B, Langley S 1977 Cultural factors and the response to pain. In: Landy D (ed) Culture, disease and healing. Macmillan, New York

Yusuf F 1986 Ethnic differences in Australian fertility. Clinical Reproduction and Fertility 4:107-116

2. Class inequalities in health and lifestyle

Jake M. Najman

The identification of social class inequalities in health in the Australian population has paralleled their observation in many of the developed, and developing, countries in the world. It is, of course, a chancy business comparing different developed countries. Accepting that one is not strictly comparing like with like, it nevertheless appears that social class health inequalities in Australia are similar in magnitude to those observed in Britain, the United States and many of the Scandinavian countries (see Broom 1984, Mackenbach & Maas (undated)). Because data detailing socioeconomic mortality inequalities in Australia are of a relatively recent origin, and morbidity data has only been obtained in the last decade or so, it is sometimes necessary to use overseas findings to fill in the gaps in our understanding of what is happening in Australia. In this paper a recourse to data from other countries is reserved for situations where comparable Australian data does not exist, and when such 'imported' data provides a reasonable indication of what is likely to be the case in Australia.

With these considerations in mind there are four issues which need to be addressed if we are to understand the association between social class and health inequalities in Australia. Firstly, we consider the variations in health inequalities over time and between different countries. Such a consideration provides us with an indication of the extent to which different social, economic, and political systems have an influence on socioeconomic health inequalities.

Secondly, we to discuss the extent of social class related health inequalities, particularly inequalities in mortality and morbidity; for various conditions; for the young, middle aged and elderly; and for such concerns as preventive behaviour and dental caries.

Thirdly, we examine why these health inequalities are believed to exist. Here the prime concern is with the extent to which health inequalities reflect individual or social group behavioural choices. Is social class inequality itself the cause of health inequalities or are there some important intervening factors?

Finally, we discuss what might be done to reduce the magnitude of social class determined health inequalities. To understand what needs to be done, one can begin with a better understanding of who the groups are with the worst health and how they differ, other than in health terms, from the rest of the community.

Changes over time and variations between countries

Data comparing health inequalities over time and between countries needs to be interpreted with caution. Not only have there been marked changes in the occupational structure of developed countries (e.g. the shift from semiskilled and unskilled work to clerical, administrative and service work), but there are differences between the developed countries in their occupational structures. Bearing these concerns in mind, the best long-term data describing class inequalities in mortality come from England and Wales.

Figure 2.1 is adapted from studies by Pamak (1985) and Wilkinson (1989). In order to deal with changes in the class structure of the population over time, Pamak (1985) has ranked the social class of a wide variety of specific occupations for which comparable data was available, over the period 1921 to 1983. Indicated as separate graph lines are the time trends for the age-standardized mortality rates for the top and bottom 1% of occupations, with professional/managerial occupations at the top and unskilled workers at the bottom. The average (for all occupations) age-standardized death rate is indicated. Overall death rates have clearly declined in a more-or-less steady trend over this period of time (note, there was little or no change in 1970–72 over 1959–63). The gap in the death rates between the top and bottom 1% of occupations decreased in 1930–32 and again in 1945–53. The contribution of the British National Health System, to this decline is, at best, a matter of

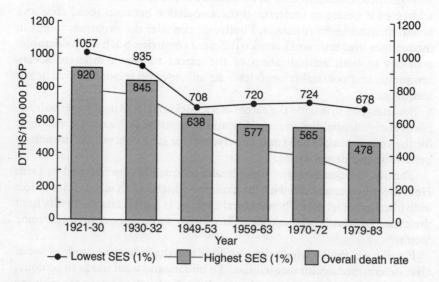

Fig. 2.1   Age standardized mortality rates in England and Wales 1921–1983.
Source: Najman 1992

speculation. However on every occasion data is available since the British National Health System was introduced, the gap between the mortality rates of the top and bottom 1% class groups has increased. Not only does the gap between the top and bottom class occupations appear to be increasing, but it is now substantially larger than it was in 1921–3, when this data first became available. Moreover as Judge and Benzeval (1993) have argued in relation to socioeconomic status (SES) inequalities in child mortality, occupational data is likely to underestimate class mortality differences as those not employed (unemployed, single parents) may have the worst health and are excluded from the above comparisons. These groups are not employed and do not receive a class score but they would usually be allocated to the lower class groups further increasing the gap between the *top* and *bottom* of society.

Only Britain is able to provide data on long term trends in mortality, but recent data from countries as diverse as the United States (Yeracaris & Kim 1978), New Zealand (Pearce et al 1983), Sweden (Lundberg 1986) and Australia (McMichael 1985, Taylor et al 1983) all confirm the existence of class inequalities in mortality. The absence of such data for other countries reflects the lack of relevant research rather than the existence of findings which question the generality of these inequalities. Depending upon how class is defined and measured, the lowest class groups have mortality rates some 50% to 100% higher than the highest class groups. For example in a recent paper examining potential years of life lost for persons aged 5–64 by socioeconomic status in Brisbane, the lowest SES group lost 53.6 years of life/1000 population per year compared to 35.7 years of life/1000 population per year, in the highest SES group (Siskind et al 1992:318). Based upon these figures it appears that persons in the lowest group lose 50% more years of life between the ages of 5-64, than do persons in the highest SES group. Another way of interpreting these differences is that persons in the lowest SES group have a shorter life expectancy, as a result of their higher age-standardized death rates, than do people in the higher SES groups.

Extent of SES health inequalities

The range of SES inequalities in morbidity and mortality is truly remarkable. With only a few exceptions persons in the lowest class groups manifest higher rates of morbidity and mortality from almost all causes of illness, disability and death. While research does suggest that in a few instances the causal process is the reverse of the one usually hypothesized (disease sometimes leads to poverty, particularly when it involves a chronic disability), the more common situation is that low social class leads to poor health.

Table 2.1 provides age-standardized mortality ratios describing SES inequalities in mortality for males and females, for specific age categories. (This uses data based on the socioeconomic status of the area in which people live).

Table 2.1 Mortality differentials for Australia 1985–1987

	Age group (years)			
	0-14	15-24	25-64	65+
Males				
SES Quintile				
1 (Highest)	1.00	1.00	1.00	1.00
2	1.15*	1.24*	1.17*	1.05*
3	1.18*	1.35*	1.33*	1.10*
4	1.28*	1.34*	1.41*	1.12*
5 (Lowest)	1.46*	1.46*	1.67*	1.13*
Females				
SES Quintile				
1 (Highest)	1.00	1.00	1.00	1.00
2	1.10*	0.96*	1.16*	1.04*
3	1.29*	1.11	1.24*	1.07*
4	1.39*	1.12	1.27*	1.07*
5 (Lowest)	1.63*	1.49*	1.49*	1.10*

* P<.05
Source: Australian Institute of Health and Welfare 1992

In the 0–14 age group the lowest SES group has mortality ratios, for males 46%, and females 63%, higher than those in the highest SES group. Similar inequalities are observed in the 15–24 and 25–64 age groups. By contrast the socioeconomic inequalities in mortality are relatively small for the 65 and over age group. It is not clear whether this latter finding reflects the 'survival of the fittest', or whether once people leave their work, their health is less subject to their social and economic circumstances (or indeed whether these inequalities diminish somewhat at retirement). The observation of substantial mortality inequalities in the young emphasizes how unequal are our 'life chances' right from birth.

While class mortality inequalities are observed for all the main causes of death, the association is stronger for some causes than others. Thus Australian data points to pneumonia/influenza (opportunistic infections?), lung cancer, diabetes and bronchitis, asthma and emphysema as categories where the lowest class group have death rates over three times those of the highest class group (Australian Institute of Health and Welfare 1992:375). For motor vehicle accident deaths the lowest class group have three times, and for ischaemic heart disease (the cause which accounts for one-third of all deaths) two times the death rate of the highest class group.

Australian data on morbidity have only recently been collected on a national basis. While it would be of considerable interest to know whether people from different class groups differ in their disease related behaviour (do some groups not obtain adequate health care?) such data is not available. Instead we have national survey data which details the extent to which there are class differences for disease conditions which have received some attention (e.g. self-medication, medical or other care). Given that specific diseases are

Table 2.2   Indicators of morbidity differentials for Australia 1989–90

Males (25-64)

SES Quintile	Serious chronic illness	Recent illness	Reduced activity	Those fair/ poor health
1 (Highest)	1.00	1.00	1.00	1.00
2	1.10	1.09*	1.25*	1.22*
3	1.13*	1.11*	1.39*	1.36*
4	1.00	1.04	1.19*	1.45*
5 (Lowest)	1.12	1.07	1.56*	1.61*

Females (25–64)

SES Quintile				
1 (Highest)	1.00	1.00	1.00	1.00
2	1.00	1.06	1.06*	1.32*
3	1.13*	1.05	1.12*	1.48*
4	1.07	1.05	0.90*	1.51*
5 (Lowest)	1.22*	1.07	0.98	1.67*

* P<.05
Source: National Health Strategy 1992

relatively uncommon, only aggregate data provides sufficient cases to enable meaningful comparisons.

As Table 2.2 indicates, the most consistent class difference is that those in the lowest class group more often self rate their health as fair or poor. Lower class males are also consistent in reporting higher rates of days when they have reduced activity. Class differences in rates of serious chronic and recent illness are relatively small and they provide a less consistent pattern.

In addition lower class groups appear to be less active in their preventive activity. For example lower class groups have poorer dental health with higher rates of decayed and missing teeth (Australian Institute of Health and Welfare 1992:222) and fewer visits to a dentist (Najman et al 1979:57). They are less active in maintaining their immunization levels (Najman et al 1979:57).

It is clear that the impact of the class health disadvantage is pervasive, beginning in childhood and extending right through and, in many instances, past working life. Children in lower class groups not only have a higher rate of a range of diseases (Bor et al 1993) but manifest higher levels of development and vocabulary learning problems even by the age of five (Najman et al 1992). They also manifest higher rates of aggressive and delinquent behaviour (sometimes labelled psychiatric morbidity) from a young age.

This health disadvantage of lower SES/class groups continues throughout life for a wide variety of diseases. Thus it could be reasonably argued that lower class groups have a lower quality of life, as well as a lesser quantity of life.

What indicators of class should be used?

Despite their theoretical and conceptual differences such concepts as socioeconomic status and class are often used interchangeably. Concepts like socioeconomic status and class need to be understood as abstractions, as ideas for organizing aspects of the social world. It is not possible, for example, to *touch* or *feel* someone's socioeconomic status, though one may observe and feel manifestations of it. Socioeconomic status or class exist as concepts which tend to be defined differently by researchers. There remains much debate about what socioeconomic status and class are (see Ch. 6), but whatever views are advanced the concepts are only meaningful to the extent that they reflect some widely held beliefs and relate to a range of behavioural variations in society.

It follows then that since class exists only as an abstraction, as a concept in the mind of the researcher, it cannot be the direct or proximate cause of disease or death. If socioeconomic or class differences are not the proximate causes of the health inequalities we have observed, then why is there such a consistent and clear association between SES/class and various measures of disease? Further some might argue that it is more important to deal with the 'real' causes of disease rather than concepts developed by sociologists for 'organizing' social reality. Both these questions need to be answered, but a short discussion of the meaning of SES/class differences serves to provide a context for the answers to these questions (see Ch. 6 for an extended discussion).

The concept of class historically preceded that of socioeconomic status. It was popularized by Marx and Marxist thinkers who believed that the economic system, and the location of individuals within the economic system, determined much if not all social behaviour. The concept of socioeconomic status was popularized by Lloyd Warner (1960) and others who developed various measures of socioeconomic inequality, for example the level of education, income, quality of housing and occupational status or prestige of respondents.

When researchers have used socioeconomic status or class as predictors of health inequalities they have often had to use whatever convenient indicator was available. Thus the British 'occupational class' inequalities we have observed are not derived explicitly from a Marxist or Warnerian approach. Rather people's occupations were ranked by the Registrar General, according to varying criteria which have changed over time. For example in the 35th annual report of the Registrar General (published in 1875), the industry in which a person worked was used to determine that person's class location, with managers and labourers working in the same industry, grouped together while persons of rank with property and school children were allocated to an 'indefinite' category (Jones & Cameron 1984:38). This makes more sense than might first appear as it might have permitted the detection of industrial or workplace hazards to health. In 1911 the then Registrar General constructed an eight category class measure based upon a person's education and culture—and it has been suggested that the subsequent 1921 revision was manipulated to provide for a class gradient in mortality (Jones & Cameron 1984:39). Thus it has been pointed out that the class categories used by the Registrar General, are used simply because they 'work', that is, they show class differences in mortality (McDowall 1983:28).

What then is the meaning of class inequalities in society? Leaving aside such considerations as the theoretical integrity of different conceptualizations of class, in part because we do not know whether theoretical integrity has empirical relevance to behaviour, it is worth recalling that despite many different approaches to class measurement, similar results are observed, particularly with respect to inequalities in mortality.

Here it may be more productive to disregard the elaborate conceptual creations of the professional academic and instead turn to the community for the meaning its members give to class inequalities. When people are asked to describe the honour, status or prestige of various occupations in their society, three facts emerge which together can be taken to convey an important statement about what class inequalities mean and why they matter. Firstly, the rankings people give are extraordinarily similar. Regardless of where they themselves appear in the hierarchy, respondents are able to rank their own and the positions of others in this hierarchy almost perfectly (correlation is over .95) (Congalton 1969). Secondly, it is extraordinary that while occupational rankings do differ a little from country to country, they remain remarkably similar—even when one is comparing such countries as diverse as the UK, West Germany, Japan, Poland and the USSR (Penn 1975:355–6). What little historical data is available suggests there has been little change in these rankings over time (Nilson & Edelman 1979:8). Thus despite political, economic, educational and occupational systems which differ widely, community perceptions of the rankings of these occupations remain similar.

Thirdly, it is clear that children acquire an understanding of the occupational status hierarchy from a very young age. Thus children as young as 8 years have conceptions of class which are similar to those reported by older youth and young adults (Lehman & Witty 1931:109).

What criteria then are being used which enable people to be so consistent in ranking the social standing of occupations? One gets two types of answers to this question depending upon how the research is done. If people are asked an open-ended question about why occupations are allocated different class locations the response tends to identify the responsibilities, service to the community, skill, autonomy, difficulty or risk associated with the job itself (Nilson & Edelman, 1979:1–2).

However a more quantitative answer is provided by the work of Coleman, Rainwater and McClelland (1979). They were concerned with understanding the relative importance of the three main contributors to socioeconomic inequalities, income, education and occupation. In their research they asked respondents to assess the ranking of a person about whom data was provided on that person's income, educational and occupation. Lists of occupations were provided such that the same income and education might be associated with different occupations, or vice versa. Thus a respondent might be told that a worker was a carpenter with a trade diploma but his income would be differently described on different occasions. Holding two criteria constant but varying the third indicated that income was clearly the major criterion used to rank occupations. Doubling income increased general status by 49%; doubling the job led to an increase in 22% in general status, while doubling education produced a 7% increase in general status (Coleman et al 1979:220).

While it is true that the relative contributions of income, occupation and education are not strictly linear across the range of general status rankings, the relative importance of each of the three criteria seems unambiguous. Coleman, Rainwater and McClelland (1979) sum up the findings by suggesting that 'income is the end, occupation the means and education the preparation' (Coleman et al 1979:68).

If these community perceptions are correct in noting the primary behavioural and social importance of income inequalities, then the categories created by the Registrar General and many other social researchers 'work', that is they identify class differences in health, largely because the class measures they use are crude approximations of income inequalities. Furthermore if it is income inequalities that really matter, then social policies to redress such inequalities are more easily identified than if the Marxist or stratification analyses are 'correct'.

What then is the basis of the argument that income inequalities are of primary importance to class inequalities in health?

Firstly, there is the extension of minimum standards of education to the whole population and the gradual increase in education levels for all social groups. This enables the lowest class groups to be more knowledgable about health related matters and to access the same mass media sources which their wealthier middle-upper class counterparts may previously have tended to monopolize. Here education can be seen to supplant familial class origins as an influence of health and behaviour.

Secondly, there is the view that the mass media have made middle-upper class culture visible, if not accessible, to all. Whereas in the past the lifestyles of groups with differing economic resource capacities were to a large extent segregated from each other, now the food, recreation, transportation and housing of the middle-upper class are visible to all class groups. While lower class groups may not be able to purchase many of these goods and services, they tend to know about them and may well aspire to obtain them.

Thirdly, there is the argument that money enables people to purchase the very goods and services which are relevant to their health. This includes food—particularly the more expensive fresh fruit and vegetables, better quality housing, safer modes of transportation and recreational activities and the recreational time needed to enjoy the greater wealth.

Fourthly and finally, with the extension of free health care to the disadvantaged (a policy implemented in Australia continuously since 1970), there have not been significant economic disincentives which limit the access of the poor to health care. Thus with health care relatively freely available to all, lifestyle differences between social and economic groups may have become the major basis of class differences in health and illness. These lifestyle differences are arguably a reflection of the education and income inequalities in society, and occupational class only appears to be important because it is a function of a person's education and income.

If education and income are the primary aspects of what is more colloquially known as class inequalities, then how do education and income influence health? The answer would appear to be that education provides knowledge, and income the means to implement that knowledge. According to this view, more educated, higher income persons are both motivated and enabled to behave in a healthier manner. While the data are not unambiguous in support of this interpretation, they do tend to, on balance, argue for its validity. Why then might education and income inequalities influence morbidity and mortality rates?

Explaining class inequalities in health

In 1977 the United States Centers for Disease Control published a report which examined the key factors which were believed to be related to the ten main causes of death (Centers for Disease Control 1977). Taking the two leading causes, heart disease and cancer—they estimated that people's lifestyles accounted for 54% of heart disease and 37% of cancer deaths; with the environment being responsible for 9% of heart disease and 24% of cancer deaths. Overall people's lifestyles were estimated to be causally related to 51% of these ten causes of death, while the environment accounted for 19% and genetics 20%. The remaining 10% of deaths was associated with the availability and use of health services. Accepting that these are approximations, it would nevertheless seem reasonable to hypothesize that if education and income influence health outcomes, they do so by having an impact on people's lifestyles.

A number of lifestyle related variables can be identified, each of which make a major contribution to morbidity and mortality. These lifestyle variables tend to be important across a range of diseases and together would account for the bulk of the impact of lifestyle on health. To what extent are these lifestyle variables associated with education, income and class inequalities in society?

Cigarette smoking

Cigarette smoking has been causally implicated in lung cancer, heart disease, stroke and other causes of death. In 1989–90 in Australia some 32% of men and 25% of women were found to be smokers (Australian Institute of Health and Welfare 1992:70). Despite steady declines in the rate of smoking since the mid–1970s, smoking remains Australia's major lifestyle factor which causes disease with around 40% of males and females in the 20–29 age group reporting they are smokers (Australian Institute of Health and Welfare 1992:70).

Australian data is consistent with overseas data in indicating that less educated and lower income males and females smoke at higher rates, (National Health Strategy 1992:2–3). Lower income Australians smoke about 40% more often than higher income Australians, and the least educated smoke, for males 85%, and females 67% more often than their most educated counterparts. German data points to even larger class differences in smoking rates though this may reflect the way class has been measured in this latter study (Helmert et al 1989:39).

Diet

Various aspects of diet have been related to health, and it is increasingly clear that diet can have a major influence on such diseases as coronary heart disease, stroke, and cancer of the digestive system. Estimates of the proportion of the population who have an unhealthy dietary lifestyle depend very much on where somewhat arbitrary dietary cut-offs are drawn. Despite the imprecision in the estimates it is clear that large sectors of the population eat high levels of saturated fats, consume excessive quantities of salt, fail to include sufficient fibre in their diet and consume inadequate quantities of fresh fruit and vegetables.

Australian data on patterns of food consumption are not readily available. However the overseas data are consistent and suggest similar patterns are likely to be found in Australia.

Thus Wynn (1987) using US data on the elderly found that those whose income was below the poverty line were substantially less likely to consume the recommended dietary allowance of vitamin C. Whichelow (1989:1–2) presents data on the consumption of polyunsaturated and low fat spreads by occupational level. He finds that the higher the occupational level (e.g. professionals vs unskilled workers), the higher the rate at which polyunsaturated and low fat spreads are used, with the highest class group being more than twice as frequent users of unsaturated/low fat spreads. Viikari (1990:16) presents similar data for Finland showing that 90% of persons with the highest education use low fat milk, compared to 59% of their least educated counterparts. A similar pattern is observed for unsaturated spreads. Full cream milk consumption shows the opposite pattern. Thus the data suggest that lesser educated, lower income persons eat less healthy foods and that they may more frequently fail to consume basic nutrients.

Cholesterol levels

While there is still some debate about what is the best indicator of cholesterol level in the blood, the data from the MRFIT project, which involved the screening of 350 000 men, show that lower plasma cholesterol levels are associated with lower heart disease rates (Martin et al 1986). As Marmot (1993) notes there is no safe cholesterol level in developed countries, and China, which has a generally lower distribution of cholesterol levels, still produces a more-or-less consistent level of association between cholesterol levels and heart disease.

Recent data suggest that specific fractions of cholesterol may be a better indicator of cardiovascular risk than total plasma cholesterol. High density lipoproteins (HDL) are the so-called 'good' fraction, while low density lipoproteins (LDL) are the 'bad' fraction of cholesterol, from a cardiovascular risk perspective. German data (Helmert et al 1989:39) point to class differences for both males and females in their HDL levels, with lower class persons having low HDL levels. There is little Australian data available on this point, though my colleague Ruth English has recently completed a PhD which, amongst other things, indicates that for women at least, the least educated and lowest occupation levels had lower mean HDL levels (English 1993).

Exercise and physical activity

Higher levels of exercise and physical activity are associated with reduced levels of coronary heart disease, stroke, diabetes mellitus and osteoporosis (Australian Institute of Health and Welfare 1992:65). With the increasing use of technology to relieve workers of the mechanical, repetitive and physically demanding aspects of their work, there has been a reduction in the extent to which work itself provides for an adequate level of activity and physical fitness. About 25% of the Australian population can be described as living a sedentary lifestyle (Bauman et al 1990).

US data points to increased levels of leisure physical activity for those in higher income groups (Caspersen et al 1986:589). This finding is to some extent balanced by Pocock et al's (1987) observation that while higher class groups much more frequently engage in regular physical recreational activity, the cardiovascular benefits of this recreation are compensated for by the more physically demanding nature of the work done by those in lower class groups. In Australia it is difficult to find studies which balance recreational and work related physical activity. Bauman, Owen and Rushworth (1990) have found that those with a tertiary education are more likely to exercise than their less educated counterparts, but whether workplace physical activity balances these differences in Australia, it is not yet possible to report.

Overweight

Being overweight is a risk factor for coronary heart disease, breast cancer and diabetes mellitus (Australian Institute of Health and Welfare 1992:65). Based on national surveys almost 50% of males and 35% of females in Australia in the age range 20–69 are overweight or obese. The percentage of the Australian population overweight or obese increases to a majority of the male and female population once persons older than 45 are considered (Australian Institute of Health and Welfare 1992:67). Being overweight is likely to reflect a combination of factors including genetic predisposition, diet and a low level of physical activity. The former, of course, cannot be changed, while the latter two factors have an association with class indicators.

Data from Germany confirm a strong association, for both males and females, between an indicator of social class and the proportion of the population both overweight and obese. There is the consistent observation that class differences are more pronounced for women than for men. Lowest class men are almost twice as likely to be overweight or obese compared to highest class men. Lowest class women are between 3.6 times as overweight and 4.0 times as obese, when compared to highest class women (Helmert et al 1989, Helmert et al 1990).

Australian data in Table 2.3 is consistent with the overseas data, but tends to point to a lesser range of differences. Least educated men are, on average, 22% more likely to be overweight while least educated women are 68% more likely to be overweight.

Hypertension

Hypertension or high blood pressure is a major cause of coronary heart disease and stroke deaths. Recent Australian data suggests that 18% of men and 14% of women are hypertensive. Hypertension increases with age, and about half those 65–69 years of age have hypertension. Only about half the men and two thirds of the women with hypertension appear to be being treated for their condition and substantial proportions under treatment do not have good control of their blood pressure (Australian Institute of Health

Table 2.3 Ratio of overweight and hypertension in Australia

Education level	Ratio of overweight		Ratio of hypertension	
	Males	Females	Males	Females
High	1.00	1.00	1.00	1.00
Middle	1.09*	1.29*	1.07	1.75*
Low	1.22*	1.68*	1.27*	1.26*

* P<.05
Source: National Health Strategy 1993

and Welfare 1992:67). This pattern of diagnosis and treatment must be a major source of concern as hypertension is relatively simply diagnosed and a. variety of effective treatments are available.

There are substantial class differences in the rate of hypertension in the community. US data from a large scale study indicate that 23.1% of the least educated group have hypertension compared to 13.5% of the most educated group, with a linear trend for the education groups in between (HDFP-Cooperative Group 1977:354). Again the Australian data are here consistent with the findings observed overseas.

Simons et al (1986:448) found that the mean systolic and diastolic blood pressures for less educated persons are greater than for more educated persons. The National Health Strategy (1992) reports that the least educated groups have higher rates of hypertension than the most educated groups. This difference is particularly marked for women with least educated women having rates of hypertension more than twice those of most educated women (see Table 2.3).

Alcohol consumption

Unlike cigarette consumption, alcohol consumption can be safe (sometimes even beneficial) at some levels. Indeed persons who drink, on average, 1–2 glasses of alcohol a day not only have reduced rates of coronary heart disease, but overall lower rates of mortality. Recent research indicates that the reduced cardiovascular disease rate evident for light drinkers may result from the impact of alcohol increasing high density lipoprotein levels ('good' cholesterol). High levels of alcohol consumption do not greatly impact on coronary heart disease rates but increase death rates from a variety of other causes (e.g. accidents, liver cirrhosis). Thus there is a J curve association between alcohol consumption and overall mortality with the highest mortality rates at the highest alcohol consumption levels, and somewhat elevated coronary heart disease rates for those who abstain from alcohol consumption (Lazarus et al 1991).

Of the Australian population about 87% of men and 75% of women report drinking alcohol. About 74% of men and 52% of women report drinking alcohol in the week prior to interview (Australian Institute of Health and Welfare, 1992:72). About 10% of men and 3% of women are believed to drink alcohol at a level which constitutes a danger to their health.

In discussing the association between social class and self-reported alcohol consumption, there may be substantial inaccuracies as people may under report what is commonly perceived as a socially unacceptable level of alcohol consumption. Further as the proportion of abstainers and heavy drinkers is relatively low, many studies with modest samples, will not produce stable, reliable estimates of alcohol consumption levels by social class.

In the only study of its type Knupfer (1989) has pooled the data from twelve different studies of social class differences in alcohol consumption.

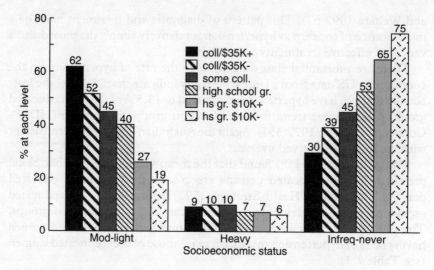

Fig. 2.2   SES and alcohol use, 12 studies, females. Adapted from Knupter 1989:1309.

She reports data separately for males and females, although only the data for females is presented in Figure 2.2. When we examine 'heavy' levels of alcohol consumption, there are no clear education/income trends. However moderate to light levels of alcohol consumption are strongly class related with the highest education/income group having the highest proportion of moderate to light drinkers. By contrast the infrequent-never drinkers are disproportionately found in lower education/income groups. Thus the healthiest level of alcohol consumption has a strong linear association with education/income while the less healthy pattern of abstaining or drinking alcohol infrequently is inversely associated with indicators of social class. There are no class differences for the least healthy pattern of heavy drinking.

In sum there are three key points which emerge from our exploration of why there are socioeconomic or class differences in health. Firstly, we have suggested that the concept of class is little more than a convenient abstraction, and education and income inequalities are the components of class which ought to receive our attention. It is education and income which are more directly associated with knowledge and with opportunities to make lifestyle choices which are of direct health relevance.

Secondly, one of the major reasons why persons who are of lower class have higher rates of disease and death is that they lead less healthy lifestyles. These lifestyle differences include (but are not limited to) higher rates of cigarette consumption, the consumption of less healthy foods, higher cholesterol levels and higher rates of high blood pressure. Lower class persons also engage in less recreational physical activity and are more often overweight and or obese.

Finally, while we have only explored some seven factors which are arguably a result of class membership, and which have direct health consequences, there are likely to be many other factors which play an additional intermediate role between social class and health.

Reducing social class inequalities in health

As there are few, if any, published evaluations of programs developed with the specific intention of reducing social class inequalities in health, what follows represent 'signposts' for action, rather than a specific program of activities. Some suggestions can be made with confidence, others are necessarily hypothetical, given our state of knowledge.

The data from England and Wales are clear in indicating that the introduction of 'free' and accessible health care has little direct impact on health inequalities. This tends to be confirmed by European data on health inequalities where 'free' health care is accompanied by class based health inequalities. Providing those in need with accessible and expensive health services may serve any of a number of functions, but it has a limited impact on class inequalities in health.

Social class health inequalities appear to be associated with the degree of income inequalities which exist in a society. As economic changes increase or decrease the extent of these income inequalities, so there is evidence of a commensurate change in health inequalities (see Najman 1992).

Social class health inequalities reflect, in part, differences in lifestyle associated with a family's income. While the evidence is somewhat incomplete, it does indicate that people driven into poverty often manifest a change in lifestyle, this change being detrimental to the individual's mental and physical health (see Najman & Western, 1993).

If we accept the above as a reasonable reflection of our present state of knowledge regarding the causes of social class inequalities in health, then what courses of action are open to those who would seek to reduce the magnitude of these health inequalities? Four categories of activity are typically discussed in the context of preventing disease. These have all been found to be effective in some circumstances and not others. Our concern here is specifically with the likely contribution of each of these strategies to a reduction in social class inequalities in health.

Individual education and/or persuasion

Whenever patients visit a doctor or have contact with other health care providers, there is an opportunity for preventive advice to be given. Studies of medical advice to 'quit smoking' have found that up to one-third of patients will act on this advice (Richmond et al 1988.)

In a clinical context it is also possible to screen patients (where appropriate), for such health problems as high blood pressure, evidence of excessive alcohol consumption and the like. It might even be argued that persons living in poverty should have their health related behaviour more intensively assessed as they are at higher risk for a wide variety of problems. A patient's underlying poverty status could serve to alert health care providers to a range of possible health problems. Such a strategy is, however, unlikely to have a major impact on class inequalities in health. Simply put it is unlikely a sufficient number of cases will be identified and that the requisite behaviour changes will be of sufficient magnitude to have a major impact on class inequalities in health. While the population's health might improve as a result of more intensive clinically based efforts to prevent disease, this strategy is unlikely to materially reduce social class inequalities in health.

Community education/persuasion

Strategies of community education and persuasion have been remarkably effective in producing health related behaviour changes. There have been substantial reductions in smoking levels, improved dietary intake and increased exercise levels as people become aware of, and respond to, advice to change their lifestyles. It has been suggested that half of the recent decline in death rates from cardiovascular disease can be attributed to such changes in lifestyle.

It can be numerically demonstrated that a small percentage change in community behaviour (say a 5% decline in the per cent of the population smoking cigarettes) can produce a substantially greater impact on health than say the routine provision of smoking cessation advice in clinical encounters. This is a reflection of the large proportions of the population that can be reached using mass media techniques.

Our concern however is not with whether mass media techniques work, but rather with whether their extension is likely to reduce class inequalities in health. Such an effect might be observed if either one or both of two possibilities are found to be the case. If a risk behaviour or practice were found to occur at higher rates in the poor and these poor were equally liable to respond to mass techniques, then they would disproportionately benefit. Alternately if the risk behaviour or practice were equally distributed by class membership but the poor were more responsive to persuasion, then they would again disproportionately benefit. However the evidence indicates that while risk behaviours are more frequent in the lowest class groups, these groups are less responsive than their more affluent counterparts to persuasion. Thus it follows that whatever the community benefits of mass campaigns, such campaigns are unlikely to reduce class inequalities in health.

Environmental/legislative initiatives

Environmental and legislative initiatives generally reflecting governmental responses to pressure groups, have been amongst the most cost-effective strategies of preventing disease. For example legislation to enforce the wearing of seat belts, the requirement for impact absorbing materials in cars and the building of separated roads and roundabouts, to prevent head-on collisions, have all contributed to a substantial reduction in road deaths. The addition of fluoride to our water supplies, and vitamin D (thiamine) to bread also represent efficient strategies for improving community health. Laws to prevent the advertising and promotion of harmful products particularly to the young, represent additional activities of government which arguably confer benefits to the community, albeit by restricting the freedom of those who profit from the promotion and sale of their harmful products.

Some legislative activities have the capacity to reduce social class inequalities in health. Strategies which focus on community development and on improving the organization and delivery of services to the poor, may reduce health inequalities. Here poorer communities could be easily identified and targeted for special programs.

Alternately those unhealthy behaviours and practices which are more common in lower class groups, could be the focus of legislation. While this legislation could impact on all economic groups, it could produce disproportionate benefits for those who manifest these unhealthy behaviours with the greatest frequency. Legislation concerned with cigarette smoking, diet or accidents and injuries would appear to have the highest priority in the above context.

Economic redistribution

Governments collect taxes and then use these to provide an infrastructure and services for the population. All governments, to a greater or less extent, act to redistribute resources. From the health perspective it is pertinent to raise the question of whether a more economically equal society could be created by allocating a greater proportion of resources to the poor, and assessing whether such an equalization might reduce the health gap between rich and poor.

Certainly there are a number of data sources which indicate that the mortality gap between classes runs parallel to the income gap between them. As income inequalities increase so have mortality inequalities been found to increase (see Najman 1993 for a more detailed discussion). Using correlation data for selected OECD countries, there is a strong correlation between the percentage of children, adults and the elderly living in poverty and infant mortality rates, while the percentage of the elderly living in poverty is strongly associated with life expectancy.

In any event if one considers the characteristics of those living in poverty, they tend to fall into one or more of five categories. These are single parents (the largest group), the aged, the unemployed, racial minorities (e.g. Aborigines) and the disabled. All these groups have large proportions of their numbers dependent upon government funded welfare benefits. In an important sense, their poverty status is a reflection of the level at which governments set benefits and the failure of successive governments in Australia to generate programs which would reduce the proportion of the population living in poverty.

Clearly programs aimed at reducing poverty would act to advantage the health of those in greatest need. Such programs should serve to reduce the mortality gap between rich and poor. At the very least the time has come to trial welfare initiatives which have the specific aim of reducing health inequalities.

Conclusion

Changes in social class inequalities in mortality over the earlier part of this century indicate that the social, political and economic circumstances in which people live have a profound influence on their health. While it is true that poverty itself cannot cause disease, poverty is associated with a lifestyle which can have profound consequences for the health of adults and children. Governments determine the level of economic inequality in a society by setting benefit levels and by initiating programs to enable the single, the unemployed and the disabled (and others) to gain employment and to re-enter the mainstream of society.

We live in a society where there remain some curious contradictions. There is public support for government action to provide equal access to health care. Few feel comfortable with a society in which the very young as well as the aged living in poverty are subject to worse health and experience disproportionately higher death rates. Yet it is curious that while governments 'tinker' with the health system in an effort to deal with health inequalities, they themselves contribute to these inequalities by their failure to eliminate or reduce the existing level of poverty in Australian society.

REFERENCES

Australian Institute of Health and Welfare 1992 Australia's health 1992: The third biennial report of the Australian Institute of Health and Welfare. AGPS, Canberra
Bauman A, Owen N, Rushworth R L 1990 Recent trends and sociodemographic determinants of exercise participation in Australia. Community Health Studies 14:19–26
Bor W et al 1993 Socioeconomic disadvantage and child morbidity: an Australian longitudinal study. Social Science and Medicine 36(8):1053–1061
Broom D H 1984 The social distribution of illness: is Australia more equal? Social Science and Medicine 18(11):907–917
Caspersen C J et al 1986 Status of the 1990 physical fitness and exercise objectives—evidence from NHIS 1985. Public Health Reports 101(6):587–592
Centers for Disease Control 1977 Ten leading causes of death in the United States 1975. Centers for Disease Control, Atlanta, Georgia
Coleman R P, Rainwater L, McClelland K A 1979 Social standing in America. Routledge & Kegan Paul, London
Congalton A A 1969 Status and prestige in Australia. Cheshire, Melbourne
English R 1993 Socio-economic status, diet and risk factors for coronary heart disease. PhD thesis, Department of Social and Preventive Medicine, University of Queensland

HDFP Cooperative Group 1977 Race, education and prevalence of hypertension. American Journal of Epidemiology 106(5):351–361

Helmert U et al 1989 Social class and risk factors for coronary heart disease in the Federal Republic of Germany, results of the baseline survey of the German cardiovascular prevention study. Journal of Epidemiology and Community Health 43:37–42

Helmert U et al 1990 Relationship of social class characteristics and risk factors for coronary heart disease in West Germany. Public Health 104:399–416

Jones I G, Cameron D 1984 Social class analysis: an embarrassment to epidemiology. Community Medicine 6(1)37–46

Judge K, Benzeval M 1993 Health inequalities: new concerns about the children of single mothers. British Medical Journal 306:677–80

Marmot M 1993 Cardiovascular disease. Journal of Epidemiology and Community Health 47(1)2–4

Martin M J et al 1986 Serum cholesterol, blood pressure and mortality: implications from a cohort of 361 662 men. Lancet ii:933–6

Knupfer G 1989 The prevalence in various social groups of eight different drinking patterns from abstaining to frequent drunkenness: analysis of 10 US surveys combined. British Journal of Addiction 84:1305–1318

Lazarus N B et al 1991 Change in alcohol consumption and risk of death from all causes and from ischaemic heart disease. British Medical Journal 30(6802):553–556

Lehman H C, Witty P A 1931 Further study of the social status of occupations. Journal of Educational Sociology 5:101–112

Lundberg O 1986 Class and health: comparing Britain and Sweden. Social Science and Medicine 23(5):511–517

Mackenback J P, Maas P J (undated) Social inequality and differences in health: a survey of principal research findings. In: Gunning-Schepers L J, Spruit I P, Krijnen J H (eds) Socio-economic inequalities in health. Ministry of Welfare, Health and Cultural Affairs, The Hague, pp. 25–80

McDowall M 1983 Measuring women's occupational mortality. Population Trends 34:25–29 OPCS, HMSO

McMichael A J 1985 Social class (as estimated by occupational prestige) and mortality in Australian males in the 1970s. Community Health Studies 9(3):220–230

Najman J M 1993 Health and poverty: past and present and prospects for the future. Social Science and Medicine 36(2):157–166

Najman J M et al 1979 Patterns of mobility, health care utilisation and socio-economic status in Brisbane. Australian and New Zealand Journal of Sociology 15(3):55–63

Najman J M et al 1992 Child developmental delay and socio-economic disadvantage in Australia: a longitudinal study. Social Science and Medicine 34(8):829–835

Najman J M, Western J S 1993 Sociology of social structures and cultural reproduction. Sociology of Australian Society: introductory readings, 2nd edn. Macmillan, Melbourne

National Health Strategy 1992 Enough to make you sick: how income and environment affect health. Supplement to Research Paper No. 1. Australian Institute of Health and Welfare, Canberra

Nilson L B, Edelman M 1979 The symbolic evocation of occupational prestige. Reprint 348. Institute for Research on Poverty, University of Wisconsin, Madison

Pamak E R 1985 Social class inequality in mortality from 1921 to 1972 in England and Wales. Population Studies 39:17–31

Pearce N E et al 1983 Mortality and social class in New Zealand II: male mortality by major disease groupings. New Zealand Medical Journal 96(740):711–716

Penn R 1975 Occupational prestige hierarchies. Social Forces, 54(2):352–364

Richmond R L, Austin A, Webster I W 1988 Predicting abstainers in a smoking cessation program administered by general practitioners. International Journal of Epidemiology 17(3):530–534

Simons L A et al 1986 Education level and coronary risk factors in Australians. Medical Journal of Australia, 145(November 3):446–450

Siskind V, Najman J M, Veitch C 1992 Socioeconomic status and mortality revisited: an extension of the Brisbane area analysis. Australian Journal of Public Health 16(3):315–320

Taylor R et al 1983 Occupation and mortality in Australia: working age males 1975–77. Department of Social and Preventive Medicine, Monash University, Melbourne

Viikari J et al 1990 Cardiovascular risk in young Finns. Acta Paediatrica Scandanavica 365:13–19
Warner W L et al 1960 Social class in America: a manual of procedure for the measurement of social status. Harper, New York
Whichelow M J 1989 Choice of spread by a random sample of the British population. European Journal of Clinical Nutrition 43:1–10
Wilkinson R G 1989 Class mortality differentials: income distribution and trends in poverty 1921–81. Journal of Social Policy 18(3):307–335
Wynn A 1987 Inequalities in nutrition. Nutrition and Health 5(1/2):79–94
Yeracaris C A, Kim J H 1978 Socioeconomic differentials in selected causes of death. American Journal of Public Health 68 (4):342–351

3. Young people, unemployment and health

Rob White

The child shall enjoy protection, and shall be given opportunities and facilities, by law and by other means, to enable [them] to develop physically, mentally, morally, spiritually and socially in a healthy and normal manner and in conditions of freedom and equality.

United Nations Convention on the Rights of the Child

Young people are often presented as being 'our future'. The rhetoric of politicians and community leaders alike is replete with grand statements about young people being 'our most valuable resource' and 'our greatest asset'. International conventions and covenants also stress the 'natural' rights of the young to all manner of protections and facilities. Yet the reality for a large and increasing number of young Australians is that society is providing them a terribly unhealthy environment within which to develop, an environment devoid of occupational and economic opportunities. And an unhealthy social environment inevitably leads to personal sickness, despair and depression for many individuals.

The aim of the chapter is to explore briefly the issue of youth unemployment and the health of young people. The essay reinforces the commonsense view that there is a strong connection between unemployment and poor mental and physical health. Rather than just state the obvious, however, the chapter plans to explore more fully the many dimensions of this relationship—including the main reasons for the existence of such an unhealthy social environment in the first instance.

In essence, it will be argued that to define 'health' in relation to the young requires that we view it in a much larger family and community context. For example, the marginalization of young people on the basis of age helps explain why and how they are treated as they are in areas of official health policy and participation in various public health campaigns. But, more fundamentally, the overall well-being of young people and the kinds of health problems they may endure is most affected by the deep social divisions in society—those based on class, gender and ethnic background. In order to see how this occurs in practice, we shall focus on the specific issue of unemployment and the ways in which different groups of young people are affected by this.

Young people, work and unemployment

The nature of work in Australia has been radically transformed over the last two and a half decades. This has been due to a range of interrelated factors, such as technological innovations, the globalization of the market system, changing trading relationships in the international arena and the restructuring of work processes themselves. For young people the impact of the changing nature of work has been particularly profound and in some instances devastating.

For example, teenage full-time employment has plummetted in the last 25 years. It has been pointed out that the 'proportion of all 15–19 year olds in full-time employment fell from 58% in August 1966 to 20% in August 1991' (McDonald 1992:18). Many young people today in this age group are in fact in some kind of training or education program. Even so, youth unemployment generally has continued to rise dramatically in recent years. Thus, in late-1992 the official national unemployment rate of young people not in training was approximately 38%.

By way of contrast, part-time employment for 15-19 year olds has increased from 3.5% in 1966 to around 23% in May 1992 (McDonald 1992:18). The majority of young people in part-time work are also students; employers appear to have a preference for these workers over the full-time unemployed (Sweet 1987, White 1989).

If out of work, and out of school, the chances of gaining employment are diminished considerably. Indeed, the 'average length of time a young person is unemployed has increased from 2.9 weeks in 1966 to 25.1 weeks in 1991' (Youth Action and Policy Association 1992:15). In terms of actual numbers, it has been noted that:

> There are currently around 230 000 young people—17% of all 15–19 year olds—who can be categorised as being 'at risk'. This includes those not in full-time education and either unemployed, employed only part-time or not in the labour force (i.e. discouraged young people who have given up looking for work or training) (McDonald 1992:19).

Hence, there is a considerable number of young people who are in a very vulnerable position indeed. And it is these young people who are also the most 'at risk' in terms of basic health problems and healthy lifestyle options.

There are of course substantial social differences which are reflected in the composition of those young people who are unemployed and therefore most 'at risk' in health terms. For example, Aboriginal and Torres Strait Islander young people have the highest rates of joblessness in the country, and are further disadvantaged by overt racist behaviour, poor educational opportunities and in many cases geographical isolation. Young people in rural and remote communities are likewise suffering greatly from lack of local job markets and lack of ready access to relevant, quality education and training options. Young people with intellectual and physical disabilities, and young non-English speaking migrants, are also two categories of young people who are particularly disadvantaged in the race for jobs. And young women have seen their job prospects diminish over the last two decades due to a combination of work restructuring and the involvement of older women in the labour force.

Overall, however, the crucial variable in determining employment chances is that of class background. The social class of one's family of origin ultimately dictates the general chances that a young person has in finding work or in undertaking further study which may lead to a job (see Jamrozik 1988). Those families with insufficient financial or cultural resources relevant to the economic structures of a capitalist society are those which cannot provide the necessary boost for their members to compete successfully in a very restricted labour market. One result of this is chronic unemployment. While young people from across a range of income backgrounds may experience varying bouts of unemployment, the main issue is whether or not they have the resources (family or otherwise) to keep their aspirations alive. This may take the form of ongoing education, or simply of having the finances to bridge temporary periods of joblessness until an appropriate opportunity emerges. It is the working class—broadly defined, and including young people of both sexes and many different cultural and ethnic backgrounds—which invariably bears the burden of economic downturn and crisis.

As the nature of the labour market changes so too does the position of these young people in the overall economy. The Australian economy can be seen in terms of four interrelated spheres of activity: the formal waged economy, the informal waged economy, the informal non-waged economy, and the criminal economy (see White 1989). Pressures in one sphere have direct and indirect consequences for activity in the other spheres.

In terms of unemployment, it can be said that a significant proportion of working class young people have effectively been squeezed out of the full-time formal waged economy. This has foisted upon them a reliance upon state benefits and/or finding income from other kinds of sources. For those young people in the paid workforce, there are strong pressures to accept low wages and poor conditions under the threat of dismissal and no future job security.

For many young working class people the lack of paid work in the formal economic sector may lead them to pursue alterative work arrangements in the informal waged economy. This includes, for example, the so called 'cash-in-hand' phenomenon where workers are paid 'under the table' for their efforts. However, here too many young people find themselves competing on unfavourable terms with others for the work at hand. The oversupply of workers in the formal economy ultimately spills over into the cash economy as well.

If paid work is not available in these two sectors then young working class people, especially young women, will in many cases be forced to be active in the informal non-waged economy. Thus, in return for lodgings and board, young women are placed in a position of having to play 'domestic servant' due to their dependant and vulnerable economic status.

In many instances poverty-stricken young people of both sexes may be forced to be active in the criminal economy. Activities in the criminal economy differ from those in the informal economy in that the latter are not in themselves different from 'legitimate' economic transactions in the formal waged economy. Income in the criminal economy, however, is generated through irregular commission of criminal offences, ranging from shoplifting to buglary.

The well-being of working class young people is intimately linked to the stresses and strains associated with movements in and out of each sphere of economic activity, and the pressures of securing an income in each particular case.

Youth lifestyle and well-being

The transformation of work has generated terrible levels of stress on the part of young people in Australia today. This has not been helped by government policies which are based upon notions of 'unemployability' rather than seeing unemployment as the main issue. That is, instead of focussing on systematic job creation, the response of governments has been to stress the individual responsibility and 'deficiencies' of young people. Labour market programs and government policies are thus structured in such a way as to train and educate young people to learn new skills, to act in certains ways, to adopt the proper attitudes, etc.—they do not grapple with the huge drop in full-time employment positions or seriously consider radical alternatives to existing work patterns (White 1990).

Young people from low-income backgrounds are most vulnerable to the deteriorating fortunes of the established labour market and the substantive changes occurring in social welfare provision. But they are not alone in feeling the incredible pressures of unemployment on both the competition for jobs and the struggle to retain work once it has been found. Unemployment is affecting virtually everyone in Australia—young and old, male and female, people from many diverse ethnic backgrounds. It is having an impact on many people in the middle layers of the established socioeconomic pyramid, as well as those with fewer economic resources and occupational choices.

Prior to entry into the labour force, the competition for entry into tertiary education courses and to successfully complete Year 12 studies has intensified. Regardless of actual skill content and level of skill required for a particular job, the educational credential has risen in value as a means to sift out potential employees. Thus the fear of unemployment is a significant factor in the lives of those young people currently in study or who are already in the workforce.

With respect to those young people in a 'job', as distinct from those in the first stages of a 'career', there is constant pressure to perform well. By their very nature, low level jobs involve the easy substitution of one worker for another. This means that any young working class person who has such work is immediately under pressure to accept the dictates of the employer. Partly as a reflection of this insecurity, it is notable that young workers constitute the highest proportion of those workers who are injured at the workplace each year (Australian Council of Trade Unions 1988).

If we further investigate the nature of these injuries, too often we find that men adopt a macho attitude toward issues of industrial health and safety due to certain media stereotyping of workers (Biggins 1987 & 1988). Women on the other hand, especially migrant women, are disproportionately subject to injuries such as 'repetition strain injury' and are among the least protected industrially and in terms of alternative employment chances (Alcorso 1988, Stewart 1986). Those who work in the informal economy would seem to be equally vulnerable due to their insecure work situations. Young workers are appreciated (and kept on) only insofar as they maintain certain degrees of productivity and are compliant in the performance of their labour.

The young unemployed and the working poor who live in low-income households used to contribute a significant amount of money to those households (Moore 1988). However, with changes in government policy, especially with respect to payments to 16- and 17-year-olds, many households are now struggling to make ends meet. This is compounded by the low wages paid to those young workers lucky enough to be in the paid workforce (Australian Council of Trade Unions 1989). The inability of many households to keep their financial resources up in relation to the costs of living puts a severe strain on families and relationships.

One consequence of this is the presence of a large number of homeless young people in Australian society (Burdekin 1989). For many young people the consequence may be to price them out of the rental and housing markets, and thus force them to return to the parental home. This may entail a process of 'infantilization', whereby young women in particular are treated like children, whose duty it is to obey the whim of the providing parent (White 1990). It also may mean that these young people are restricted by financial means and household chores to spend most of their time in the home, rather than outside with friends, doing activities of a more recreational and creative nature. Thus, the question of social isolation looms large in this kind of situation. So too, do the issues of sexual abuse, incest and exploitation of child labour.

If one is without financial resources in a consumer society, then trouble can be anticipated. For the young unemployed and the working poor a compounding problem many experience is the lack of a venue or public space which they can call their own. Indeed, much of contemporary 'law and order' policy is precisely geared to monitor and police the young unemployed—the non-consumers who frequent our malls and shopping centres (White 1994). Youth crime is subject to periodic 'moral panics' in the mass media, and the activities of all young people are increasingly subject to scrutiny and control by various officials of the state. Thus, to be homeless, to be poor, to be without paid work, to be cooped up inside one's parent's house, are all compounded by the constant harassment and hassles associated with street life in Australian cities today.

Obviously the changes occurring in the lives of young working class people will have profound effects on their lifestyles, life opportunities and on their immediate health. The usual definition of 'health' in the contemporary period is along the lines of 'health is not the absence of disease or infirmity; it is a state of complete physical, mental and social well-being' (see Youth Affairs Council of Australia 1991). To this we might add that health 'is considered in terms of the ability to achieve one's potential and to respond positively to the challenges of the environment, that is, as a resource for everyday living' (National Health and Medical Research Council 1992:1). Given the incredible difficulties briefly outlined above, it is clear that many of these young people are growing up in an environment which is far from conducive to health and well-being. Many are struggling simply to cope with life on the margins.

Social and health costs

Unemployment and poverty, and the stresses related to these, are apparent in a range of social indicators of well-being. These show a significant impact in terms of mortality rates (i.e. death) and morbidity rates (i.e. illness). For example, it was reported at the first Australian conference on Unemployment and Health at the University of Sydney in November 1992 that unemployment had strong links with both mortality and mental health. One study found that unemployed young people were more likely to commit suicide or die in a car accident than those with a job; another study found that young unemployed people had psychiatric disorders at least three times the national rate (Connolly 1992:9).

It would certainly appear that suicide rates among young people have changed in accordance with changed economic circumstances. For the categories of 15–19 year old males and 20–24 year old females there has been a 100% increase in suicides recorded since the mid-1960s (Mason 1990:20). In monetary terms, the costs of youth suicide have been estimated to be in the range of between $100–$200 million a year (Mason 1990:24). While not simply reducible to unemployment alone, increasing youth suicide does correlate strongly with the increasing rates of youth unemployment. If we take into account the ways in which males and females are differentially socialized with regard to the techniques of 'successful' suicide (e.g. use of guns), and the particularly threatening impact of unemployment on young men's sense of masculinity (especially where personal identity is tied up with work status), then we gain some sense of the reasons why young men are statistically over-represented when it comes to suicide.

A major study into mental health and young people also provides findings which are of interest to the present discussion. For example, while not specifying the experiences of the young unemployed per se, the researchers found that young people identified a range of factors which cause mental health problems. The most frequently cited were 'stress' and 'family issues'. It was pointed out that:

In general, the category 'stress' included a range of potentially stressful events arising at home and at school including 'peer pressure', 'stressed out because of pressure from school', and 'society beating down upon you'. Some of the issues in the category labelled 'family issues' included, 'not being looked after by your parents', 'what's left over from an abusive childhood', 'marriage breakups', 'misunderstanding between parents and children', 'not raised to be confident', and 'trouble with parents understanding you're becoming an adult'. (Sawyer et al 1992:40-41).

Earlier in this report the authors indicated the importance of biological factors in mental illness as well. Nevertheless, even where biological predisposition may occur, the fact is that young people themselves see stress as a major factor in their overall mental health. Again, it needs to be reiterated that while all young people may experience the 'normal stresses' of growing up (e.g. biological changes), wider social and economic circumstances will have a profound impact on the character of the stresses experienced by particular categories of young people.

For example, we might consider the specific kinds of problems which present themselves in the case of young homeless people (see Burdekin 1989). Low self-esteem, feelings of hopelessness and social isolation may be aggravated by the stress of homelessness; and a vicious circle may arise where such feelings and perceptions manifest themselves in destructive personal behaviour, ranging from self-mutilation through to substance abuse of various kinds (e.g. alcohol, tobacco, cannabis, amphetamines, heroin, glue).

The marginalization of young people who are poor, unemployed and possibly homeless has a compounding impact on their immediate mental and physical health. For instance, low income and low self-esteem is associated with poor nutrition, weight loss, skin infestations and infections, and respiratory and gastrointestinal infections (National Health and Medical Research Council 1992, Watkins 1991). Lack of economic and social resources, however, reinforces the condition which the young person may be experiencing. That is, the primary health problems are often accompanied by lack of preventive health care (e.g. dental checks, pap smears, chlamydia testing, use of contraceptives), and poor care of chronic illnesses such as diabetes, and a lack of or a failure to use appropriate aids such as spectacles (National Health and Medical Research Council 1992:4-5).

Young working class women are particularly 'at risk' in a situation of little family or community support. In addition to the issue of sexual abuse, which an astonishing proportion of all young women endure in Australian society, there are other issues associated with power and sexuality. Teenage pregnancy, as a means to escape poverty, is not an unknown phenomenon. Nor are the dilemmas associated with young women attempting to use abortion services, especially if they are under 16 years of age. The high, and gender specific, cost of sanitary pads, much less contraceptive devices, has an impact on both the financial position and health requirements of these young women as well. Problems of low self-esteem coupled with media images of the ideal woman can also lead to various eating disorders, such as anorexia nervosa. Thus, the idea of thin is beautiful may, in these circumstances, have a basis in actual economic conditions.

The unemployed are also susceptible to poor sexual health. This may be due to multiple sexual partners, from abuse or prostitution. A 1991 Western Australian report found that:

> Poverty has been recognised as a contributing factor to the risk of HIV infection among young men and women. It has been established that economic pressure, often exacerbated by homelessness, can lead to some young people engaging in prostitution, often offering unprotected intercourse in exchange for money, shelter, food or drugs. Such young people are at a high risk for HIV infection. (Watkins 1991:24).

Significantly, those young people with less social resources are also those who are less likely to know about at risk behaviour, or the nature of various physical and psychological symptoms.

Young gay men and lesbian women who may be unemployed and poor also have to cope with the fact that homosexuality remains relatively taboo in Australian society. In a hostile context, the chances of engaging in at risk behaviour are increased, and this is especially so when driven by economic necessity. Legal sanctions and negative media portrayals, as well as direct attacks on the street (see Gay and Lesbian Rights Lobby 1992), create enormous problems for those gay and lesbian young people who are trying to survive economically in any way they can because they have not been able to get paid work in the formal economic sector.

In general, health and welfare services are not available equally to all young people. This is partly a question of class and income background; it is also related to geographical location and gender. For instance, it is well known that young women in rural areas are particularly disadvantaged in terms of choice of doctor, confidentiality of treatment, and procurement of preventive health care aids (Omelczuk et al 1990). The frequency of contact with health officials depends a great deal upon family resources and general social background.

As an indirect indicator of inequalities in family and household resources, and of the disparity in medical and general health services available to different groups in society, we can take a look at what happens when one is unemployed and black. Membership of and identification with an oppressed 'minority' group is definitely bad for one's health and this is especially so in the context of entrenched racist attitudes and institutionalized inequalities. In Western Australia, for example, it was reported in 1991 that 'some 68% of youth incarcerated in this state are Aboriginal and 86% of these were neither employed nor attending school prior to their incarceration' (State Government Advisory Committee on Young Offenders 1991:6). The phenomenon of high detention rates and high levels of unemployment among Aboriginal young people has been well documented, as have high levels of police harassment and violence directed at Aborigines (see, for example, Gale et al 1990, Cunneen 1990).

What is less discussed in matters of this nature is the general well-being and health status of those young people who are put into detention. Some indication of this is provided in figures relating to young people held in the Longmore Detention Centre in Perth. It has been reported that:

Between 1983 and 1990, nursing staff administered 8176 treatments to inmates. In 1990, 20 960 treatments were administered. There was a consistency in the number of inmates over this time. Nursing staff maintain that young people are coming to Longmore in a poorer state of health and that this is reflected in the greatly increased number of treatments needed. Common health problems among this group include: poor nutrition, weight loss, drug abuse, the effects of car accidents, scabies, ringworm, and sexually transmitted diseases. (Watkins 1991:38).

Given that the majority of these inmates are in fact Aboriginal, these figures represent yet another indication of the low and deteriorating conditions of life for young Aborigines generally. Colonization has been devastating to Aboriginal people, severely affecting their economic base, family unit, social organization and cultural heritage. That Aboriginal health status is the worst of any sector in the community is confirmed by the data and discussions contained in the Report of the Royal Commission into Aboriginal Deaths in Custody (Johnston 1991). The Commission Report, for example, demonstrates the far greater prevalence of illness conditions and diseases, such as leprosy and trachoma, among Aboriginal people than non-Aboriginal people. It further documents things such as the impact of malnourishment among Aboriginal people, and the extent among young Aboriginal people of advanced ischaemic heart disease, a health problem relatively uncommon among young non-Aboriginal people.

The marginalization of young people economically and socially directly and indirectly contributes to the illnesses and decline in well-being of young people. Many of these young people are also denied or lack information and access to medical and health services, and few know of their rights in claiming such services. While inequality in community resources underpins the ill health experienced by these young people, specific types of health problems are associated with particular groups of young people (e.g. eating disorders and young women; petrol sniffing and young Aborigines).

Government reponses to youth ill health

The predominant government response to the health needs and health related issues of the young unemployed has been to focus on the symptoms rather than the causes of the problem. Certain assumptions are continually made regarding the 'causes' of 'deviant' or 'unhealthy' behaviour, and these are used to inform various campaigns and service delivery strategies. For instance, much state attention has been directed at anti-drug programmes (such as the 'Respect Yourself—Drink Safe' campaign), and on the propagation of materials on issues relating to AIDS and sexuality.

The problem with these measures is threefold. First, they tend to imply that 'prevention' is simply a matter of education and/or coercion. Secondly, the stress on 'morality' and 'pathology' in constructing responses to the issues leads to inadequate and inappropriate campaigns for the young people most in need of correct information. Thirdly, they fail to address the reasons why young people, especially the young unemployed, may engage in particular 'at risk' practices in the first place.

A classic instance of this kind of government response to youth health needs is the federal government's cutting of funds to the New South Wales Family Planning Association (FPA) in 1992 after it had printed the *Fact and Fantasy File Diary*, information that was distributed to high school students as part of the FPA's Making Sense of Sex project for young people. Deemed to be too explicit, to endorse homosexuality as socially legitimate, and to be non-judgemental across a range of sexual and social matters, the *Diary* was initially criticized via a concerted public campaign orchestrated by sections of the Sydney media. In response to the government's knee-jerk and somewhat belated efforts at censorship, copies of the *Diary* were reproduced and distributed nationally by the socialist youth organisation Resistance, where it was, by all accounts, received enthusiastically by high school students from around the country.

Some positive discussion has taken place over attempts to design services to meet the special needs of some groups of young people. This is so, for example, with respect to the health and welfare of young homeless people (Burdekin 1989, National Health and Medical Research Council 1992). In a similar vein, government reports at both state and federal level now regularly take note of the range of social factors affecting youth health—such as poverty, unemployment, family breakdown, sexual abuse, racism and so on. Inequality is formally acknowledged and very often lip service is paid to the notion of providing social justice in the health area.

But funding for research and for service delivery has still tended to concentrate on specific illnesses and specific health related social behaviours (i.e. drug use and abuse) rather than wider structural inequalities (Boland & Jamrozik 1989). In essence, prevailing approaches tend to focus on the effects of deeper structural processes affecting young people, instead of enhancing the overall well-being of the young people concerned. 'Health issues' are thus constructed in policy terms as self-contained problems which can be dealt with adequately in terms of specific institutional changes or interpersonal interventions in the lives of the young. As such, the issues are seen more as problems of circumstance and policy, rather than as fundamentally related to the basic economic and social structures of society.

The basic dimensions of the relationship between youth health and youth unemployment presented in this chapter are shown in the box. It is suggested in this that underlying structural inequality and social division means that unemployment and poverty will impact upon different groups of young people and be experienced differently depending upon their social background. The actual experiences of unemployment—involving lack of financial resources, and fears and insecurities generated by the situation—in turn give rise to a wide range of health problems. These are the direct effect of the unequal distribution of community resources and of the prior existence of deep social divisions in Australian society.

Social structure and young people's health

Health and well-being (social effects)
- Mortality rates e.g. suicide, car accidents
- Mental health e.g. psychiatric disorders, low self-esteem, stress, depression, anorexia nervosa
- Physical health e.g. poor nutrition, substance abuse, sexually transmitted diseases, weight loss, skin infections
- Preventive health care e.g. dental checks, pap smears, use of contraceptives, chlamydia testing

Unemployment and poverty (situational factors)
- Effects of lack of financial resources e.g. homelessness, social isolation, infantilization, abuse and exploitation, police harassment, less access to health and welfare services
- Effects of fear of unemployment e.g. stress, insecurity, powerlessness, work injury, credentialism; plus the added burdens of racism, sexism and discrimination of various kinds based on age, disability, etc.

Social context (structural conditions)
- Inequality and social divisions of capitalist society e.g. unequal distribution of community resources on the basis of class, gender, ethnicity, age, disability, geography
- Transformations in nature of work e.g. changes in pay, opportunities and personal control in the formal and informal economic sectors, particularly for young working class people, Aborigines, non-English speaking background migrants, young people in detention, and young people in rural and isolated areas

---

An appropriate and adequate response to the health needs of the young unemployed will thus require significant reform and change at a number of levels. First, major efforts have to be made to transform the conditions which set the limits of, and pressures on, each individual's health condition and his or her ability to take a full and active part in society. This means that meaningful employment and a secure adequate income is a must for these young people. Youth homelessness and unemployment do not affect all groups the same way. Indeed, there is substantial evidence that young people's position in society is closely related to the class position of their family of origin (Boland & Jamrozik 1989). For substantive changes to occur, therefore, much more needs to be said and done about the fact that the present social structure rests upon deep class divisions and inequalities.

It is essential, for example, that state intervention in the economy be directed at meeting working class community needs. Expanded social services, innovative job creation projects and the redistribution of wealth and income via taxation are just some of the measures which would enhance the immediate health prospects of many unemployed young people. In a similar vein, improvements in the health and well-being of Aboriginal young people ultimately demands acknowledgement of the centrality of self-determination, including land rights, in any reform agenda, and action to redress and compensate Aborigines for injustices which continue up to the present day.

A second area where concerted reform is necessary is that of the health system itself. As Jamozik and Boland (1991:29) point out: 'while some health issues are clearly of concern mainly to young people, or even solely of concern to young people, most such issues are also of concern to other age groups'. Given this, then any changes in policy should also reflect the interests of wider groups in our society, particularly those who are presently among the most disadvantaged and who are often excluded from mainstream services—Aborigines, migrants, women and the unemployed and working poor.

It has been noted that while the overall health of the Australian population relative to other countries is good, serious inequalities in health and access to quality care nevertheless persist (Sharp 1991). To a certain degree such inequalities reflect changes in the relationship between public and private interests in medical and health service provision. Recent years have seen a substantial growth in entrepreneurial medicine, the orientation of health care toward the making of private profit, the deregulation and privatization of health and medical systems, and a severe shortage of resources put into preventive and community health programs. Alternatively, the development of a democratic, interventionist, inclusive and wholistic health care system is one pre-condition for the removal of the inequalities in this area. For young people specifically, this means the 'development of a community style approach to health services which cater for and are accessible to young people—this will require the consultation of young people in the decision making, developmental and management process'. (Youth Affairs Council of Australia 1991:16–17). Only in this way will the present deficiencies in service provision start to be addressed in any sort of constructive and viable manner.

The stresses and tensions experienced by young unemployed people in Australian society are not unusual, whether this be in terms of people in similar situations or with regard to the dynamics of poverty and unemployment in the first instance. It has been argued that unemployment itself is part and parcel of the present economic system, not an aberration. Thus, as Novak (1984:23) observes:

> Poverty is a fundamental fact of life under capitalism. Its system of wage labour and its private ownership of productive wealth has created for the mass of the population a dependence on the labour market and on wages for survival. It is the fundamental insecurity of wage labour which lies at the root of poverty, and it is the need of capitalism for this insecurity as the ultimate discipline and incentive to work which makes the abolition of poverty under capitalism impossible.

This kind of statement raises several important questions for those people concerned about the health of the young unemployed. It makes one wonder about the nature of the manipulations of body and mind by unemployed young people (e.g. use of alcohol, eating disorders), by putting such responses to health issues in the context of an unhealthy social environment. Fundamentally, however, it puts on the agenda the importance of political action and political campaigns for social change. For if the structure of society is implicated in the reasons why some people get sick, then the cure must lie in changing that very structure.

REFERENCES

Alcorso C 1988 Migrant workers and workers' compensation in New South Wales. Social Welfare Research Centre, University of New South Wales, Sydney
Australian Council of Trade Unions 1988 Young people are the most likely victims of industrial accidents. ACTU Bulletin, November:11–13
Australian Council of Trade Unions 1989 Youth strategy. ACTU, Melbourne
Biggins D 1987 The politics of occupational health. Current Affairs Bulletin 64(3):27–31
Biggins D 1988 Focus on occupational health: what can be done? New Doctor 47:6–10
Boland C, Jamrozik A 1989 Young people and health: an overview of current research. National Clearinghouse for Youth Studies, Hobart
Burdekin B 1989 Our homeless children: report of the national inquiry into homeless children by the Human Rights and Equal Opportunity Commission. Australian Government Publishing Service, Canberra
Connelly A 1992 Youth unemployment linked to violent death. The Weekend Australian November 7–8:9
Cunneen C 1990 A study of Aboriginal juveniles and police violence. Human Rights and Equal Opportunity Commission, Sydney
Gale F, Bailey-Harris R, Wundersitz J 1990 Aboriginal youth and the criminal justice system: the injustice of justice? Cambridge University Press, Melbourne
Gay and Lesbian Rights Lobby 1992 The off our backs report: a study into anti-lesbian violence. Report by the Lesbian and Gay Anti-Violence Project, Sydney
Jamrozik A 1988 Young people, the family and social class: issues for research and social policy. Youth Studies 7(1):26–32
Jamrozik A, Boland C 1991 Health issues for young people (to be taken in context). Youth Studies 10(4):24–29
Johnston E 1991 National report of the Royal Commission into Aboriginal Deaths in Custody, vols 2–4. Australian Government Publishing Service, Canberra
Mason C 1990 Youth suicide in Australia: prevention strategies. Department of

Employment, Education and Training, Canberra

McDonald B 1992 Unemployment statistics—figure it out. Social Welfare Impact August:18–19

Moore T 1988 Young people face cash crisis. Social Welfare Impact May:10–12

National Health and Medical Research Council 1992 Health needs of homeless youth. Australian Government Publishing Service, Canberra

Novak T 1984 Poverty and social security. Pluto Press, London

Omelczuk S, Underwood R, White R 1990 Issues confronting youth in remote communities. Conference Proceedings, Future shock into future health: the challenge of change for young Australians in the 90s, The biennial conference of the Australian Association for Adolescent Health, November, Perth

Sawyer M, Meldrum D, Tonge B, Clark J 1992 Mental health and young people. National Clearinghouse for Youth Studies, Hobart

Sharp R 1991 Justice and medical practice: misdiagnosis and maltreatment of a chronic disorder. In: O'Leary J, Sharp R (eds) Inequality in Australia: slicing the cake. William Heinemann Australia, Melbourne

State Government Advisory Committee on Young Offenders 1991 Juvenile justice. Committee response for the Premier on initiatives in programme provision, Perth

Stewart D 1986 Workers' compensation and social security: an overview. Social Welfare Research Centre, University of New South Wales, Sydney

Sweet R 1987 The youth labour market: a twenty-year perspective. Curriculum Development Centre, Canberra

Watkins J et al 1991 Health and welfare (discussion paper no.1). Select Committee on Youth Affairs, Legislative Assembly, Perth

White R 1989 Making ends meet: young people, work and the criminal economy. Australian and New Zealand Journal of Criminology 22(2):136–150

White R 1990 No space of their own: Young people and social control in Australia. Cambridge University Press, Melbourne

White R 1994 Street life: police practices and youth behaviour. In: White R, Alder C (eds) The police and young people in Australia. Cambridge University Press, Melbourne

Youth Action and Policy Association (NSW) 1992 A living income: income support for young people. YAPA, Sydney

Youth Affairs Council of Australia 1991 Health. YACA Discussion Paper, Melbourne

4. Occupational stressors: an insidious form of assault

Dennis McIntyre

This chapter is located within the field of occupational health and presents a case study which examines aspects of a protracted struggle between Newcastle bus operators and State Transit Authority management around the issue of occupational stressors. The project is ongoing action research, and teasing out the manifold connections between the parts and the whole is still in progress. None the less, substantive research demonstrates that in periods of crisis the relationship between production and health appears most lucid.

In response to an apparent increase in debilitating illnesses that were rendering Newcastle State Transit Authority (STA) bus operators unfit for driving duties, the Australian Tramways and Motor Omnibus Employees Association (ATMOEA) invited me to survey its members (June 1990) and produce a report (released in October 1990). Two years later (June 1992) working conditions remained unaltered, bus operators continued to be medically retired, and central issues such as recovery times ('rest' breaks) remained unresolved.

Management insisted that bus operators were 'at risk' because stress is inherent to the occupation (i.e. coping with traffic and passengers), whereas the union contended that stress was not inherent to the occupation, but was imposed through the organization of production—a task controlled by management. For Newcastle bus operators, occupational health became a terrain of contestation where technical and legal imperatives (timetables and changes to awards), rather than workers' health outcomes, were the focus of debate. The problem of occupational stressors became a struggle around competing definitions of efficiency: staffing levels, pace and hours of work, and how production was to be carried out.

Bus operators addressed the problem of occupational stressors through sponsoring research; calling for the establishment of a stress steering committee; numerous forays into the Australian Industrial Relations Commission; revitalization of the workplace occupational health and safety committee; and extensive media exposure of the problem. Management consistently rejected the bus operators interpretation of the situation: workers are not health 'experts', their knowledge is subjective; they are malingerers in search of compensation. The standard management response to worker's initiatives was a reiteration of the managerial prerogative:

State Transit alone has the responsibility for the health, welfare and safety of its employees and cannot cede that responsibility to the Union. Equally, State Transit is fully committed to its obligations under the legislation in respect to occupational health and safety. Whereas State Transit is prepared to work with the Union in this very sensitive area, it must be stressed that it cannot surrender its responsibilities in this area to the Union (McIntyre 1991:9).

The first section of the case study summarizes themes that have shaped my analysis of the struggle between Newcastle bus operators and STA management around the issue of occupational stressors. In this section the relationship between the labour process, especially the issue of managerial control, and occupational health is emphasized. The next section deals with substantive issues; namely the conflictual nature of labour and management perspectives on occupational health, and responses to the problem of occupational stressors. It is contended that the union was not challenging management's responsibility to control the labour process, but was contesting the notion that management could continue to assault bus operators through the current, and proposed, organization of production. Finally, it is proposed that management by successfully sabotaging progress on the stress issue actively supported the continued maintenance of an unhealthy work place. This is why I maintain that occupational stressors are an insidious form of assault.

A parable for health workers

The salient features of the argument presented here are described in the following parable (see Ratcliffe et al 1984).

A group of health workers standing by a river sighted a person who was obviously drowning. Several of them plunged into river, rescued the person in distress; the rest rallied around and commenced resuscitation. Then it was noticed that there were also others drowning: two, three, and soon scores. In spite of an heroic effort, the health workers were unable to rescue everybody, and of those dragged to safety not all could be resuscitated.

Later, when analysing this human disaster, one health worker suggested that all who go in or near the river should learn how to swim. It was agreed that education was a strategy for survival, but how would swimmers cope with rips and undercurrents, sharks, and other hazards. Another health worker then suggested that they should set off up-stream to discover who or what had pushed so many people into the river; and, if possible, to put a stop to it.

The health workers were actually debating the effectiveness of health strategies. First, they had tried heroic intervention—and not all could be saved. Second, they had discussed risk avoidance—and had identified problems. Third, they had raised the question of risk imposition—and had set out to investigate this issue. The first strategy, tertiary health care, is focused entirely on the person in trouble. The second strategy, secondary health care, is largely concerned with changing the behaviour of persons deemed to be at risk. Whereas the third category, primary health care, deals with removing risk imposition through structural change. A labour process perspective on occupational health provides the means of looking up-stream.

The labour process perspective on occupational health

This analysis of the struggle between Newcastle bus operators and STA management around the issue of occupational stressors derives from the work of Michael Quinlan (1988), David Biggins (1988), and Evan Willis (1989) who use, and/or advocate the use of, the labour process perspective in their various critiques of occupational health issues. Their work is in the critical tradition pioneered by Karl Marx and builds on studies by Harry Braverman and Michael Burawoy. By using a labour process approach, it can be demonstrated that occupational stressors are shaped by the nature of labour and management relations.

Historical materialism as a method of social analysis takes into account modes of production, consumption and exchange at several levels—economic, political and ideological. What is produced, how it is produced and how it is distributed forms the basis of any society. Marx ascribed two elements to production: the labour process—any process of transformation of an object into a product via human activity using instruments of labour, and the social relations of production. Braverman (1974) reformulated the Marxian labour process thesis to take account of monopoly capitalism (as a mode of production) by arguing that notions of control and efficiency are inseparable; that managerial strategies, technological innovation, and the organization of production are not neutral—they are part of a social process that includes coercion.

Other analysts such as Burawoy (1979 & 1985) have investigated the 'manufacturing of consent' that occurs concurrently with the production of goods and services, and look beyond the workplace to civil society and the state to better understand how struggles of contestation and resistance between labour and capital are shaped by, and in turn shape, the labour process. To Burawoy, the production and reproduction of interests is a central aspect of the labour process.

Quinlan (1988) critically assesses both psychological and sociological research upon occupational illness. He argues that industrial psychology and its offshoot ergonomics have provided an important intellectual foundation for 'victim blaming' explanations of work-related illness because of the central focus on individual worker behaviour. However, while recent sociological research has provided a counter to this, significant problems still remain to be addressed—the political economy of health, for instance. He further argues that there is a need for sociological research to make more use of the insights emanating from the labour process debate, and to move beyond authority structures, negotiated orders, and payment systems. He concludes that it is within the context of the labour process that the historical role of industrial psychology as a managerialist response to the problems of worker discipline, productivity and health can be more readily understood.

In essence, Quinlan contends that bio-medicine, industrial psychology, and management via their various reductionist techniques seek out pathologies located in individuals, blame the victim, and invite the intervention of the 'expert' and the submission of the victim in order to cure the problem.

Biggins (1988) claims that the social aspects of occupational health have been largely ignored by health workers. He maintains that bio-medicine ignores social determinants of health, encourages changes in lifestyle rather than workstyle and concentrates on curing disease. He also points out that only three of the 17 members of the National Occupational Health and Safety Commission are representative of workers organizations (unions) and suggests that occupational health is managed by political institutions of capitalist society: corporations and the state (itself a major employer). Biggins argues that science has been used ideologically—levels and standards of toxicity are not absolutes but social constructs reached after negotiation. And that the media reinforces the lack of support given to occupational health and focuses on road accidents and strikes; however, two to three times more working hours are lost through injuries at work.

According to Biggins the institution of medicine is an important mechanism of social control (doctors are the 'experts') and assists in maintaining the dominant/subordinate relationship between labour and capital. This is not part of a conspiracy but instead represents the middle class background of most doctors, their ignorance of working class needs and issues, a lack of training in occupational health, and employment opportunities. Few doctors are employed by working class organizations, whereas significant numbers are retained by corporations and insurance companies.

Biggins considers that the various occupational health and safety acts have not engendered 'real' worker participation. Rather, the state has incorporated occupational health (e.g. Workcover) into existing structures and neutralized the potential for social change.

Utilizing what he terms 'Labour Process Theory', Willis (1989:319) maintains that speeding up the pace of work, technological innovation, and so forth are directed not towards reducing the need to labour—but towards control and efficiency; managerial strategies are not neutral, they are designed for the maximization of efficiency and as labour is treated as a production cost, there has existed the tendency to regard health and safety in economic rather than ethical terms. At the same time, however, it has been the cost of compensation that has shaped occupational health.

According to Willis, occupational health and safety have been presented as a technical issue to be resolved through consensus by panels of experts— but it is political. When occupational health and safety committees address cause rather than effect, they have the capacity to intervene in and shape the labour process. Although management may present the issue as a struggle for control, essentially it is around competing definitions of efficiency: staffing levels, pace and hours of work, and how production is to be carried out (the essence of the labour process).

Willis argues that the ideological separation between occupational health and industrial relations is being overcome as health and safety increasingly becomes an arena for contestation and resistance—with responses from labour, capital, and the state. Here, he takes issue with the neutralization hypothesis advocated by Biggins (1988); but does recognize emerging problems as union resources hitherto directed to occupational health and safety issues are rediverted to award restructuring. He maintains that occupational health is not a neutral issue: it is a contested terrain between labour, capital, and the state.

Australian stress research

Stress is explained via a collection of competing perspectives and, although not a disease state (where a specific pathology or malfunction of a tissue, organ or system is evident—e.g. cancer), it is part of an illness process. Over time the process can engender harmful physiological changes. Heart disease and gastric disorders are two known outcomes (see Quinlan & Bohle 1991 for a critical review of the competing perspectives).

Yossi Berger (1991:19-20) maintains that occupational stress has been understood in four distinctive ways:

These four ways are based on four different definitions of the word 'stress'. The main distinction being a shift in emphasis in cause and effect, where in one perspective 'stress' identifies a cause, in another a consequence.

These four definitions are:
(a)   Those focussing on the demand imposed on the worker, eg. a demand for faster production is stress;
(b)   Those focussing on the responses (reactions), where the faster heart rate or the anxiety resulting is stress;
(c)   Those referring to a mix of both of the above where the interpretation of workload demands and the inner response are the stress;
(d)   Those identifying the entire process of reacting and adapting as a single stress process.
The one I [Berger] prefer and the one recommended by the ACTU/VTHC [Australian Council of Trade Unions/Victorian Trades Hall Council] Occupational Health and Safety Unit to unions as a useful model, is the fourth one. This recognises that many constantly interacting events affect people over time. This is a process of perceiving, understanding, reacting, coping and constantly changing. This approach recognises that human behaviour is complex and rich, and events of the body and mind are not like single matches in a matchbox, but rather like pockets of water in a river.

A wide range of relevant events should be referred to as Candidate Stressors. Many events at the workplace are conditions that may lead to harsh demands and difficult workloads. Some candidate stressors will cause every one problems. For example, high levels of noise, unrealistic production targets, primitive operating condition or long hours of work. Others will cause problems to particular groups of workers or individuals. For example, older or younger workers or untrained workers.

Australian stress research has focused on a diverse range of occupational groups: urban transit bus operators (Shapiro 1983, Borthwick 1989), air traffic controllers (Tesh 1984), flight cabin attendants (Lessor 1985), sea pilots (Berger 1986), process workers (Otto 1985) and nurses (Linder-Pelz 1986). In every instance there was evidence which indicated that stressors had origins in the physical and/or mental strains resulting from the nature of work and/or working conditions (e.g. posture, physical exertion, temperature, noise, ventilation, concentration, monotony, pace of work, irregular hours, degree of autonomy, nature of labour and management relations). Thus, the implicit premise that occupational stressors are shaped by the labour process is not of recent origin, and managers in all industries have had ample time to note and respond to this assertion.

Working on the Newcastle buses—the drivers' interpretation of the situation

The study began with the implicit hypothesis that unsatisfactory working conditions were stressors resulting in symptoms for which bus operators frequently sought relief. The questionnaire was therefore designed to test this hypothesis. There were questions on stress as defined by the health literature and questions on working conditions. Persons with specialist knowledge of the situation, bus operators themselves, were active in designing the survey. The subsequent high response rate (71%) and the extent to which participants were prepared to reveal their feelings about everyday working life indicate that the issues addressed were of central concern to Newcastle bus operators. It was research for *bus operators conducted by bus operators*.

The report, released in October 1990, revealed patterns of evidence suggesting that restructuring the organization of work on the Newcastle buses has produced a more alienating, hence less healthy, work-place for bus operators. A survey, as the name implies, is an overview and only seeks to identify the existence of predetermined features—in this case, the relationship between occupational stressors and the organization of bus operators work—and makes no claim to represent the total experiences of the population. Nonetheless, when a majority, or significant minority, of an occupational group are reporting similar experiences, shared meaning about a situation can be claimed. Bus operators reported that certain aspects of the job were stressful (traffic conditions, cutting corners, timetables, passengers, rosters, and management). They also reported that cutting corners (breaking rules), especially where this related to problems with traffic and passengers, had been generated through the imposition of unrealistic timetables and rosters. The current timetables and rosters had been in existence since 1988.

The labour process on the Newcastle buses over the past forty years has not been static. First of all, bus operators became multi-skilled (before the term was coined); that is, over time they had absorbed the work previously performed by conductors and had at the same time lost a means of social support. Successive governments trimmed down the workforce and at the same time intensified the pace of production.

With the election of the Liberal-National Party government (March 1988) the pace of restructuring increased. There were subsequent job cuts and a radical reorganization of the management structure as part of a corporatization process. There had not been a parallel change in transport technology (e.g. total off-bus ticket sales), and consequently the pace of work was intensified. In capitalist enterprises and state services that have adopted the logic of capitalism (corporatization), maximizing the extraction of labour power (actually productive labour) is synonymous with efficiency.

A key strategy in the quest for maximizing the extraction of labour power has been, so called, *scientific management* or *Taylorism* (see Braverman 1974), and involves the separation of the control and execution of production (i.e. bus operators drive the bus, management plans and controls the rosters, routes, and timetables). Accompanying an intensification in the pace of production there had been attempted changes in the character of the work force, replacing full-time workers with part-time workers—thus reducing the need for bus operators to be on duty during off-peak periods, a period when bus operating was less demanding—in the name of efficiency.

The management's logic of efficiency involved maintaining services while reducing costs; not just through technological change, but also through intensifying the pace of production and changing award conditions (i.e. hours of duty, meal breaks, and penalty rates). The bus operators' logic of efficiency involved getting through the day with the minimum of fuss and at the same time providing a safe and reliable service to customers. The survey revealed that a major restructuring of the labour process, rosters and timetables in 1988 had been accompanied by a heightened experience of occupational stressors. A job which to some had been endurable had become unbearable. Consequently, bus operators contended that intensifying or ameliorating the problem of occupational stressors was within the control of management.

In the conclusion to the report I stated 'The temptation to list a series of recommendations that may eliminate or diminish the impact of stressors has been resisted. Managerial control over the organization of work has been identified as the central issue. Getting management to take note of and act upon what bus operators have to say is another matter' (McIntyre 1990). This was a sincere recommendation, not an escape clause. The finding of the survey demonstrated that workers as a group have a collective memory and experience that places their interpretation of a situation, their reality, in an historical perspective. They know what is going on in their work environment and for how long it has been going on. They also have first hand experience of how their participation in the labour process has impacted on their health, individually and collectively (Navarro 1986).

Union and management responses to occupational stressors

There is a considerable social dimension to research, such as the propensity for a group to embrace one report as scientific, and denounce another report as rhetoric premised on ideology. Literature concerning the sociology and philosophy of science is full of instances of the science/ideology dichotomy: that which lends support to the ideology of the group is scientific, whereas that which does not is rhetoric (Mulkay 1979, Navarro 1986). The issue of rhetoric can be resolved—are the reported findings supported by evidence? Is there a link between theory and evidence? Theory does shape research by suggesting approaches, research questions, and hypotheses, but in the final instance—the finding stated in the report must depend on the evidence from the empirical research (Rose 1982).

The hypothesis, that unsatisfactory working conditions were stressors resulting in stress symptoms for which bus operators frequently sought relief, was supported by the evidence (McIntyre 1990, 1991). Management consistently maintained that the occupational health of bus operators was of the utmost importance. Yet, progress on the stress issue was sabotaged by them through recourse to legal mechanisms, the Australian Industrial Relations Commission, and attempts to individualize the problem via the introduction of a medical assessment. Two issues, the recovery time dispute and the medical assessment dispute, highlight the operation of sabotage.

The recovery time dispute

The survey identified timetables as a central problem. First, many routes could not be covered in the allocated time and bus operators were being harassed by passengers for late running. Second, because of the tightness of schedules, an operator could work for up to 4 hours without a paid rest break (recovery time). The union and local management reached and ratified a formal agreement on a formula for recovery times (13 November 1990). New timetables were released (3 December 1990) which the union claimed departed from the agreement (management defined unpaid meal breaks as recovery time). The dispute was taken to the Labor Council of New South Wales for possible resolution. The Council found in favour of the union, and management rejected this decision. To undo this impasse the union then referred the issue of recovery times to the Australian Industrial Relations Commission (AIRC) for conciliation. In the meantime management advised the union that it was disengaging from the agreement (3 January 1991).

At the AIRC (16 January 1991) management argued jurisdiction and the issue was moved to a hearing by a Commissioner (22 January 1991) for arbitration. Management claimed that as any local industry agreement made with the Newcastle bus operators had the potential to flow on to state and national spheres it was a matter of grave concern that ought to be adjudicated at the appropriate level (Australian Industrial Relations Commission 1991a).

This new interpretation of a local industry agreement was a repudiation of management's previous position because the formal agreement on recovery times endorsed by labour and management commenced with the preamble:

The following Agreement applies to the running and standing times for bus operations within the Newcastle Division only of the State Transit Authority of New South Wales, and reflects the Division's special and unique circumstances...

[And concluded] The parties acknowledge that the terms of this agreement will not establish precedent for similar work practices to be claimed elsewhere. Should either party seek to implement any such practice elsewhere in the future, the need for such a practice will be argued on its merits only.

A lengthy and costly legal dispute over the status of a local industry agreement then ensured. Finally, Mr Justice Maddern (AIRC President) ruled that the issue of recovery times was outside the Commission's jurisdiction, and should not have been processed: not because the Commission was unwilling to hear occupational health matters, but because an actual industrial dispute that had crossed state boundaries was not in progress (Australian Industrial Relations Commission 1991b).

One union approach to reforming the labour process has been through application to the AIRC. Carson and Henenberg (1989) note that there is a reluctance by the AIRC to make a ruling on occupational health, especially when the employer is the state (as in this case, New South Wales). Quinlan and Bohle (1991) maintain that disputes which relate to control of the labour process are seen as impacting on the managerial prerogative, and the AIRC has been ambivalent about the managerial notion that a distinct ideological separation exists between occupational health and industrial relations. In this case the AIRC upheld management's contention that industrial relations, not occupational health, was the issue.

The issue of recovery times, as an aspect of occupational stressors, remains unresolved. At a conference (Newcastle 5 December 1991) management refused to alter the timetables unless the union agreed to the loss of 45 full-time positions, the introduction of part-time staff, longer shifts and fewer restrictions on the working of overtime. Eventually, in July 1992, the union was forced to concede these changes to the award under the threat of privatization.

The medical assessment dispute

At the NSW state election (May 1991) the Liberal-National parties were returned, albeit as a minority government. Would the politics of economic rationalism be pursued with a greater urgency? A general meeting of bus operators (Sydney, 9 July 1991) roundly rejected a STA proposal for massive voluntary redundancy and the introduction of part-time work. One week later, STA attempted to cull the workforce through the imposition of a medical assessment.

The assessment failed at the levels of ethics, theory and method: intrusive questions were asked (sexually transmitted diseases) and confidentiality was at risk; the instrument was disease oriented, ignored the issue of stress, and was not specifically tailored to suit the occupation of bus operating; finally, a pre-employment instrument was touted as an assessment for current employees, and employees who failed to comply fully with the assessment procedure were threatened with stand down.

The assessment was so appalling that, other than its authors, not one health professional could be found to defend it, and it was eventually withdrawn for redesigning after substantial amendments. Yet, in spite of an obvious poverty of ethics, theory, and method, public condemnation from people and organizations (David Christie, Professor of Occupational Medicine at Newcastle University; AIDS Council of NSW, and the Council for Civil Liberties), and sustained and intensive criticism in the media (e.g. *Newcastle Herald* 2 August 1991), management consistently maintained that it was motivated by concern for bus operators' health.

In a letter to the *Newcastle Herald* (3 August 1991) the Chief Executive Officer of State Transit wrote:

The [assessment] has been fast-tracked in Newcastle because of some serious claims, made by the Newcastle ATMOEA, about the well-being of bus operators in that area and the effect this may have on public safety. The Newcastle branch seems to be doing all in its power to thwart the State Transit medical assessment program. After so much discussion and disruption to Newcastle bus passengers, is the ATMOEA in Newcastle now concerned about the credibility of its assertions? The medical assessment criteria used were developed and endorsed by occupational physicians to meet State Transit's requirements. State Transit has a responsibility to ensure the health and safety of its employees and the safety of its passengers. This responsibility cannot be ceded to any party, including the ATMOEA.

The recovery time and medical assessment disputes are more complex than I have presented them, but they serve to demonstrate that management actively sabotaged progress on the stress issue. Changes to procedures, such as recovery times and periodic health assessment, will produce changes in the labour process that will have positive or negative implications for bus operators' health. The union had not attempted to invalidate the State Transit's responsibility for the health and safety of its employees and the safety of its passengers. Nor had the union challenged management's responsibility to control the labour process. The union was challenging the notion that management has the prerogative to produce ill health through the current, and proposed, organization of production.

Conclusion

Under the New South Wales Occupational Health and Safety Act there is no notion of victim or perpetrator. The Act recognizes that a fundamental conflict of interests exists between labour and management, and that all groups in society have their particular interests to protect. The theory is that the neutral state will intervene and, via a tripartite sharing of power, unions, employers, and governments will work together to bring about change.

For the Newcastle bus operators this has not been the case. The state is also the employer, and it is here that a notion of power relations and the non-neutrality of occupational health becomes glaringly evident. STA management was able to use its power to sabotage progress on the stress issue, whereas a federal union with 11 000 members could financially bleed to death in a struggle around better health for its members in Newcastle. By sponsoring the management interpretation of occupational health, the state actively supported the maintenance of an unhealthy workplace.

While management continues to reject explanations of occupational health which are shaped by the labour process perspective, the notion of risk imposition will remain marginal, and it will be the effect, rather than the cause, that continues to receive major attention. Other than quitting their jobs, actual and potential victims will be obliged to seek treatment from the clinician who seeks out disease and sick workers rather than healthy working environments; the counsellor who seeks to change individual behaviour rather than the work place; and, the health promoter who seeks to change lifestyle rather than workstyle.

While management responses to health and illness in the workplace continue to be defined by the managerial prerogative, the rhetoric of concern for workers welfare will dominate, the opportunity for change will be restricted, occupational stressors will remain an insidious form of assault, and the casualty list will continue to grow longer.

REFERENCES

Australian Industrial Relations Commission 1991a State Transit Authority of New South Wales and Australian Tramways and Motor Omnibus Employees Association. Commonwealth Reporting Service C No 20042
Australian Industrial Relations Commission 1991b The New South Wales government bus traffic employees' award 1981. Commonwealth Reporting Service C No's 20582 & 20588
Berger Y 1986 Sea pilots: the problems of irregular hours. Proceedings of seminar, Brain Behaviour Research Institute, La Trobe University, Melbourne, symposium 8:13–16
Berger Y 1991 Occupational stressors: some myths and legends. In: McIntyre D (ed) 1991 Bus driving—a terminal occupation? Proceedings of an occupational health seminar. University of Newcastle, Department of Psychosocial Health Studies & The Centre for Human Ecology and Health Advancement, Newcastle NSW, pp 19–23
Biggins D 1988 Focus on occupational health: what can be done? New Doctor (47):6–10
Borthwick K 1989 Occupational health and safety psychosocial evaluation for ATMOEA. Sydney hospital: occupational health & safety unit
Braverman H 1974 Labor and monopoly capital: the degradation of work in the twentieth century. Monthly Review Press, New York
Burawoy M 1979 Manufacturing consent: changes in the labour process under monopoly capitalism. University of Chicago Press, Chicago
Burawoy M 1985 The politics of production: factory regimes under capitalism and socialism. Verso, London
Carson W, Henenberg C 1989 Social justice at the workplace: the political economy of health and safety laws. Social Justice 16(3):124–140
Lessor R 1985 Consciousness of time and time for the development of consciousness: health

awareness among women flight attendants. Sociology of Health and Illness (7):191–213

Linder-Pelz S 1986 Occupational stress in nurses in an Australian general hospital. Community Health Studies (10):307–316

McIntyre D 1990 Working on the Newcastle buses: the drivers' interpretation of the situation. University of Newcastle, School of Health, Newcastle NSW

McIntyre D (ed) 1991 Bus driving—a terminal occupation?: proceedings of an occupational health seminar. University of Newcastle, Department of Psychosocial Health Studies & The Centre for Human Ecology and Health Advancement, Newcastle NSW

Mulkay M 1979 Science and the sociology of knowledge. Allen & Unwin, London

Navarro V 1986 Crisis, health, and medicine: a social critique. Tavistock, New York, pp 103–140

Otto R 1985 Health damage through work stress: is stress management the answer? New Doctor (35):13–15

Quinlan M 1988 Psychological and sociological approaches to the study of occupational illness: a critical review. The Australian & New Zealand Journal of Sociology 24 (2):189–207

Quinlan M, Bohle P (eds) 1991 Managing occupational health and safety in Australia: a multidisciplinary approach. Macmillan, Melbourne, Ch. 10

Ratcliffe J, Wallack L, Fagnani F, Rodwin V 1984 Perspectives on prevention: health promotion vs health protection. In: de Kervasdoue J, Kimberly J, Rodwin V (eds) The end of an illusion: the future of health policy in western industrialized nations. University of California Press, Berkeley

Rose G 1982 Deciphering sociological research. Macmillan, London

Shapiro R S 1983 The driver driven. New Doctor (29):43–45

Tesh S 1984 The politics of stress: the case of air traffic control. International Journal of Health Services 14 (4): 569–587

Willis E 1989 The industrial relations of occupational health and safety: a labour process approach. Labour & Industry 2:317–333

5.   Health impacts of work: the case of Broken Hill miners[1]

Murray Couch

In the public discussion of occupational health and safety two themes commonly recur. The first is the awesome dimension of the human and economic cost of work-related injury and disease. The second theme is the constitution of occupational health and safety as a predicament not amenable to easy or agreed solutions.

Below are extracts from a statement in 1991 by Dr Ted Emmett, Chief Executive of Worksafe Australia (the National Occupational Health and Safety Commission), which illustrate the point:

> Let me give you a few indications of the sort of human burden imposed by Australia's relatively poor record on occupational health and safety:
> - there are over 16 000 compensated occupational injuries in Australia each year requiring at least 5 days off work
> - a total of between 600 000 and 900 000 are compensated nationwide each year
> - 500 Australians are killed in work related accidents each year
> - and probably more die from occupational disease—to take just one disease, deaths from asbestos-related mesothelioma have risen from 100 annually in 1980 to 300 annually last year, and are still rising.
>
> And occupational disease is likely to be an increasingly significant problem in the future.
>
> (Emmett 1991:24)

Emmett then moves on to the difficult task of quantifying the problem economically.

> - the direct cost of workers' compensation claims was $4.8 billion in 1989–90
> - the total costs of workplace deaths, injuries and disease is estimated to be over $9 billion annually
> - the direct workers' compensation costs constitute 1.5% of GNP and around 20% of total health care costs
> - the direct costs of workers' compensation in constant dollar terms was three times as much in 1986–87 as in 1978–79
> - the number of working days lost through employment injuries in 1986–87 was ten times that lost through industrial disputes.
>
> (Emmett 1991:24)

This chapter will reflect on why preserving and protecting the well-being of workers is conceived of, and may well be, an intractable problem. Further, the chapter will propose a sociology of morality in relation to occupational health and safety which goes beyond expressions of outrage couched in economic terms.

The sociological study of occupational health and safety does not yet have available to it a comprehensive body of developed theory. This chapter will move towards a theoretical account which makes links beyond the workplace, to domestic and social life, and which attempts connections with the market, the state, gender and worker subjectivity.

The theoretical story so far...

Twentieth century social science research into occupational health and safety has been dominated by industrial psychologists and ergonomists, and this has led to a dominant view of an individual, rather than a systemic, notion of injury and disease causation. Layman (1987:2), in a review of the Australian literature on occupational health, comments on the surprisingly narrow conceptual base on which most of the explanations rested: 'a psychological model of workers dysfunctional behaviour'.

Hopkins and Palser (1987:26) note the more recent development of theories of industrial injury and disease causation falling into two broad types, which they characterized as 'blaming the victim' and 'blaming the system'. The later includes 'those which focus on the routine production process,...those which stress the pressures placed on workers to engage in unsafe practices when normal production processes are interrupted, those which point to the impact of productivity bonuses and so on.'

The level of complexity and subtlety of which systems explanations are capable (and their inherent limitations) is demonstrated in a systems model of accident causation[2] developed by Laflamme (1990). She examined the existing models of accident causation most often quoted in the literature, and her analysis of these models led Laflamme to develop a systems approach which she argues stresses that multi-dimensional mechanisms of influence rather than simple linear causes must be sought in order to reconstitute the causal chain of injury and disease outcomes.

Laflamme's model uses four levels: work organization, the working situation, the causal sequence, and the incident itself. The strength of this model is its rejection of single linear causal explanations, and its recognition of multi-dimensional influences within the system. However, its inherent weakness is that it takes no account of the wider social, political, economic and cultural influences in which the system itself is embedded.

Occupational health and safety literature has been influenced by the classic sociological traditions coming from Karl Marx, Max Weber, and Emile Durkheim, and also by 'social constructionist' theorists.

The most developed and consistent Marxist sociological literature comes from Vicente Navarro and other historical materialist theorists associated with the International Journal of Health Services. Navarro (1980) argues that the fight for the realization of health is central to the workplace conflict between capital and labour. In Navarro's account, bourgeois ideology legitimates and facilitates the reproduction of the power relations of capitalism through medicine based on a science/ideology dichotomy, which in turn, generates an expert/layman dichotomy. These dichotomies mirror the dominant/dominated relations of the workplace. Medical science, formulated in this way, has focused on the microcausality of disease, while ignoring 'the analysis of macrocausality, i.e...the power relations of that society' (Navarro 1980:541).

Gersuny (1981) examines conflicts over work hazards by comparing the climate of industrial hazards in the United States around the turn of the century with the reforms pertaining to work hazards enacted from 1960 to 1970 and culminating in the Occupational Safety and Health Act, 1970. In this examination of class conflict Gersuny's makes imaginative use of Weber.

In Weber's analysis, class situation means the typical probability of procuring goods, gaining a position in life, and finding inner satisfactions, a probability which comes from some control over goods and skills, and from their income producing potential (Weber 1978:302). Thus, class situation for Weber has to do with 'the typical chance for a supply of goods, external living conditions, and personal life experiences, in so far as this chance is determined by the amount and kind of power, or lack of such, to dispose of goods or skills for the sake of income in a given economic order.' (Weber 1977:181)

Gersuny (1981:4) takes the view that 'work injury and occupational disease impair market capacities for future earnings and impair life chances, which include chances for health and survival.' Employment in a hazardous occupation, then, with all the present and future uncertainty, is related to class position because it influences life chances.

Durkheim's view of values and beliefs as emerging from particular societies has had some impact on theoretical reflection of occupational health and safety. In particular this has been through the social anthropologist Mary Douglas (Douglas & Wildavsky 1984), who proposes that beliefs about risk are embedded in a complex social system of beliefs and values. As Nelkin (1985:16) puts it, 'judgements about risk are in effect political statements expressing points of tension and value conflicts in a given society.'

Nelkin (1985) argues that disputes over occupational risk divide labour and management, with each playing out traditional adversarial roles. In her view it is not only economic territory which is at stake in assumptions and beliefs about risk, but also professional ideologies, bureaucratic routines, career pressures, and political predilections.

The fourth, and most recent thread in the sociological literature on occupational health and safety can be termed 'social constructionist'. This approach argues that medical knowledge is produced socially within a highly specialized combination of social practices and discourse.

One example of a writer using this approach to examine work-related medical conditions is Karl Figlio (1979, 1980, 1984, 1985). He (Figlio 1984:176) links the creation of medical knowledge with power, which he sees as diffuse and beyond the commonsense notions of actor and acted upon, oppressor and oppressed, ruler and ruled. He recognizes that his view of power and the production of knowledge comes close to that enunciated by Foucault (1980, 1984).

Figlio has examined the history and social function of the syndrome 'miner's nystagmus' [3] between 1890 and 1940, and recorded the process by which the condition was constituted within the social relations of production, and the medical and legal practices associated with compensation, along with the way the government and medical profession used the condition to mediate the relations between miners and employers.

To summarize, there have been developments in the social science literature on occupational health and safety from explanations grounded in dysfunctional individual behaviour, to explanations located in organizational systems through to explanations taking into account social, political and cultural structures, and social practices which produce knowledge.

The fundamental paradigm, however, remains that of conflict between competing interests. The dominant conflict is still characterized as that between capital and labour. Given the workplace related nature of the case this might be expected. However, fuller account needs to be taken of other dimensions, such as gender, the state, and morality.

Future theoretical development requires a vision which can at once make more subtle distinctions about processes and experiences located in the workplace and identify linkages between the workplace and social, political and cultural life beyond the workplace.

I have undertaken research on workers' well-being in the Broken Hill mining industry. The following section of the chapter will call upon that research to look at ways in which a two way interaction between the workplace and the world beyond it needs to be built into any social theory of occupational health and safety.

Distinctions and broadening vision

What is being proposed here is an elaboration of the concept of 'occupational health and safety'—a stretching of the concept—which will expand the possibilities for theoretical elaboration by identifying elements and linkages which need to be taken into account.

I propose that theorizing about the well-being of workers requires an analysis with two complementary and interacting trajectories. On the one hand there are multi-dimensional pressures from the workplace and beyond which have an effect on the well-being of workers, the consequences of which are experienced *in the workplace*. Examples are market-driven pressures to cut costs, and the amount of personal control workers have over their jobs, within the organization of any work process, which in turn will be determined by the technology being used.

On the other hand there are multi-dimensional pressures arising from the workplace which have an effect on well-being experienced in the domestic and social spheres *beyond the workplace*. An example is an effect on a worker's fertility from a workplace exposure to a hazardous substance such as lead.

In this two layered scheme, the first is concerned with threats to well-being which are experienced in the workplace. The focus of the analysis here is the workplace itself, and the analysis is concerned with all of the structures and dynamics which impinge on the well-being of workers while they are at work which determines the shape and incidence of workplace injury and disease.

The second is concerned with threats to well-being which arise in the workplace but which are experienced beyond the workplace. The focus of the analysis is as broad as society itself, and is concerned with reverberations which begin in workplaces, spread wider and which have consequences for the well-being of more than just the workers, for example partners, families, the physical environment and so on.

Having separated these two sets of multi-dimensional and bi-directional pressures, a further set of distinctions can be made by separating injury from disease, and further separating out effects on subjective well-being apart from injury and disease.

This allows for a two-by-three analytical matrix within which different phenomena can be located (Fig. 5.1).

	From the workplace and beyond to the workplace	From the workplace to beyond the workplace
Injury		
Disease		
Subjective well-being		

Fig. 5.1 Two-by-three analytical matrix of threats to well-being within and beyond the workplace.

	From the workplace and beyond to the workplace	From the workplace to beyond the workplace
Injury	Musculoskeletal damage	Domestic violence
Disease	Diesel exhaust emissions: respiratory and carcinogenic	Threats to reproductive health Blood lead levels in children
Subjective well-being	The experience of working in diesel exhausts	Alcohol abuse

Fig. 5.2 Examples of perceived potential threats to well-being from the Broken Hill mining industry.

This matrix can now be used to separate out some examples of perceived potential threats to well-being of the mining industry in Broken Hill (Fig. 5.2).

These examples cannot be elaborated in detail. However, the following comments on each cell in the matrix are offered, to indicate that deleterious effects on health are located within linkages between the workplace, and domestic and community domains, and are shaped to some degree by market decisions, intervention of the state, and gender.

Musculoskeletal injuries are a major category in all forms of mining. As corporate extractive strategies have moved substantially in the direction of becoming capital intensive, rather than labour intensive, there has been some change in the shape of musculoskeletal injuries. Traditionally musculoskeletal injuries in mining have been the result of manually intensive work over a long period. The use of extractive techniques which employ very large units of mechanical equipment produces injuries to the musculoskeletal system which are more directly experienced, and associated with vibration and the sharp movements involved in operating the large equipment.

Other health problems which are experienced globally in mechanized mining (and in many other industries) are commonly associated with diesel fume emissions. This problem is exacerbated when the exhaust is in combination with dust. Contention about the effects of diesel fumes on conditions such as chronic bronchitis, respiratory function and the occurrence of cancer goes on (Sampara 1986). The state has an enforcement function in relation to the acceptable standards of exposure to airborne contaminants, dust and ventilation.

There are, however, other sub-acute effects of working in diesel fumes: effects which can be characterized as assaults on subjective well-being. These include eye and respiratory irritation. I have reported (Couch 1992) accounts from Broken Hill miners of the barely tolerable experience of working in conditions when the level of diesel fume emission is high. The following are typical:

- Diesel fumes burn my bloody throat and eyes. I can't stand it. It makes me bloody vomit actually.
- You can't tell me blokes can go down there a shift and then cough up bloody big black googlies, and not be doing something to their chest.
- There are still blokes in the shower that cough up big black bloody phlegm and so you can't say that's not affecting their lungs and whatever.

(Couch 1992:1150)

Elsewhere (Couch 1991), I have argued that the mining industry in Broken Hill has contributed to the construction of a masculinity with particular features. Traditionally the principal conduit available to young men to appropriate masculinity for themselves in this community, and mining communities around the world, is initiation into a masculine job, the benchmark of which is the job of mining itself. Within mining communities the beginning of a working life takes on the quality of a rite of passage: at once, the 'blooding' into work and masculinity. Masculinity thus constituted with its roots in the workplace, seems to be implicated in a relation to a range of local psychopathologies as described by Yellowlees and Kaushik (1992): high levels of alcohol abuse, domestic violence, sexual assault and incest.

Health outcomes, which demonstrate links between the workplace and the domestic sphere, include the potential threat to miners' reproductive health and capacity associated with working with lead,[4] and the dangerously high blood lead levels which are now being measured among children in some sections of this community.

These examples lead to a discussion of the market, the state, and gender in relation to the deleterious health effects of work; and further on to a discussion of the relevance of Bauman's (1990) work on morality to this issue.

The market and the state

At the level of macro-analysis, there is some evidence of a relationship between industrial injuries and the level of economic activity and business cycles. That is, periods of high economic growth and periods of recession will produce different injury outcomes. However, there is little agreement about the interpretation of these co-relations.

Nichols examined the business cycle and industrial injuries in British manufacturing over the 25 years 1960–1985, and reports that 'the business cycle does have an effect on the fatality rate; that this remains after operative hours at risk are taken into account; and that the association is a pro-cyclical one'. (Nichols 1989:547). He makes the point however that it does not follow from saying that the level of injury is a pro-cyclical one that the level of safety in factories is 'unaffected by the balance of power between capital and labour or by the extent to which the state protects, or attacks, labour' (Nichols 1989:547).

Wallace (1987) moves beyond concern with the forces of the market alone in an attempt to explain the long-term decline in both fatal and non-fatal injury rates in the American coal mining industry from 1930-1982. His analysis identifies the impact of the industrial business climate and state regulation and industrial relations on the changes in injury rates.

He concludes (Wallace 1987:336) that the collective capacities of miners to organize effectively against unsafe conditions and the business climate are equally or more important than state regulatory efforts for the improved health and safety conditions in American coal mining.

Market fluctuations and the intervention of the state are implicated in the construction of occupational safety and health outcomes. However, the ways in which the market and the state, individually and in interaction, shape workers' well-being has not been theorized.

Gender

Jan Lucas (1991), before her untimely death, blew the whistle in a most original way on the gender blindedness of the occupational health and safety discourse. She did this in part by demonstrating that workplace sexual harassment, clearly implicated in a relationship between health and work, could find no place in the available theoretical structures. She advocated, as I have done in imitation above, that the occupational health and safety literature needs to be elaborated and refined by adding dimensions other than the capital labour conflict. She argues that gender is one of those dimensions.

Lucas (1991) argued that an appropriate representation of occupational health and safety would need to be able to deal with the incidence of occupational illness and injuries which result from the fact that women overwhelmingly perform the domestic labour in Australian society, and the stress which women encounter in having often to cope with two occupations, homemaker and primary parent. She also argued that account be taken of stress resulting from the feminization of poverty and specific occupational health risks encountered by women in the workplace resulting from the division of labour in Australian occupations and problems associated with sexual harassment.

The integration of gender into occupational health and safety theory in the comprehensive way called for by Lucas is yet to happen. The matrix developed above may be a contribution to such a project, for a core restriction of the masculinist construction of occupational health and safety has been the forcing of all phenomena into the two categories of injury and disease. It is not surprising that women engaged in emotional labour, for example, could not construct deleterious effects of their working life into the confines of either injury or disease.

An adequate incorporation of gender into a theory of occupational health and safety will take patriarchy into account, and in particular the ways in which organizational structures within patriarchy assume that the normative worker is a man.

Hartmann (1981:14) defines patriarchy as a 'a set of social relations between men, which have a material base, and which, though hierarchical, establish or create interdependence and solidarity among men that enable them to dominate women.' An examination of these social relations, which Sedgwick (1985) elaborates as 'homo-social', and their attendant social practices, may open up possibilities in theorizing how gender shapes injury, disease and subjective well-being in the workplace, and beyond in ways affected by the workplace.

Acker (1990) argues that this bonding of men in the interests of the maintainance of their power is partly masked through the obscuring of the embodied nature of work and organizational structures. She argues that organizational structure is not gender neutral, but assumptions about gender underlie the documents and contracts used to construct organizations.

> Abstract jobs and hierarchies, common concepts in organisational thinking assume a disembodied and universal worker. This worker is actually a man; men's bodies, sexuality, and relationships to procreation and paid work are subsumed in the image of the worker. Images of men's bodies and masculinity pervade organisational processes, marginalising women and contributing to the maintenance of gender segregation in organisations (Acker 1990:139).

Unravelling the implicit gendered nature of organizations, workplaces and work processes under patriarchy may be a way to begin to locate the lived experience of women (and men) within theories of occupational health and safety.

Sociology of morality

Having established that any theoretical account of worker's well-being must account for the structures and dynamics of the market, the state, and gender, attention can now be turned to the issue raised at the commencement of this chapter—the question of morality, and its legitimate place in such theorizing.

This attempt to locate 'morality' within a sociology of occupational health and safety begins with Bauman's endeavour to construct a sociology of morality.

In Bauman's (1990) view morality is innate. That is, humans are born with a morality, or natural ethical impulse, and this belief is the foundation of Bauman's attempt to construct a sociology of morality. To suppose that a moral tendency is innate or inborn, in Bauman's terms, means simply that humans are inclined to behave morally towards others unless they are forced to do otherwise (Bauman 1990:14). Humans do not have to consciously take on responsibility, but responsibility comes from a natural closeness (or 'proximity' in Bauman's terms) to others (Bauman 1990:18).

Bauman's project is to trace the demise of moral proximity by looking at how forms of social life developed which have left us 'less room for the face-to-face situations in which proximity grows' (Bauman 1990:22). He investigates aspects of communities living together 'that favour distance over proximity and the contract over unconditional responsibility' (Bauman 1990:22–23).

A sociology of occupational health and safety requires a theory of morality. All that is possible here, however, is to signal two points at which such a project could begin, drawing on Bauman's notions of 'responsibility for' and 'moral proximity'. The first is an examination of what the fundamental work contract in our society implies about workers' well-being. The second is an examination of Threshold Limit Values (TLVs), which are measures used to establish standards for workplace contaminants.

It is not unreasonable to characterize the fundamental assumptions of the work contract in our society as containing an inherent (and therefore unspoken) assumption that to engage in work is to bear some degree of the risk of injury and some possibility of a degree of health loss or even shortening of life. This is possible because of the commodification of labour and therefore the impersonalizing—the moral distancing—of the relationship between the employer and the employed.

Giddens (1987:173) argues that the association between capitalism and the nation state, 'can be prised open by concentrating upon some specific and distinctive features of the capitalist labour contract. Giddens points out that Marx claimed that the capitalist labour contract differs in a basic way from modes of exploitation of surplus production found in pre-capitalist societies. In the latter, the exploiter is in some sense an agent of the state and possesses the means of violence, or its threat, as a principal instrument ensuring the compliance of the subordinate class or classes. However the capitalistic labour contract does not involve the exploitation of surplus production or labour; it depends upon the extraction of surplus value, an exploitative relation that is hidden in the overall system of production and distribution. The capitalistic labour contract establishes a purely economic relation of mutual dependency between employer and worker.

The work contract then, may prove a useful point of reference to an understanding of how social practices of power within a fundamentally economic relationship, preclude, mask, or at least makes difficult the framing of questions of responsibility in relation to workers' well-being.

At a far less abstracted level, TLVs, used to determine standards for workplace contaminants, may provide another useful point of inquiry in the construction of a sociology of morality in the case of occupational health and safety. The determination of TLVs provide an example of the way in which scientific and technical knowledge is created and applied in a way which mitigates against moral proximity.

TLVs have been developed by the American Conference of Government Industrial Hygienists, a private professional organisation, and have formed the basis for exposure in a number of countries, including Australia.

Quinlan and Bohle, citing Douglas et al (1986) make the point that 'the relationship between the extent of the exposure or dose and its effects are often difficult to quantify and are, in any case, based on the assumption that there is a *harmless* level of exposure which can be practically distinguished from a *harmful* one.' (Quinlan & Bohle 1991:150)

Campbell, a defender of the use of TLVs, indicates how the risk inherent in the work contract is built into occupational health discourse:

Assessment of risk involves at least two dimensions: probability of harm, and if harm does eventuate, the likely extent of that harm. A reasonable assessment of the total risk, both probability and consequence, is clearly necessary if a sound judgement is to be made. The credibility of such assessments, however, often remains annoyingly elusive despite the authoritative testimony of scientific research. Then there is the problem of substances where any deleterious effect may only become evident long after the initial exposure.

If it is agreed that in general there cannot be absolute safety, we must consider the level of risk that is deemed 'acceptable'. In the work environment that may mean a level of exposure to a contaminant that will do the least harm consistent with its utility. Hopefully that would be a level that is unlikely to cause harm to the workers so exposed—the threshold that may be accepted.

(Campbell 1988:320)

Campbell acknowledges that TLVs do have major problems: taking no account of individuals who are hyper-susceptible to particular substances; those whose health makes them either permanently, or temporarily, more susceptible to some harmful substances; and synergist reactions with the exposure to more than one substance (Campbell 1988:322).

In the process of establishing workplace standards, then, TLVs remove decision making to what purports to be a scientific, objective, and impersonal domain, and in which there is no moral space in which questions of 'responsibility for' can be framed between local employers and employees at a workplace level.

Conclusion

This chapter set out to reflect on why preserving and protecting the well-being of workers is conceived of as, and may well be, an intractable problem.

Emerging from the chapter is the proposition that the seemingly intractable nature of the problem is related to its fundamental location in the nature of western industrial society. The commodification of labour, and the economic nature of the labour contract, masks the contest over risks implicit in the very nature of work. Without a recognition of this contest, solutions are applied to occupational health and safety problems which do not function at a sufficiently fundamental level. Partial 'solutions', or even 'solutions' which may work against the prevention of work related injury and disease in the long term, operate at the level of individual behaviour and attitudes, organizational arrangements, or the dictates of technical and scientific considerations.

A second intention of this chapter was to investigate the possibility of a sociology of morality in relation to occupational health and safety which goes beyond expressions of outrage couched in economic terms. It has been suggested here that the structures of working life and the dominance of technical rationality remove social actors from the possibility of accepting responsibility for workers' well-being in a way in which moral proximity would allow.

This chapter has recognized difficulties in effecting any significant reduction to the cost in human and economic terms of work-related injury and disease in Australia. It has also made a claim for a sociology of morality in relation to occupational health and safety. This recognition and this claim reveals the need for continuing development of theoretical reflection in this field. Such development will need to add to insights about conflicting workplace interests, the mediating impact of gender, the operation of the market, and the role and function of the state.

NOTES

1   I acknowledge useful comments by Dr Stephanie Short made on an earlier draft of this chapter.
2   Most commentators and theorists in this field would avoid the use of 'accident', as it suggests outcomes which are arbitrary and not amenable to management control.
3   This is characterized by an oscillation of the eyes.
4   Although there are no studies linking lead mining with infertility specifically, there are studies linking other forms of mining (involving other hazards) with infertility (Weise & Skipper 1986), and exposure to lead with infertility (Henderson, Baker & 1986).

REFERENCES

Acker J 1990 Hierarchies, jobs, bodies: a theory of gendered organizations. Gender & Society 4 (2):139–158
Bauman Z 1990 Effacing the face: on the social management of moral proximity. Theory, Culture & Society 7:5–38
Campbell I B 1988 Thresholds: fact or fiction. Journal of Occupational Health and Safety— Australia and New Zealand 4(4):319–323
Couch M 1991 Production and reproduction of masculinity in a mining community. Paper presented at 'Research on Masculinity and Men in Gender Relations' (Conference sponsored by The Australian Sociological Association), Macquarie University, 7–8 June 1991

Couch M 1992 Workers' health and safety in the Broken Hill mining industry: the generation of competing rationalities. In: Tendfelde K (ed) Towards a social history of mining in the 19th and 20th centuries. Verlag C H Beck, Munchen

Douglas D, Ferguson D, Harrison J, Stevenson M 1986 Occupational health and safety. Australian Medical Association, Canberra

Douglas M, Wildavsky A 1982 Risk and culture. University of California Press, Berkley

Emmett T 1991 OHS speeds micro-economic reform. Worksafe Australia (A publication of the National Occupational Health and Safety Commission) 7(1):24–25

Figlio K 1979 Sinister medicine ?: a critique of left approaches to medicine. Radical Science Journal 9:14–68

Figlio K 1980 Second thoughts on 'sinister medicine'. Radical Science Journal 10:159–166

Figlio K 1984 How does illness mediate social conditions: workmen's compensation and medico-legal practices, 1890–1940. In: Wright P, Treacher A (eds) The problem of medical knowledge: examining the social construction of medicine. Edinburgh University Press, Edinburgh

Figlio K 1985 Medical diagnosis, class dynamics, social stability. In: Levidow L, Young B (eds) Science, technology and the labour process. Marxist studies, vol 2. Free Association Press, London

Foucault M 1980 Power/knowledge: selected interviews and other writings, 1972–1977. Pantheon, New York

Foucault M 1984 The history of sexuality, volume 1: an introduction. Penguin, Harmondsworth

Gersuny C 1981 Work hazards and industrial conflict. University Press of New England, New Hampshire

Giddens A 1987 Social theory and modern sociology. Polity, Cambridge

Hartmann H 1981 The unhappy marriage of Marxism and feminism: towards a more progressive union. In: Sargent L (ed) Women and revolution: a discussion on the unhappy marriage of Marxism and feminism. Pluto, London

Henderson J, Baker H W G, Hanna P G 1986 Occupational-related male infertility. Clinical Reproduction and Fertility 4(2):87–106

Hopkins A, Palser J 1987 The causes of coal mine accidents. Industrial Relations Journal, 18 (1):26–39

Laflamme L 1990 A better understanding of occupational accident genesis to improve safety in the workplace. Journal of Occupational Accidents 12:155–165

Layman L 1987 The study of occupational health in Australia. Labour History 52:1–14

Lucas J 1991 Sexual harassment: current models of occupational health and safety and women. Australian Feminist Studies 13:59–70

Navarro V 1980 Work, ideology, and science: the case of medicine. International Journal of Health Services (10):523–550

Nelkin D (ed) 1985 The language of risk: conflicting perspectives on occupational health. Sage Publications, Beverley Hills

Nichols T 1986 Industrial injuries in British manufacturing in the 1980s: a commentary on Wright's article. Sociological Review 34:290–306

Nichols T 1989 The business cycle and industrial injuries in British manufacturing over a quarter of a century: continuities in industrial injury research. Sociological Review 37(3):538–550

Quinlan M, Bohle P 1991 Managing health and safety in Australia: a multidisciplinary approach. Macmillan, South Melbourne

Sampara P 1986 Do diesel exhaust emissions cause cancer or respiratory disease? Canadian Centre for Occupational Health and Safety, Hamilton, Ontario

Sedgwick E 1985 Between men: English literature and male homosocial desire. Columbia University Press, New York

Wallace M 1987 Dying for coal: the struggle for health and safety conditions in American coal mining, 1930–82. Social Forces 66(2):336–364

Weber M [Gerth H, Mills C W (ed)] 1977 From Max Weber: essays in sociology. Routledge & Kegan Paul, London

Weber M, [Ross G, Wittich C (ed)] 1978 Economy and society: an outline of interpretive sociology. University of California Press, Berkeley

Wiese W H, Skipper B J 1986 Survey of the reproductive outcomes in uranium and potash mine workers: results of first analysis. Annals of the American Conference of

Governmental Industrial Hygienists 14:187–192
Yellowlees P M, Kaushik A V 1992 The Broken Hill psychopathology project. Australian
and New Zealand Journal of Psychiatry 26:197–207

6. The measurement of social class in health research: problems and prospects

Gavin Turrell   John S. Western   Jake M. Najman

Social class is an important and extensively used concept in Australian health research. During the last two decades, social epidemiologists, public health researchers and medical sociologists have employed a variety of measures of the concept based mainly on occupation, education and income. These researchers have consistently demonstrated that those class groups with the least access to material and economic resources are significantly disadvantaged in terms of their health status. Compared with affluent and educated groups, socially disadvantaged groups have higher age-standardized mortality rates for almost all known causes of death, their morbidity profile indicates that they experience more acute and chronic ill health, and their use of immunization and preventive health care services suggests that they are less likely to prevent disease or detect it at an asymptomatic stage (Dobson et al 1985, Broadhead 1985, Lee et al 1987, Health Targets and Implementation Committee 1988, National Health Strategy 1992).

While the available indicators of class have been able to discriminate among social groups in terms of their health status, there are nevertheless many unresolved problems associated with the measurement of class in health research. The general aim of this chapter is to examine some of these problems as they pertain to the Australian situation.

The concept of class can be seen as having consequences for the broader and more encompassing concept of social justice. A ubiquitous feature of developed societies is the unequal distribution of resources and material wealth among their members and one form by which this social inequality is manifest is via the class structure. Australian society has a clearly definable class structure (Baxter et al 1991) which produces (and reproduces) educational, income and health inequalities, with some groups experiencing relatively unrestricted access to these 'necessary' resources and other groups having very limited access. That Australian society is socially and economically differentiated on the basis of class is in itself evidence that social justice is an unrealized ideal in this country. An important assumption underpinning this chapter is that social justice in terms of health is more likely to be realized if we are able to accurately measure and interpret health inequalities among class groups: this latter objective will in part be achieved by theoretical and empirical advances in the area of class measurement.

The chapter is divided into three sections. The first identifies the types of measures of class most widely used in health research and examines some of the problems which characterize each specific measure. This section also provides an overview of the research findings which have been associated with each measure. The second section examines a number of problems which are common to all measures of class currently used in health research. The third section outlines two recent developments in the measurement of class. These newly developed measures may overcome some of the problems which characterize class measures used in health research, although they too have their limitations.

Class measures used in Australian health research

Occupational-based measures of class

The most commonly employed measures of class in Australian health research are based upon occupational categories. This is not surprising, since sociologists have consistently argued that occupation is the most reliable single indicator of social and economic position (Coxon & Davies 1986). A variety of measures based on occupation have been used by health researchers. For the purposes of this paper however, these can be categorized into two groups: industry or skill-based occupational classifications, and measures of occupational prestige.

Australian health researchers, until very recently, employed an industry-based occupational measure known as the Classification and Classified List of Occupations (CCLO). During the 1970s and 1980s, the CCLO provided an important baseline of data on the health of different occupational groups in Australia. Using this measure researchers have shown that persons employed in professional, technical, administrative, executive and managerial occupations experience lower rates of mortality (Gibbered et al 1984, McMichael & Hartshorne 1982, Dobson et al 1985), morbidity (Broadhead 1985) and risk factor prevalence (Opit et al 1984, Hill & Gray 1984, English & Bennett 1985) when compared with those in mining, transport and communication, trades and production.

Although the CCLO was able to demonstrate that occupational differences in health status existed, the measure was deficient in a number of respects. Firstly, the CCLO was characterized by significant misclassification problems that stemmed in part from the fact that the measure was constructed by grouping occupations according to industrial sector. For example, people who were doing similar work in different industries were often placed in different occupational categories and conversely people in the same industry but at different levels of qualification, skill and responsibility were placed in similar occupational categories (Najman 1988:32). In short, the CCLO generated occupational categories which were not mutually exclusive in terms of their work-based characteristics. Secondly, the measure lacked a clearly discernible occupational hierarchy. Thirdly (and directly related to the foregoing), the CCLO is likely to have produced statistical associations which less than adequately represented the 'true' occupational differences in health outcomes. Fourthly, the measure generated results that were rarely straightforward or easily interpreted.

The CCLO has now been superseded by a skill-based occupational classification known as the Australian Standard Classification of Occupations (ASCO). A skill-based occupational classification, such as ASCO, is derived by grouping together occupations which require similar levels of education, on-the-job training and experience, to form a number of discrete occupational categories. These occupational categories are then ordered in a hierarchy based on their different skill levels, with those occupations having the most extensive skill requirements located at the top of the hierarchy. Ideally, each of the occupational categories forming the classification should be unambiguously defined and mutually exclusive in that they group together occupations which have similar work-based characteristics. If these measurement criteria are not sufficiently met (as was the case with the CCLO) then this is likely to dilute statistical relationships and produce results which are, at best, difficult to interpret and, at worst, misleading.

Although the ASCO classification is not devoid of problems (Najman 1988) it appears to be an improvement over the CCLO in that the occupational categories are more homogeneous with respect to the characteristics which define the employees' location within the hierarchy.

ASCO is now being used for census, death certificate and health data collections and undoubtedly will be used extensively by researchers as a measure of class in future health studies. Table 6.1 presents the broad categories used in the CCLO and ASCO occupational classifications.

Table 6.1 CCLO and ASCO occupational classifications

	CCLO		ASCO
0	Professional, technical and related workers	1	Managers and administrators
1	Administrative, executive and managerial workers	2	Professionals
2	Clerical workers	3	Para-professionals
3	Sales workers	4	Tradespersons
4	Farmers, fishermen, hunters, timber getters and related workers	5	Clerks
5	Miners, quarrymen and related workers	6	Salespersons and personal service workers
6	Workers in transport and communication	7	Plant and machine operators and drivers
7/8	Tradespersons, production process workers and labourers	8	Labourers and related workers
9	Service, sport and recreation workers		
10	Members of the armed services		
11/12	Occupation inadequately stated or not in the workforce		

In a number of studies researchers have used a method of occupational classification which is broadly similar to that used by most British health researchers. Najman et al (1979), Broom (1984) and Hill and Gray (1984) all used an occupational skill scale, the basis of which was derived from the British Registrar-General's (BRG) occupational classification. Table 6.2 illustrates the skill-based occupational classifications used by these researchers.

To date, studies using skill-based occupational classifications have produced inconsistent findings. Najman et al (1979) found few significant relationships between their skill-based occupational measure and health beliefs, reported morbidity and levels of health care utilization. Similarly, Broom (1984) found no clear or consistent relationship between occupation and rates of morbidity in her study of the social distribution of illness in Australia. Hill and Gray (1984) however, found significant occupational differences in their study of tobacco smoking and related health beliefs: males and females in semi-skilled and unskilled occupations were significantly more likely to smoke cigarettes.

It is important to note that while these researchers used the same types of skill-groupings, they defined their groups in different ways. Najman et al aggregate the skilled and semi-skilled groups whereas Broom, and Hill and Gray collapse the semi-skilled and unskilled groups. Similarly, Najman et al and Hill and Gray aggregate professionals and managers whereas Broom keeps these groupings separate (see Table 6.2). While there are clear inconsistencies among these researchers in terms of their respective methods of categorization, the differences are not great. However, it should be pointed out that there are a number of potential problems associated with using similar measures that are categorized differently. These problems have been highlighted by Teevan (1985). Using similar single indicator measures of class but with different cut-off points and categories, Teevan found a marked degree of variation in the relation of each measure with three health outcome variables: number of visits to a doctor; extent of depression; and degree of reported pain. More particularly, the correlations between each measure of

Table 6.2 Skill based occupational classifications

Najman et al	Broom	Hill & Gray	BRG Scale
Professionals and managers	Professionals	Professionals and managers	Professionals
Clerical and sales	Managers	Clerical and sales	Managers
Skilled and semi-skilled	Clerical and sales	Skilled	Intermediate
Unskilled	Skilled	Semi-skilled and unskilled	Skilled manual
	Semi-skilled unskilled		Semi-skilled
			Unskilled

class and health ranged from 0.05 (a very weak relationship) to 0.36 (a moderate relationship) depending on how each measure of class was categorized.

One undesirable consequence of this degree of variability in results is that conclusions drawn by health researchers would also be variable and thus our understanding of the relationship between class and health would not be furthered. Moreover, if these results are typical of the distorting effects that are associated with different operational definitions then health researchers will need to exercise greater consistency when measuring their variables.

Partly in response to the inadequacies of the CCLO, and as a result of a demand for a sociologically meaningful ranking of occupations (Najman 1988), Australian social scientists developed a number of measures of occupational prestige.

With a prestige measure the general public ranks occupations according to the level of esteem they perceive each occupation has in the wider society. All occupations are differentially vested with power and privilege and each occupation's incumbents possess varying levels of education and expertise and receive incomes that reflect the possession or otherwise of these traits. It is presumed that individuals use these and other characteristics when assessing the prestige of an occupation and hence are able to rank them accordingly (Daniel 1978, 1984, Coleman & Rainwater 1978).

The two most widely used measures of occupational prestige in Australian health research are those devised by Congalton (1969) and more recently Daniel (1983). Both of these measures rank occupations on a scale ranging from 1 to 7 with the lower scores denoting high status occupations (professionals, managers, senior civil servants, etc.) and the higher scores denoting lower status occupations (clerks, sales staff, drivers, labourers, etc.). Congalton however, also produced a four category rating of occupational prestige (ABCD) and this has been used on occasions by health researchers (Najman et al 1979, McMichael 1985).

Studies employing measures of occupational prestige have demonstrated that incumbents who occupy prestigious occupations have lower rates of mortality (McMichael 1985), they have nutrient intakes and eating patterns more in line with recommendations for the prevention of cancer (Baghurst et al 1990) and their children engage in fewer risk-taking behaviours such as smoking (Leeder et al 1973, 1977) and have higher levels of knowledge about health, nutrition and fitness (Simons et al 1982).

In recent years, criticism has been directed at measures of occupational prestige because they are generated solely on the basis of subjective assessments made by a variously informed general public. As Liberatos et al (1988:97) have noted, prestige ratings reflect 'averages of judgements made by persons having various degrees of familiarity with each occupation'. Such criticisms are used as the basis for suggesting that prestige measures fail to capture accurately a person's objective structural position in society. However, these criticisms overlook the fact that overseas and Australian researchers have demonstrated that measures of occupational prestige do have a clearly defined structural basis (Reiss et al 1961, Jones 1989). Jones for example, regressed a large number of socio-economic census variables against Daniel's (1983) measure of occupational prestige. The results of this regression analysis suggest that an increase in units of prestige are positively associated with indicators such as income, education and employment status. As Jones (1989:192) notes:

> being in the highest income category raises the prestige of a worker's job by between one-half to one full rank in the Daniel scale...Having a degree has an even larger effect, while being an employer or a self-employed worker also enhances the prestige of the job.

The evidence presented by Jones has three important implications for Australian health research. First, measures of occupational prestige now have a demonstrated structural basis in that occupations having high levels of prestige are also imbued with objective structural characteristics such as being an employer, being highly educated and earning a high income. Second, occupations not included in Daniel's original scale can now be given a prestige score. Third, knowing that measures of occupational prestige have a structural basis may facilitate the interpretation of research findings.

Educational-based measures of class

Class measures based on educational attainment can be operationalized either in terms of the number of school years completed (quantitatively) or in terms of discrete categories such as 'completed primary school', 'completed high school' and 'completed tertiary studies' (qualitatively). To date, Australian health researchers have employed the latter approach almost to the exclusion of the former. Using such measures, researchers have demonstrated that higher levels of educational attainment are significantly associated with lower smoking rates (Gray & Hill 1977, Hill & Gray 1984), lower rates of recent self-reported illness and mental instability (Broadhead 1985), lower systolic and diastolic blood pressure (Simons et al 1986) and a lower body mass index and levels of obesity (English & Bennett 1985).

Despite their predictive validity, educational-based measures of class are shrouded by a number of problematic issues which have yet to be adequately resolved. First, it is clear that educational attainment varies by the age cohort of the individual (Liberatos et al 1988). Many more persons completed secondary school and tertiary studies in the 1980s than in any previous period, yet it is uncertain whether, as a consequence, these persons should be assigned a higher position in social and economic hierarchies. Second, education is usually assumed to be a precursor to income and occupational attainment (Hauser & Featherman 1977). However, evidence compiled by Liberatos et al (1988), and Susser et al (1985) suggests that high levels of educational attainment do not necessarily lead to well paid, high status occupations. Third, and relatedly, Morgan (1983) and Haug (1973) have noted that western populations are becoming more homogeneous in terms of their educational attainment: this will become more common as youth are encouraged to continue their education beyond the minimum school leaving age. A net effect of an increase in educational homogeneity will be decreasing variability in years of education relative to other indicators of class such as income (Liberatos et al 1988).

Income-based measures of class

Of the 25 Australian health-related studies reviewed for this paper only three employed income-based measures. Najman et al (1979) used a measure of total gross household income in their study of the relationship between socioeconomic status and patterns of morbidity and health care utilization. These researchers measured income as a four-level categorical variable (e.g. less than $4000; $4000–7999; $8000–11 999; and $12 000 or more) but made no adjustment for the number of people comprising the household unit. Using this measure they demonstrated positive associations between SES level, health and health behaviour. Occupation and education were also employed but on the whole, these produced inconsistent findings for most health measures.

Broadhead (1985) used an income-based measure in his national study of the relationship between social status and morbidity. Using data from the 1978 Australian Health Survey, he devised a measure of 'relative affluence' which consisted of an estimate of net annual income adjusted for family size and standardized for age. This measure was then divided according to the 1977–78 simple Henderson poverty line (HPL) to produce the following categories: below HPL, 100–200% HPL and greater than 200% HPL. Confidentiality restrictions imposed on the data structure by the ABS limited the extent to which Broadhead was able to devise more sensitive income categories.

Despite its limitations, this measure was able to clearly distinguish among the three income groups in terms of health status. For both males and females (aged 15 years or older) there was a strong significant relationship between the measure of relative affluence and rates of morbidity. More particularly, those respondents below the poverty line experienced significantly higher rates of recent self-reported illness and chronic conditions, they had significantly higher General Health Questionnaire scores and they reported more days of reduced activity.

Like Najman et al (1979), Broadhead also used occupation and education based measures. In keeping with the pattern established by Najman et al, Broadhead found that 'the most striking (social status) differences occur when relative affluence, based on income adjusted for family size, is used as the discriminatory variable' (Broadhead 1985:87).

Broom (1984), in her secondary analysis of the Gosford/Wyong study (Shiraev & Armstrong 1978), used an income based measure similar to that of Broadhead. Her analysis showed a significant increase in 'chronic illness among middle-aged men and women, and among men over 65. The predicted pattern was also evident for recent illness among young men and for consulting among elderly respondents, but these associations were not statistically significant' (Broom 1984:909). The discriminatory power of income based measures relative to occupation and education was also evident in Broom's analysis. Of the three measures she employed, income was the most consistent in terms of its predictive capacity while occupation was the least consistent.

In Australian health research, measures of class based on education and income have not figured as prominently as occupational based measures. This is surprising as both measures have a number of advantages when compared with occupation based measures. First, the collection of education and income related data is relatively simple and is usually accomplished using a single straightforward question. Occupation based measures however, can require a number of detailed questions to be asked if the responses are to be reliably coded. Second, measures based on education and income allow groups such as the unemployed and those outside of the occupational structure to be assigned a position in a stratificationist hierarchy. These groups are often included in occupation based measures but they usually constitute anomalous categories such as 'other' or 'not easily classifiable': rarely do these categorizations yield results that are meaningful or readily interpretable. Thirdly, income based measures, and to a lesser extent education based measures, have a high degree of face validity (Najman 1988). In other words, these measures provide a relatively unambiguous and easy to understand estimate of inequality: these properties are not as apparent with occupation based measures.

Area-based measures of class

The construction of an area-based measure of class usually involves ranking geographic regions in terms of their mean score on variables such as income, education and occupation. A separate mean value is calculated for each geographic region and then researchers are able to compare regions differing in social and economic composition in terms of health outcome variables. Studies employing area-based measures have consistently demonstrated that socially disadvantaged regions have disproportionately high rates of infant mortality (Dasvarma 1980, Siskind et al 1987a), adult mortality (Fisher 1978, Gordon et al 1989, Siskind et al 1987b) and morbidity (National Health Strategy 1992).

Despite their predictive value, there are a number of problems which characterize area-based measures. The most well known of these is the 'ecological fallacy' where the results of area-based correlations are interpreted as if they were correlations between individual characteristics of persons. A second and related problem is that of interpretation. When a significant association is observed between the social characteristics of an area and a health outcome, it is difficult to account for this finding except in very broad and tentative terms.

Finally, area based studies and studies at the individual level have produced, on occasion, different patterns of results for the same disease outcomes (Pukkala & Teppo 1986, Hakama et al 1982). These studies examined the relationship between class and breast and cervical cancer and gastrointestinal cancer using individual and area based measures and found differences in the strength and direction of some associations depending on which measure was used. These discrepancies clearly need to be examined further, as they raise important questions about what area based indicators are actually measuring, and how and why they sometimes produce results that differ from measures used at the individual level.

Problems common to most measures of class

During the 1980s researchers highlighted a number of methodological and substantive problems which are common to many measures of class (Abramson et al 1982, Illsley & Baker 1991, Jones & Cameron 1984, Liberatos et al 1988, Najman 1988); the most important of these are discussed below.

One fundamental yet unresolved problem concerns the most appropriate means of assigning a class position to women. The vast majority of empirical studies which use class measures have tended to either exclude women from the analysis or women have been assigned a class position on the basis of the class location of the male 'head' of the family (Baxter 1991a). This 'conventional' means of assigning women to a class position is often defended on the grounds that women, by virtue of their private sector orientation, have only an attenuated and intermittent connection with the labour force (see Goldthorpe 1980, 1983). Thus by default, the class position of women can only be accurately determined by their partner's or father's class position, as their connection with paid work is consistent and continuous over the life-course. Increasingly however, social researchers, and feminist writers in particular, are pointing to a number of theoretical and empirical flaws in the rationale underpinning the conventional method of assigning a class position to women (e.g. Crompton & Jones 1984, Walby 1986). For example, they argue that the conventional method fails to take account of gender inequalities which militate against women's continuous involvement in paid work, and also that this method fails to consider the changing characteristics of the labour force, particularly the large increase in the number of women entering and remaining in paid work. Although there is no consensus as to the most appropriate means of assigning a class position to women, the accumulating evidence is increasingly calling into question the validity of assuming that the male's occupation is the most appropriate criterion by which to assign a class position to women (Baxter 1992).

A second criticism often directed at measures of class is that they are adequate only as descriptive labels (Illsley & Baker 1991). In other words, class measures are able to discriminate among social groups in terms of their health status, but beyond this they are clearly inadequate: class measures point to a socially related health problem but they do not greatly advance our understanding of why the problem exists.

A third and related problem concerns the issue of measurement validity. In short, what is the underlying phenomenon which indicators of class purport to be 'capturing' and measuring? At present, this question remains largely open to speculation. Given that few measures of class are adequately conceptualized (i.e. have emerged from a well developed and clearly articulated body of theory), it is difficult to know, except in vague and tentative terms, what class indicators are actually measuring. In addition, a lack of conceptualization makes it difficult to explain or understand the results from empirical studies, as research findings often have meaning and significance only when located within a broader theoretical context.

Fourthly, there is the problem of which measure of class is most appropriate in any given research situation, as it may be the case that some measures are more applicable in certain health contexts than in others. For example, education based measures may have greater predictive value than income or occupation based measures when addressing issues relating to preventive health. The choice of any particular measure also has policy implications. Income related health inequalities may suggest ameliorative responses through the redistributive potential of the welfare system and education related inequalities raise the possibility of education based initiatives such as health promotion strategies (Najman 1988).

Finally, an often neglected issue which needs to be considered is the important interdependency that exists between measures of class and the data collection source. Ultimately, the availability of conceptually grounded, non-sexist and meaningful measures of class will in part be a function of the demographic and social information that is recorded when health data are collected.

Many researchers examining the relationship between class and health use data that has been compiled by independent data collection agencies such as the Australian Bureau of Statistics and the National Heart Foundation, or they obtain their data from routinely recorded statistics. Examples of the types of secondary data sources available to health researchers include the Australian Health Survey, the Risk Factor Prevalence Study, census data and unit record death certificate information. These sources however, are often limited with respect to the type and amount of social data they record. For example, death certificates typically make provision only for the collection of occupational data and this is only 'recorded with any reliability for males aged between 25 and 64 years' (Gibbered et al 1984:26).

The limits imposed by the available data collection methods have had and continue to have important consequences in terms of the types of measures of class that can be devised and employed by health researchers. In short, the nature and extent of the social data that is presently collected by government agencies are not sufficiently detailed or sensitive and the measures of class that are being constructed from such data reflect this deficiency.

Recent developments

As was demonstrated earlier, most studies which examine the relationship between class and health rely on measures of occupational status or prestige, educational attainment or income level. Even though health researchers employ the term 'class' when using these measures they are more appropriately seen as being measures of social stratification in that they assume a hierarchical ordering of occupation, income and education rather than a relational understanding of social structure (Baxter 1991b). In other words, classes have not been conceptualized as discrete groupings within the economic structure, with each group being related on the basis of inherent characteristics such as the ownership or non-ownership of productive capital, or the possession of skills, expertise and experience. Consequently, more theoretically based models of class such as those developed by Wright (1985, 1987, 1988), Wright et al (1989) and Goldthorpe (1980, 1981, 1982, 1983) are missing from the health literature. This absence is unfortunate, as the measures developed by Wright and Goldthorpe may overcome some of the problems discussed earlier. The particular advantage of these measures is that they are theoretically informed. Importantly, studies using general social science data indicate that Wright and Goldthorpe's measures have predictive value (Baxter et al 1991) and they may have descriptive and explanatory utility when applied in the health context, although this has yet to be empirically demonstrated. It should be pointed out however, that these two measures also share a number of the problems and limitations which currently beset many class measures used in health research. For example, the perennial problem of allocating women to a class position remains to be adequately resolved, although recent work (Baxter 1992) has suggested a strategy to be adopted. In addition, 'true' class measures, by their very definition, may exclude from their design persons who are located outside the paid workforce (e.g. young people, the unemployed and pensioners). Ongoing research however, is providing a solution to this problem (Baxter et al 1993).

We would argue therefore, that the two models of class outlined below have theoretical and empirical advantages over other measures of class, particularly single indicator measures based on occupation. For these reasons their inclusion in future health studies is warranted.

Wright's conceptualization of class is premised on the notion that those participating in economic or productive activities possess different kinds of productive assets which are a source of income. In modern industrial capitalist society the major productive asset is property. However, there are also two other kinds of productive assets which generate income. The first is the ability to control the technical processes of production. This asset is typically possessed by managers and bureaucrats who control and co-ordinate production, as exemplified by their position within the hierarchy of a business enterprise. Organizational assets are unequally distributed, with managers possessing a greater share than supervisors, who in turn possess a greater share than workers. The second kind of productive asset which generates income is skills or talents. These are seen most clearly when the possession of skills is associated with credentials (degrees, diplomas, etc.). Again those operating in the economic sphere will vary with respect to the skills or credentials they possess.

Variability in the possession of productive assets, organizational assets and skill or credential assets leads, in the first instance, to a relatively complex twelve-category class model (Fig. 6.1) consisting of three ownership or property classes (owners of large and small businesses and the petty bourgeoisie), and nine non-ownership classes differentiated on the basis of relative possession of organizational and skill/credential assets (indicated as 'high', 'medium' and 'low' in the figure).

For research purposes, the schema presented in Figure 6.1 can be reduced to a six-level class model comprising owners of the means of production, petty bourgeoisie, expert managers and supervisors, experts and workers. The advantage of this classification is that it distinguishes important class groups from one another. First, there is the distinction between owners of large businesses from self-employed workers and those employing no one other than family members, namely, the petty bourgeoisie. Next, three major groups within what is generally regarded as the middle class are identified: expert managers, largely top managers with tertiary qualifications, a second group of managers and supervisors lacking the qualifications of the expert managers, and lastly a group comprising experts who are largely professionals employed in staff rather than line positions in both the public and private sectors. Finally, a working class comprising semi- and unskilled white and

Fig. 6.1 Wright's multiple assets model of social class

Owners	Non-owners (wage labourers)			
1. Bourgeoisie	4. Expert managers	7. Skilled managers	10. Unskilled managers	+
2. Small employers	5. Expert supervisors	8. Skilled supervisors	11. Unskilled supervisors	0
3. Petty bourgeoisie	6. Expert workers	9. Skilled workers	12. Proletarian	-
	High	Medium	Low	
	Skill/credential assets			

Table 6.3 The Australian class structure based on Erik Wright's multiple assets model

	% in paid workforce
Employers	2
Petty bourgeoisie	12
Expert managers	18
Non-expert managers and supervisors	18
Non-managerial experts	8
Workers	42
Number	1196

Adapted from Baxter et al 1991

blue collar workers lacking organizational responsibility and possessing only minimal formal skills completes the class structure. The distribution of the Australian work force across these class locations is shown in Table 6.3.

An alternative to Wright's model, which is based on the social relations of production, is the neo-Weberian approach by John Goldthorpe. The theoretical rationale for Goldthorpe's class model was based on the aggregation of occupations according to their shared objective work and market situations. Specifically, the aim was to:

combine occupational categories whose members would appear...to be typically comparable, on the one hand in terms of their sources and levels of income, their degree of economic security and chances of economic advancement; and on the other in their location within systems of authority and control governing the process of production in which they are engaged and hence their degree of autonomy in performing their work tasks and roles (Goldthorpe 1980).

The result of this aggregation of occupations is a sevenfold class scheme (see Table 6.4). Classes I and II consist of salaried and self-employed individuals in professional occupations, managers and administrators, and proprietors of large establishments differentiated on the grounds of skill and managerial responsibility. Together they make up the service class. Class III comprises white collar workers, routine non-manual clerical and sales employees. Class IV are small proprietors and the traditional petty bourgeoisie. Class V are lower level technical workers and supervisors of manual employees. Class VI consists of skilled manual workers while Class VII is made up of semi- and unskilled blue collar workers. If more detailed class groupings are required, Goldthorpe's scheme has the capacity to be extended up to eleven categories.

The immediate advantages of Wright and Goldthorpe's models of class are twofold. First, they are grounded in a theoretical tradition which provides for the establishment of meaningful relations between class location and other aspects of the social and economic environment (Baxter et al 1991). Within a health context, these two measures would provide for the meaningful allocation of individuals to clearly defined and theoretically informed positions within the class structure. In turn, a detailed knowledge about a person's

Table 6.4 The Australian class structure based on John Goldthorpe's seven category class model

	Class	% in paid work force
I	Upper service	10
II	Lower service	23
III	Routine non-manual	22
IV	Small proprietors, self-employed workers	11
V	Lower grade technical non-manual supervisory	8
VI	Skilled manual	12
VII	Semi- and unskilled manual	14
	Number	1196

Adapted from Baxter et al 1991

position within the class structure, if related to an adverse health outcome, may facilitate and promote a fuller understanding of why the relationship existed. At present, this degree of explanatory power is not possible with existing class measures.

Second, Wright and Goldthorpe's measures are based on a small number of structured questions relating either to the nature of paid work, extent of managerial responsibility and level of skill, or occupation. These questions can be readily coded from a self-administered questionnaire.

Clearly, judgements about the predictive value and explanatory utility of the measures proposed by Wright and Goldthorpe must await the results of systematic investigations where the two measures are contrasted with the more empirically based measures of socio-economic status derived from occupation, income and education.

Conclusion

The first section of this chapter identified the types of class measures most commonly employed in Australian health research. Class is usually measured on the basis of occupation, education, income and geographic region. Overall, these measures were able to discriminate among social groups in terms of their health status. Those individuals in unskilled or low status occupations, those who have limited education, and those existing on incomes close to or below the poverty line experience disproportionately high levels of mortality, they report higher morbidity rates and they manifest a higher incidence of disease risk factors. The evidence presented in this first section clearly demonstrates that social justice in terms of health status remains an unrealized ideal.

The second section briefly discussed a number of methodological and substantive issues associated with the measurement, selection and explanatory potential of class. First, it was found that a satisfactory method of allocating women to a class position has yet to be devised. A number of alternative approaches have been suggested but as yet no consensus has been reached. Second, it was argued that class measures are able to delineate the extent of health inequalities in society but they provide few substantive insights into why these inequalities exist.

Thirdly, it is not exactly clear what current measures of class are actually measuring. In all likelihood, the measures used in health research are multi-dimensional rather than uni-dimensional in nature, tapping both material/ economic and affective/behavioural differences between social groups.

Fourthly, it was suggested that the inclusion of any particular measure of class in a health study should be carefully considered as each measure may have different predictive strengths and policy consequences.

Finally, this second section noted that many health data sources contain a limited amount of social and economic information, or the information that is available is often compressed to meet confidentiality requirements. Either of these situations limit the types of measures of class that can be devised and employed by health researchers.

The third section of the chapter briefly reviewed two recent developments in the conceptualization and measurement of class. It was argued that these measures may overcome some of the deficiencies which beset those currently in use, although these measure also have limitations. The measures, developed by Eric Wright and John Goldthorpe, are theoretically grounded. They can be easily constructed on the basis of a small number of questions which could be readily incorporated within existing data collection procedures. Most importantly, these two measures could possibly facilitate the interpretation of results, as any finding can be understood against a well developed theoretical backdrop. If these measures are employed in future health studies, they may contribute to an improved understanding of the social determinants of health and illness. At present, our understanding of the relationship between class and health is largely limited to the description of empirical findings.

REFERENCES

Abramson J H, Gofin R, Habib J, Pridan H and Gofin J 1982 Indicators of social class: a comparative appraisal of measures for use in epidemiological studies. Social Science and Medicine 16:1739–1746
Baghurst K I, Record S J, Baghurst P A, Syrette J A et al 1990 Socio-demographic determinants in Australia of the intake of food and nutrients implicated in cancer aetiology. Medical Journal of Australia 153:444–452
Baxter J 1991a The class location of women: direct or derived? In: Baxter J et al (eds) Class analysis and contemporary Australia. Macmillan, Melbourne
Baxter J 1991b Work and family: class and the household division of labour. In: Baxter J et al (eds) Class analysis and contemporary Australia. Macmillan, Melbourne
Baxter J, Emmison M, Western J, Western M 1991 Class analysis and contemporary Australia. Macmillan, Melbourne
Baxter J 1992 Is husband's class enough: class location and class identity in the United States, Sweden, Norway and Australia. Paper presented at the American Sociological

Association conference, Pittsburg, USA

Baxter J, Western J, Western M 1993 Personal communication

Broadhead P 1985 Social status and morbidity in Australia. Community Health Studies 9:87-98

Broom D H 1984 The social distribution of illness: is Australia more equal? Social Science and Medicine 18(11):909-917

Coleman R, Rainwater L 1978 Social standing in America: new dimensions of social class. Basic Books, New York

Congalton A A 1969 Status and prestige in Australia. Cheshire, Melbourne

Coxon A, Davies P 1986 Images of social stratification: occupational structures and class. Sage Publications, London

Crompton R, Jones G 1984 White collar proletariat. Macmillan, London

Daniel A E 1978 A researcher's reflections on the Blaikie contribution. Australian and New Zealand Journal of Sociology 14(1):81-87

Daniel A E 1983 Power, privilege and prestige: occupations in Australia. Melbourne, Longman Cheshire

Daniel A E 1984 The measurement of social class. Community Health Studies 8(2):218-222

Dasvarma G L 1980 Socio-demographic correlates of infant mortality in Australia. Social Science and Medicine 14D:151-164

Dobson A J, Gibbered R W, Leeder S R, O'Connell D L 1985 Occupational differences in ischaemic heart disease mortality and risk factors in Australia. American Journal of Epidemiology 122(2):283-290

English R M, Bennett S 1985 Overweight and obesity in the Australian community. Journal of Food and Nutrition 42(1):2-12

Fisher S 1978 Relationship of mortality to socioeconomic status and some other factors in Sydney in 1971. Journal of Epidemiology and Community Health 32:41-46

Gibbered R W, Dobson A J, du Ve Florey C, Leeder S R 1984 Differences and comparative declines in ischaemic heart disease mortality among sub-populations in Australia, 1969-1978. International Journal of Epidemiology 13:25-31

Goldthorpe J H (with Llewellyn C, Payne C) 1980 Social mobility and class structure in modern Britain. Clarendon Press, Oxford

Goldthorpe J H 1981 The class schema of 'social mobility and class structure in modern Britain': a reply to Penn. Sociology 15:272-280

Goldthorpe J H 1982 On the service class, its formation and future. In: Giddens A, Mackenzie G. (eds) Social class and the division of labour: essays in honour of Ilya Neustadt. Cambridge University Press, LondonGoldthorpe J H 1983 Women and class analysis: in defence of the conventional view. Sociology 17(4):448-65

Gordon I, Christie D, Robinson K 1989 Social class as indicated by area of residence: a mortality study within an Australian industrial population. Community Health Studies 13(2):170-176

Gray N J, Hill D J 1977 Patterns of tobacco smoking in Australia. Medical Journal of Australia 2:327-328

Hakama M, Hakulinen T, Pukkala E, et al 1982 Risk indicators of breast and cervical cancer on ecologic and individual levels. American Journal of Epidemiology 116:990-1000

Haug M R 1973 Women's occupational roles. Social Forces 52:86-98

Hauser R M, Featherman D L 1977 The process of stratification: trends and analyses. Academic Press, New York

Health Targets and Implementation (Health for All) Committee 1988 Health for all Australians. AGPS, Canberra

Hill D, Gray N 1984 Australian patterns of tobacco smoking and related health beliefs in 1983. Community Health Studies 8(3):307-316

Illsley R, Baker D 1991 Contextual variations in the meaning of health inequality. Social Science and Medicine 32(4):359-365

Jones I G, Cameron D 1984 Social class analysis: an embarrassment to epidemiology. Community Medicine 6(1):37-46

Jones F L 1989 Occupational prestige in Australia: a new scale. Australian and New Zealand Journal of Sociology 25:187-199

Lee S, Smith L, d'Espaignet E, Thompson N 1987 Health differentials for working age Australians. Australian Institute of Health. AGPS, Canberra

Leeder S R, Woolcock A J 1973 Cigarette smoking in Sydney schoolchildren aged 12 to 13 Years. Medical Journal of Australia 2:674–678

Leeder S R, Peat J K, Woolcock A J 1977 Cigarette smoking in Sydney schoolchildren aged 12 to 13 years: 1971–1975. Medical Journal of Australia 1:325–329

Liberatos P, Link B G, Kelsey J L 1988 The measurement of social class in epidemiology. Epidemiologic Reviews 10:87–121

McMichael A J, Hartshorne J M 1982 Mortality risks in Australian men by occupational groups, 1968-1978: variations associated with differences in drinking and smoking habits. Medical Journal of Australia 253–256

McMichael A J 1985 Social class (as estimated by occupational prestige) and mortality in Australian males in the 1970s. Community Health Studies 9(3):220–230

Morgan M 1983 Measuring social inequality: occupational classifications and their alternatives. Community Medicine 5:116–24

Najman J M. et al 1979 Patterns of morbidity, health care utilisation and socioeconomic status in Brisbane. Australian and New Zealand Journal of Sociology 15(3):55–63

Najman J M 1988 The measurement of socioeconomic inequality and social class in Australia: a review of past practices and recent developments. Community Health Studies 12:31–41

National Heath Strategy 1992 Enough to make you sick: how income and environment affect health. Research Paper No 1, September

Opit L J, Oliver R G, Salzberg M 1984 Occupation and blood pressure. Medical Journal of Australia 140:760–764

Pukkala E, Teppo L 1986 Socioeconomic status and education as risk determinants of gastrointestinal cancer. Preventive Medicine 15:127–38

Reiss A J et al (eds) 1961 Occupations and social status, New York, Free Press

Shiraev N, Armstrong M 1978 Health care survey of Gosford-Wyong and Illawarra, 1975. Division of Health Services Research, Health Commission of New South Wales

Simons L A, Andersen N, Simons J, Whish P 1982 Health attitudes and knowledge and coronary risk factors in high school children: Sydney and Inverell. Medical Journal of Australia 2:178–183

Simons L A, Simons J, Magnus P, Bennett S A 1986 Education level and coronary heart risk factors in Australians. The Medical Journal of Australia 145:446–450

Siskind V, Najman J M, Copeman R 1987a Infant mortality in socioeconomically advantaged and disadvantaged areas of Brisbane. Community Health Studies 11(1):24–30

Siskind V, Copeman R, Najman J M 1987b Socioeconomic status and mortality: a Brisbane area analysis. Community Health Studies 11(1):15–23

Susser M, Watson W, Hopper K 1985 Sociology in medicine. Oxford University Press, New York

Teevan J J 1985 Socioeconomic status is significantly related to... In: Liberatos P, Link B G, Kelsey J L (eds) The measurement of social class in epidemiology. Epidemiologic Reviews 1988 10:87–121

Walby S 1986 Patriarchy at work. Polity, Cambridge

Wright E O 1985 Classes. New Left Books, London

Wright E O 1987 Reflections on classes. Berkeley Journal of Sociology 32:19–49

Wright E O 1988 Exploitation, identity and class structure: a reply to my critics. Critical Sociology 15:91–110

Wright E O, Howe C, Cho D 1989 Class structure and class formation: a comparative analysis of the United States and Sweden. In: Kohn M L (ed) Cross national research in sociology. Sage, Newbury Park

7. The engendering of hormonal difference

Margie Ripper

It is not difficult to understand that inequality in health status and in health care can result from unfair or discriminatory treatment of individuals or groups. It is more difficult to grasp the idea that inequality can result from the fundamental definitions and assumptions that we hold about the nature of bodies and their physiological processes. This chapter will investigate how one group of people have come to be seen as inherently disabled by an aspect of their physiology. It will trace the origins of medical and societal belief in, and concern about, the allegedly disabling impact of reproductive hormones on the health of women.

An extreme form of the belief that women's well-being is determined by reproductive hormones is seen in the contemporary medical definition of the post menopausal period of life as a hormonal deficiency disease. This medical construction of women as inherently diseased/deficient for three to four decades of their lives has prompted me to reflect upon how it is that women came to be thought of as hormonally determined in the first place. In this chapter, I explore the origins of the belief that women's well-being and capabilities are determined by hormones, in a way that men's are not. This exploration is important theoretically, politically and subjectively.

Theoretically, it illuminates the way in which the concept of universal women is constructed in contemporary folklore, and shows the centrality of bio-reductionist medical 'facts' in that construction. It also shows the key role that research activity has played in constructing the facts that it claims to be investigating. In this case constructing the menstrual cycle as dysfunctional and women as inherently disabled.

Politically, it identifies the way that the belief in a biologically defined difference between women and men continues to be used to explain and to justify women's limited status and capabilities. It provides another example of an aspect of women's everyday life which has been medicalized and pathologized.

Subjectively, it forces us to reconsider our own experience. Women have come to feel, and to live, the disorders which have emerged since the discovery of hormones. There is no doubt about the 'reality' of the symptoms of disorders such as Pre-menstrual Tension (PMT): they can have a profound impact on well-being. The emergence of new disorders challenges the belief that biological processes are fixed in a human physiology which is separable from social processes. Similarly the disappearance of disorders such as hysteria (Smith-Rosenberg 1972), miner's nystagmus (Figlio 1982), chlorosis (Hudson 1977) or involutional melancholia suggest that the diseases possible within bodies are socially and historically constructed. The discovery that physiological processes are experienced differently in different social and historical milieu, challenges that idea that subjective consciousness or experience has an authenticity separate from the cultural context. This presents a caution to those who assert that 'lived experience' is a valid measure of well-being in a way that the traditional medico-scientific reliance on measurable signs and symptoms is not. The notion of a socially constructed biology forces us to confront the idea that subjective experience of our own physiology is inextricably intertwined with dominant discourses through which social relations (including gender relations) are negotiated.

Within this chapter I will trace the 'biography' of the menstrual cycle and its chief disorder PMT. PMT is an example of a disorder whose emergence has played a crucial role in the contemporary construction of gender. The next paragraph indicates how I have structured this biography.

First I outline in bald form, eight claims about the construction of the menstrual cycle and its central disorder PMT before providing evidence in support of those claims. Then I identify the conjunction of social, political, ideological, medical, technical and commercial factors that have made the menstrual cycle and PMT possible. Finally I reflect upon the intersecting web of factors that have made it possible for women to be constructed as 'hormonal' and relate this to the construction of menopause as a deficiency disease.

The eight claims which constitute my argument are as follows:

1. The emergence of a hormonal model of women's reproductive system represents a paradigm shift within medical knowledge away from an 'organistic' model towards a 'bio-chemical' model of women's (but not men's) reproductive system. By 'organistic' model I mean one which locates the central or driving force of reproduction in a specific organ (penis, brain, uterus, ovaries). This shift is recent and peculiar to western medical discourse.
2. Women's reproductive organs have long been said to cause and explain her limited status and capacity. The shift to a bio-chemical model of women's reproductive system, has substantiated that belief whilst locating the disabling factor in hormones rather than organs.
3. The menstrual cycle and its disorders have only been an object of medical interest since the demise of the organistic model of women's reproductive system. There has long been a medical fascination with menstrual bleeding but not with the issue of cyclicity.
4. There is no evidence of medical interest in, or concern about, the

premenstrual phase of the menstrual cycle until the mid 1930s, by which time the cyclic nature of menstruation was manifest and had been linked to the secretion of ovarian hormones.

5. An emphasis upon psychological ill-effects of the menstrual cycle (including the disorder PMT) was made possible by the belief that women's brain/mind/reasoning was inextricably linked to her reproductive system. This belief followed the discovery of the symbiotic interaction between pituitary and reproductive hormones which, in women, was interpreted to mean that the pituitary 'controlled' ovarian hormone production.

6. Despite hundreds of studies which have attempted to do so, there has never been any measurable hormonal difference found between women who experience PMT and women who don't.

7. Medical interest in the premenstrual phase of the menstrual cycle has been influenced by social, political, and commercial contexts in addition to the professional debates and 'discoveries' about women's reproductive system.

8. Menopause was not viewed as a hormonal deficiency until the 1960s. That is until such time as women's reproductive system had been firmly established as hormonal and commercial products made available to control and replace normal hormonal production.

Evidence in support of these claims

The following material is drawn from a content analysis of the medico-scientific literature indexed in the *Index Medicus* for the years 1900–1985. This publication indexes the contents of all major journals in the fields of medical science. It provides references to research articles, clinical opinion, letters to the editors and proceedings of some professional conferences. The data selected for this content analysis were all references to what is now known as menstruation, the menstrual cycle, menopause and PMT. (Terms have emerged and changed during the 85 years under review. A description of these changes in terminology and their meaning in the naming of new disorders can be found in Ripper 1992).

At the turn of the century medical knowledge offered an 'organistic' model of gender difference. Women's 'being' was located in her uterus whilst men's was centred in his brain (Erenreich & English 1979). Some of the clearest statements of this model of physiology are to be found in late 19th century medical treatise about the detrimental effects of education and public life on women's reproductive functioning (Barker-Benfield 1976). Conversely men's reasoning capacity and physical well-being were seen to be readily damaged by excess or 'unnatural' sexual activity, particularly masturbation.

Within the organistic reproductive system the centrality of the uterus to women's well-being placed enormous significance upon menstruation.

Unwomanly activities (including education, employment or remaining unmarried) were seen to produce structural changes in the placement, size and functioning of the uterus and to disturb the menstrual flow. Unwomanly activities were said to 'unsex' women by displacing or shrivelling the womb. (Donnison 1977).

Not surprisingly in this context there was an overwhelming fascination within the medical/scientific literature as to the 'purpose' of menstruation and with problems associated with menstrual bleeding. Three themes preoccupied medical thought at the turn of the century:

- The role of menstruation in women's health. Menstrual bleeding was *known* to be accompanied by weakness, ill-health and vulnerability. Yet menstrual flow was considered to be toxic and its elimination was seen to be essential to good health. Bleeding, purging and stimulants were utilized to remedy 'obstructed' (or failed) menstruation.
- The role of menstruation in fertility. It was generally accepted that the reproductive systems of all female animals were equivalent. Menstruation was thought to equate with oestrus as the period of fertility and sexual 'receptiveness'. This belief was consistent with 19th century Social Darwinist theories which ranked women, non-human species, and non-European 'races' as lower on the evolutionary hierarchy than Caucasian men (Gould 1981). Women were thereby constructed as reproductive units, having more in common with females of other species than they did with men.
- The role of menstruation in the survival of the species. The oestrus model of menstruation gradually gave way in face of increased focus on the role of the ovaries in women's fertility (Ehrenreich & English 1979). This change was accompanied by a great deal of dispute and conjecture within medical and scientific community as to what 'function' menstruation played in the survival of the species. A continuing theme within the literature is the meta-significance that menstruation gains when it is constructed as symbolic of women's capacity to reproduce and therefore to ensure the survival of the human race.

The custodians of medical knowledge about women's reproductive system during this organistic era were obstetrician/gynaecologists. The gynaecological therapies for reproductive and menstrual disorders were predominantly mechanical, they included surgical removal or adjustment of the uterus or ovaries, or the use of pessaries to align the pelvic organs correctly in the body.

Women's mental health was also considered to be uterus dependent, with displacement or 'disappointment' of the womb being a major cause of insanity and of women's peculiar nervous 'suggestibility'. The organistic model of human physiology asserted that the correct functioning of each organ of the body depended upon its proper connection through nerve supply to the brain. Insanity in women was said to occur because the nerve supply to women's reproductive organs was susceptible to disruption by unwomanly activities which either stimulated her brain/imagination (and starved her uterus/ovaries) or which displaced her organs thereby interfering with proper nerve supply.

The peculiar mental instability and suggestibility of women was common knowledge, women were said to be particularly vulnerable to insanity and disorders such as hysteria during puberty, pregnancy and menopause. Within the medical literature of this era menopause was classified as a form of insanity. 'Involutional insanity' and 'involutional melancholia' were the two main diseases which menopause, (conceptualized as the loss of one's essential womanhood) could produce.

The discovery of hormones

The discovery of ovarian hormones in the late 1920s altered the medical definition of women's reproductive physiology. But the new hormonal model of women's reproductive system left the negative ideology intact. It did provide new explanations for women's inherent vulnerability, and made possible new disorders of the menstrual cycle.

The existence of ovarian hormones was established during the second and third decades of this century. Initially there was spirited resistance from clinicians to the idea that women's menstrual and reproductive system was not controlled by nerves but by an essence which was produced and excreted by the ovaries. This ovarian extract was initially referred to as 'the female essence' or 'the female sex hormone' (Frank & Goldberger 1928). So fully had medical science constructed women as reproductively driven that these expressions were coined as if they were neutral descriptions.

The discovery of 'the female essence' challenged the gynaecologist's claim to reproductive medical expertise. The explanations and interventions which were the tools of trade of the obstetrician/gynaecologist all involved the cutting and sewing of pelvic organs. These interventions were being supplanted by those of the newly emerging medical specialty of endocrinology who depended not on surgical expertise but on the prescription of various ovarian extracts. The new ovarian extracts were accessible only to clinicians who had access to laboratories which could extract the ingredients from pregnant mares' urine or blood, or from surgically removed ovarian tissue. The therapeutic effectiveness of these early ovarian extracts was notoriously unreliable. The products varied in concentration depending upon their source and the method used to extract them. Further inconsistency occurred depending on whether the substance was ingested, injected, or implanted. The unreliability of early endocrine therapies created disputes between clinicians and researchers, as well as inter-disciplinary rivalry between gynaecology and endocrinology.

The full acceptance of an endocrine model of women's reproduction did not occur until the development at the end of the 1930s of synthetic hormones to replace the organic extracts. Until that point there was very little medical interest in the cyclicity of menstruation. Most of the early hormonal interventions were to alter the characteristics of menstrual bleeding that was considered too profuse, scanty, obstructed or was accompanied by pain, nausea or anaemia.

The emergence of the menstrual cycle

A number of social and demographic factors contributed to the conditions of possibility for the emergence of menstruation as a cyclic event and for cyclicity to become an object of medical interest. Since the turn of the century women were spending fewer and fewer years pregnant and lactating. Smaller families was especially marked amongst middle class and wealthy women: the very people who made up the bulk of doctor's clientele. With less years spent pregnant and lactating more occasions of menstruation were being experienced, and the cyclicity and predictability of menstruation became more clearly observed.

The pre-menstrual phase as a site of disorder

The predictability of menstruation was a necessary condition for the identification of a premenstrual phase of the cycle. There is no evidence of medical interest or concern with the premenstrual phase of the menstrual cycle until the 1930s, by which time the cyclic nature of menstruation was manifest and had been linked to the secretion of ovarian hormones. The existence of cyclicity did not necessarily lead to the pre-menstrual phase being thought of as problematic; this interpretation depended upon a number of other contextual factors. Central amongst these were new discoveries that reinforced and gave an endocrine explanation for the belief that women's reproductive health was influenced by her mind. This deepened the belief that much of women's illness (especially reproductive disorders) were psycho-somatic. The deeply entrenched negativism about menstrual bleeding made it logical to assume that when women could anticipate menstruation they would do so with dread and through their peculiar 'suggestibility' would experience pre-menstrual emotional disorders. The emphasis upon psychological ill-effects of the pre menstrual phase of the menstrual cycle was made possible by discoveries in the mid 1930s that 'the female sex hormone' was not a single essence generated from within the ovaries. Two ovarian hormones (those now known as oestrogen and progesterone) were distinguished and their production was found to cycle in a symbiotic relationship with hormones produced in the pituitary section of the brain. Concentrations of ovarian hormones in the blood influence the production of pituitary hormones and vice-versa. This interrelationship was grasped as bio-chemical evidence that women's brain/mind/reasoning was inextricably linked to her reproductive system; her pituitary hormones were said to 'control' ovarian hormone production. Within the brain the pituitary gland is located at the base of the hypothalamus, the section characterised as the centre of the emotions.

Women were already 'known' to have a peculiar mind/body connection which had accounted for their suggestibility, hysteria and problems with puberty, menstruation, pregnancy and menopause. In this ideological context the 'discovery' of an ovarian/pituitary link made biological sense of existing beliefs about women. Two quotations from influential medical researchers on the menstrual cycle, provide clear illustrations of the belief in a peculiar (hormonally determined) female physiology, which is unlike male physiology.

In 1945 Willard Cooke, President of the American Association of Obstetricians Gynaecologists and Abdominal Surgeons asserted that:

Up to a certain point, the mental processes of man and woman are alike, but beyond this point there is divergence to an ultimate degree. In women far more than men, ideation and mental activities are dominated by the reproductive factor and its side issues. *Reproduction is the central physiologic raison d'etre of woman...* The hypersensitization of the nervous system which occurs during the pre-menstrual phase of the cycle...[and the resulting] alteration of personality during this stage, is a matter of common observation, of tradition, and of history (Cooke 1945:457-458, emphasis added).

In the late 1980s the same belief was expressed in its hormonal guise by Dr Myra Steiner when describing a new psychiatric form of severe PMT which was being defined at the time by the American Psychiatric Association.

Because, as it is widely assumed, [that] the mind/body relationship is closer in women than it is in men—for some reason. It is expected that the hormonal changes that accompany cyclicity are bound to have negative consequences (Steiner 1987).

The assumption that hormonal variation has negative consequences for women is the central hallmark of medical and scientific research into the 'effects' of the menstrual cycle. Since the end of the second world war extraordinary research effort has gone into measuring cyclic variation in women's physiological states. Performance measures such as reaction time, eye-blink rate, pain sensitivity and various tests of cognitive functioning have been studied exhaustively. See Sommer (1973) for a review of these studies. But what are most commonly assessed are cyclic variation in *negative* moods (tension, irritability, vulnerability, anger, incompetence, forgetfulness, and general unwomanly behaviour) (Ripper 1991).

Two features predominate in menstrual cycle research. First, the assumption that variation is inherently dysfunctional. The 'low' points in cyclic variation are thereby constructed as disabling, 'effects' of the menstrual cycle. This construction is only possible within a paradigm where health is equated with constancy and stasis and variability is constituted as dis-order (illness). In men, physiological stasis is *presumed* to be the normal hormonal, psychological and behavioural state. So fully accepted is this assumption that the mood, performance and hormonal variation in men has not been considered worthy of investigation. The one exception was the work of

Houser which showed that fluctuations of testosterone production in men was consistently related to mood fluctuations (Houser 1979).

It is almost as rare to find studies which offer a practical measure of whether or not low points in cyclic variation are experienced by the woman as a problem. Nor has there been research effort put into assessing the strength of the effect of the menstrual cycle, compared with the impact the many every day factors which influence mood and well-being. (For example, whether it is a weekday or a weekend, whether one has enjoyed a restful night's sleep, or whether the children squabbled throughout breakfast.)

Second, the overwhelming effort has been to find negative effects of the cycle. So pervasive is the belief that cyclic variation is dysfunctional that, in the vast majority of studies, only negative phenomena have been investigated. This tendency is characterized within the influential research instrument the Moos Menstrual Distress Questionnaire which investigates 47 symptoms, 42 of which are negative (Moos 1968). Just as the late 19th century physicians catalogued the disabling impact of menstruation, so mid-20th century medicine has chosen the pre-menstrual phase as the one most disabling to women and most responsible for defining the quintessential womanly mood and behaviour.

The credibility of a hormonal model of PMT

Despite hundreds of studies which have attempted to do so, there has never been any measurable hormonal difference found between women who experience PMT and women who don't. Since the second world war a bewildering number of hormonal and biochemical explanations for the existence of PMT have been proposed (Ripper 1992:287–327). These include levels of oestrogen, progesterone, lutenizing hormone, ratios between these, number of receptor sites for each, interactions with neuro-transmitters, sodium/potassium balance and so on. Medical science never has been able to agree upon, or demonstrate, a convincing hormonal, biochemical, behavioural, or physiological explanation for PMT. Despite the undermining of an hormonal aetiology, in post second world war popular culture PMT is known to be 'caused' by hormones.

The social construction of PMT

Medical interest in the pre-menstrual phase of the menstrual cycle has been influenced by social, political, and commercial contexts in addition to the professional debates and 'discoveries' about women's reproductive system which I have already sketched.

The influence of these social factors is illustrated in Figure 7.1 which graphs the number of journal articles on PMT across the lifespan of the disorder. This biography of PMT begins with its conception in 1926 through its troubled infancy, until its 'coming of age' and gaining of a popularly

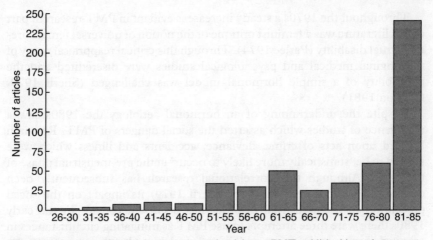

Fig. 7.1 Number of English language journal articles on PMT published in each 5-year period 1926–1985.
Source: Index Medicus

acknowledged identity in the 1950s. A stimulus to growth occurred with the mass marketing of synthetic hormonal preparations in the 1960s. Its real blossoming into adulthood has only occurred in the decades 1970s and 1980s. Major milestones in the lifespan of the disorder PMT can be identified, which coincide with the booms in research activity which are evident in Figure 7.1.

Synthetic oestrogen was first produced in 1938 and progesterone a few years later. This created the possibility for therapies which could be dispensed by general practitioners or gynaecologists to remedy pre-menstrual problems.

The social climate following the second world war was one in which women's hormonal variability was grasped as evidence of her unsuitability for the workforce (Cooke 1945, Rubin 1956). Medical research on PMT was a central element in the armory of evidence which showed that women's place was in the home. Ironically during the war research had been published which showed that the menstrual cycle was not disabling to women (Holtz 1941, Seward 1944).

A further contribution to the rise in the amount of research in the 1950s was the apparent spread of PMT beyond North America. Prior to that time all the research and opinion on PMT that had been published in English had emanated from the USA and to a minor degree from Canada. In England in 1952 Dr Katharina Dalton discovered British women to be suffering from this previously unheard of disorder, and soon after that Australian doctors began to notice it too.

A further burst of medical interest in PMT coincided with the mass marketing of hormonal contraceptive pills in the early 1960s. Not only did 'the pill' promise effective contraception it was also offered as a cure for PMT. The pill promised to replace women's fluctuating hormones with a regulated dose of synthetic hormones, thereby removing variability and disorder.

Throughout the 1970s a steady increase is evident in PMT research, part of this literature was a feminist critique of the notion of universal female pre-menstrual disability (Parlee 1974). Through this critical reappraisal many of the original medical and psychological studies were discredited and the plausibility of a simple hormonal model was challenged (Sherif 1979, Gannon 1981).

Despite the undermining of an hormonal aetiology the 1980s saw a resurgence of studies which asserted the social dangers of PMT. Research focused upon acts of crime, deviance, accidents and illness which were alleged to be 'statistically more likely to occur' in the pre-menstrual phase of the cycle. Although this correlational research has subsequently been discredited (Wilcoxon et al 1976, Sherif 1979) its impact on the social perception of pre-menstrual disorder has been widespread. In the early 1980s there were three attempts to use PMT as mitigating circumstances in criminal charges against women. The most celebrated of these was a murder case in which Katharina Dalton gave expert evidence in defence of the accused woman. The diagnosis that the accused woman was suffering from PMT at the time of the killing was based on the fact that her menstrual period began immediately following the homicide about which she was being questioned by police (Borse 1978). Dr Dalton told the court that such pre-menstrual loss of control was well known and was (in her judgement) caused by a progesterone deficiency. The accused woman was found guilty of manslaughter rather than murder, and the court ruled that her sentence be suspended on condition that she undergo progesterone therapy with Dr Dalton. Many issues are raised by the PMT court cases which cannot be explored here. The important cultural impact that they had was in galvanizing the public perception that women's behaviour is governed by her reproductive hormones. (No clearer demonstration of this axiom could be imagined than a court's prescription of progesterone to prevent criminal behaviour.)

The emphasis in the late 1980s literature was upon the extreme social and personal dangers that the pre-menstrual phase of the cycle is alleged to create for a small but extremely disabled group of women. In 1985 the American Psychiatric Association carried out extensive discussions with menstrual cycle researchers during their process of defining a psychiatric disorder of the pre-menstrual period. This severe pre-menstrual psychological dysfunction, called Late Luteal Phase Dysphoric Disorder (LLPDD), has been included in the appendix of the Diagnostic and Statistical Manual 111 (American Psychiatric Association 1987). This manual catalogues and provides diagnostic criteria for all accepted psychiatric disorders. The inclusion of LLPDD in the appendix designates it as a diagnostic category which is in need of further research, prior to its incorporation as a legitimate psychiatric disorder. Not surprisingly, there has been a burgeoning of research interest in LLPDD in the years since it has been designated as a research priority. The important practical consequence for psychiatrists of having LLPDD on the books is that pre-menstrual problems can now be diagnosed and treated by psychiatrists and the cost to the client will attract reimbursement from health insurance companies as it does if clients are treated by a medical practitioner. Again competing professional interests help structure the possibilities for disease.

Hormones and menopause

Within the medical literature, surveyed menopausal problems had been categorized either as insanity or as a loss of social role up until the 1960s. That is, until such time as women's reproductive systems had been firmly established as hormonal, and commercial products were commercially available to control and replace normal hormonal production. The literature of the 1970s increasingly focused upon hormone 'replacement' to combat specific and systemic problems associated with menopause. Since that time the emphasis within the literature has gradually changed to the point that menopause itself (rather than its symptoms) came to be described as a disorder.

The earliest attempts to promote hormone 'treatment' for menopause made no mention of its alleged therapeutic effects upon bone density. Rather synthetic oestrogen was promoted in the mid 1960s as a means of allowing women to remain 'feminine forever'. By the mid 1970s, Estrogen Replacement Therapy (ERT) was shown to increase the likelihood of endometrial cancer and also to fall short of its promise to reverse the physical or emotional correlates of ageing. Consequently the sales of ERT dropped dramatically (Bell 1987). It was at this stage that synthetic progesterone was added to the tablets to counteract the carcinogenic effects of unopposed oestrogen.

The combined Hormonal Replacement Therapy (HRT) had the effect of causing cyclic bleeding (pseudo-menstruation) which was not welcomed by post-menopausal women. Attempts were made to counteract the unpopularity of HRT by marketing it as more 'natural' than ERT because it more accurately mimicked the hormonal profile of the menstrual cycle (and therefore of women during the phase of their lifespan when they are 'true' women capable of reproduction). This logic was insufficient to convince many women to go on having periods forever (Seaman & Gideon 1977). HRT was also promoted as being 'protective against' endometrial cancer. This claim is true only by comparison with ERT, not when compared with normal ageing. None of this improved sales until it was discovered that HRT maintained bone density and therefore (allegedly) protected against osteoporosis.

The current promotion of HRT as 'preventive medicine' has succeeded in defining women as hormonally deficient following menopause. The inevitable consequence of this state of deficiency is said to be the development of individual health problems such as 'dowagers hump' and brittle bones. Also the cost to the community has been emphasized through images which portray elderly women as fragile, bedridden burdens on their loved ones and on the public health system. The horror of being immobilized and a burden to others appears to have succeeded in bringing large numbers of women, aged 40 onwards, to accept their inherent deficiency and to compensate for it with hormone 'replacement therapy.'

Conclusion

In summary the following are the conditions which made possible the belief that women's health and capabilities are determined by hormones in a way that men's are not, and that women's post-menopausal years constitute a state of deficiency. The irony is that post menopausal women are constructed as deficient because of the lack of a hormone (oestrogen) which is virtually absent in male physiology. The recent equation of menopause with osteoporosis has left osteoporosis in men bereft of an aetiology.

The hormonal model of women's reproductive system has been accepted because of its consistency with commonsense beliefs about women and about biological difference. These beliefs are reproduced within medical and popular folklore, they include the assumptions that:

- Women are inherently reproductive in a way that men are (presumed) not.
- Women are vulnerable and variable in a way that men are (presumed) not.
- Women's reproductive system is a danger to society.

In the past this took the form of menstruation causing impotence in men and turning wine to vinegar. Currently PMT makes women a danger to themselves and to their workmates and their children. Furthermore the domestic and economic stability of the society is endangered by the brittle bones and consequent dependency of frail, 'unproductive' old women.

Clinical and scientific interests were served by the development of a hormonal reproductive system for women which:

- Explained existing beliefs in biochemical terms.
- Provided therapies which were readily utilizable within medical consultation. In a typical medical encounter the practitioner's task is to elicit a description of symptoms which are recognizable as a disease entity. The appropriate drug regime is then prescribed to alleviate the symptoms. The marketing of synthetic hormonal preparations has allowed the symptoms of pre-menstrual and menopausal distress to be treated within this mode of medical practice.
- Reinforced the belief that normal aspects of women's physiology are inherently pathological and require medical control. Parallels can be drawn between the medicalization of the menstrual cycle, menopause, childbirth, pregnancy and control of fertility.

It was technologically possible to intervene in the menstrual cycle because of the distillation and later the synthesis and marketing of hormonal substances.

This produced an economic imperative for the commercial marketing of hormonal substances.

Disorders of the menstrual cycle are 'embodiable', by which I mean they can be experienced in bodies because the symptoms are an extension of subtle but identifiable fluctuations in normal bodily sensations. Given an appropriate cultural context it is possible for women to sense cyclic variation in their bodies and to experience it negatively. Clearly is it possible for people to identify quite subtle changes in physiological state. For example the effect of a cup of coffee, or of feeling hungry or sleepy. It is not peculiar that ovulation, premenstrual changes, and hot flushes can be identified. It is my contention that men would also be able to sense the ebb and flow of their testosterone levels if as much was at stake in relation to their gender identity.

Finally the construction of the belief that women are hormonally driven in a way that men are not has depended upon the complete absence of research investigating hormonal correlates of male behaviour. (The one exception has Houser's which was discussed previously.) The premise that male behaviour is not hormonally driven remains an article of faith against which women's difference is constructed. There has been research which tests an hormonal explanation for deviant behaviour in men, for example the (unsuccessful) attempt to attribute pathological violence to abnormal testosterone production (Persky et al 1979). Normal men's behaviour is presumed to be determined by rational and/or pragmatic considerations rather than biochemistry. Male sexual activity is seen to follow from desire/decision rather than hormone levels. Thus the male reproductive system remains 'organistic': men's brains and genitals are considered to determine their sexual/reproductive behaviour. A biochemical explanation for men's behaviour seems absurd, this is illustrated by considering the implausibility of any suggestion that men's urge to reproduce, to father a child, is hormonally rather than rationally derived. Yet such a suggestion would be entirely consistent with the belief that women's behaviour and reproductive system are hormonally driven. I do not wish to suggest that a hormonal model of male reproduction would advance human knowledge in any way. Rather I make this contrast to illustrate the extent to which hormones are gendered and gender has come to have an hormonal explanation which lodges women's 'otherness' and her disability in every cell of her being.

REFERENCES

American Psychiatric Association 1987 Diagnostic and Statistical Manual 111-R
Barker-Benfield G J 1976 The horrors of the half-known life: male attitudes towards women and sexuality in nineteenth-century America. Harper and Row, New York
Bell S 1987 Changing ideas: the medicalization of menopause. Social Science and Medicine 24 (6):535–542
Borse C 1987 Pre menstrual syndrome and criminal responsibility. In: Ginsberg B, Carter B

(eds) Premenstrual syndrome: ethical legal implications in a biomedical perspective. Plemum Press, New York

Cooke W 1945 The differential psychology of the American woman. Presidential address, September 7th 1944 to the American Association of Obstetricians, Gynecologists and Abdominal Surgeons. American Journal of Obstetrics and Gynecology 49:455–472

Dalton K 1964 The influence of menstruation on health and disease. Proceedings of the Royal Society of Medicine 57:262–264

Donnison J 1977 Midwives and medical men: a history of inter-professional rivalries and women's rights. Schocken Books, New York

Ehrenreich B, English D 1978 For her own good: 150 years of the expert's advice to women. Anchor Books, New York

Figlio K 1982 How does illness mediate social relations? Workmen's compensation and medico-legal practices 1890–1940. In: Wright P, Treacher A (eds) The problem of medical knowledge. University Press, Edinburgh

Frank R T, Goldberger M A 1928 Clinical data obtained with the female sex hormone blood test. American Medical Association Journal 90:106–110

Gannon L 1981 Evidence for a psychological etiology of menstrual disorders: a critical review. Psychological Reports 48:287–294

Gould S J 1981 The mismeasure of man. Penguin Books, Harmondsworth

Holtz R S 1941 Should women fly during menstrual period? Journal of Aviation Medicine 12:300–305

Houser B B 1979 An investigation of the correlation between hormonal levels in males and mood, behaviour and physical discomfort. Hormones and Behaviour 12:185–197

Hudson R 1977 The biography of disease: lessons from chlorosis. Bulletin of The History of Medicine 448–63

Index Medicus US Department of Health and Human Services: Public Health Services, National Institute of Health. ISSN No. 0090–1423

Laws S 1983 The sexual politics of premenstrual tension. Women's Studies International Forum 6(1):19–31

Moos R 1968 The development of a menstrual distress questionnaire. Psychosomatic Medicine 30:853–867

Parlee M B 1974 Stereotypic beliefs about menstruation: a methodological note on the Moos menstrual distress questionnaire and some new data. Psychosomatic Medicine 36(3):229–240

Persky H, Smith K D, Basu G K 1971 Relation of psychological measures of aggression and hostility to testosterone production in man. Psychosomatic Medicine 33:265–277

Ripper M 1991 A comparison of the effects of the menstrual cycle and the social week on self reports of performance, mood and sexual interest. In: Taylor D, Wood N (eds) Menstruation health and illness. Hemisphere Press, New York

Ripper M 1992 The engendering of hormones: the role of the menstrual cycle and its disorders in the contemporary construction of gender. PhD thesis, Flinders University of South Australia

Rubin I 1956 The changing concepts in gynecology problems and goals: presidential address to the 79th annual meeting of the American Gynecological Society. American Journal of Obstetrics and Gynecology 72:701–711

Seaman B, Gideon 1977 Women and the crisis in sex hormones. Rawson Associates, New York

Seward G H 1944 Psychological effects of the menstrual cycle on women workers. Psychological Bulletin 41:90–102

Sherif C W 1979 A social psychological perspective on the menstrual cycle. In: Parsons J E (ed) Gender roles: a dialectical, biopsychological perspective. Hemisphere, Washington DC

Smith-Rosenberg 1972 The hysterical woman: sex roles and role conflict in nineteenth-century America. Social Research, xxxix:652–678

Sommer B 1973 The effect of menstruation on cognitive and perceptual-motor behaviour; a review. Psychosomatic Medicine 35(6):515–534

Steiner M 1987 Premenstrual dysphoric disorder. Seminar presentation, Flinders University of South Australia

Wilcoxon L A, Schrader S L, Sherif C W 1976 Daily reports of activities, life events, moods, and somatic changes during the menstrual cycle. Psychosomatic Medicine 38:399

8. Aboriginal ill health: the harvest of injustice

Dennis Gray   Sherry Saggers

The inequalities in health faced by Aborigines are dramatically demonstrated in their life expectancy. At birth this is 15 to 17 years less than for non-Aboriginal Australians (Australian Institute of Health and Welfare 1992). Prior to the 1970s, infectious diseases such as diarrhoea and respiratory infections were the most common cause of morbidity and mortality among Aborigines and these were exacerbated by wide-spread malnutrition. Since the 1970s chronic diseases, including heart disease and diabetes mellitus type II, have also emerged as a significant cause of illness and death. In this chapter, we argue the pattern of Aboriginal ill health cannot adequately be understood apart from the history and continuing consequences of the non-Aboriginal colonization of Australia, the political and economic context in which Aborigines now live, and the injustice this entails.

Aboriginal ill health

Despite improvements in the early 1970s, particularly in relation to infant mortality, Aboriginal people continue to die at rates considerably higher than non-Aboriginal people, and there has been little change in the past decade. The most frequent causes of death among Aborigines are diseases of the circulatory system, respiratory disease and external causes such as accidents and violence (Australian Institute of Health and Welfare 1992, Gray A 1990). These trends are illustrated in a review of mortality in Western Australia over the period 1983-1989 (Veroni et al 1992). Table 8.1 is based on this study and compares the 10 most common causes of death among Aborigines and non-Aborigines.

Among Aboriginal and non-Aboriginal men, apart from a minor difference in ordering, the five leading causes of death were the same. These are diseases of the circulatory system, injury and poisoning, diseases of the respiratory system, neoplasms, and diseases of the digestive system. Among Aboriginal and non-Aboriginal women, four of the five most common causes of death were the same. Among Aboriginal women these were diseases of the circulatory system, neoplasms, endocrine and metabolic disorders (primarily diabetes mellitus type II), diseases of the respiratory system, and injuries and poisoning. Although these causes of death are the same, with the exception of neoplasms,

119

Table 8.1 Cause specific, age standardized mortality rates (deaths per 100 000 person years) for Western Australian males and females 1983–1989.

Cause of death	Male		Female	
	Aboriginal	Non-Aboriginal	Aboriginal	Non-Aboriginal
Diseases of the circulatory system	606.1	261.4	373.5	153.0
Injury and poisoning	232.0	61.0	85.0	20.6
Diseases of the respiratory system	214.7	49.4	85.4	19.9
Neoplasms	144.1	170.0	147.2	107.0
Diseases of the digestive system	95.4	20.8	71.5	12.5
Mental disorders	64.7	6.3	23.4	4.3
Diseases of the genitourinary system	59.6	7.0	83.6	4.9
Endocrine, nutritional and metabolic disorders	57.0	10.3	96.9	7.9
Diseases of the nervous system and sense organs	44.7	12.0	27.8	9.2
Symptoms, signs and ill-defined conditions	44.3	6.2	28.7	4.6

Source: Veroni et al 1992.

Aborigines die from them at rates between 2.3 and 4.6 times greater than do non-Aborigines.

Additionally, Aborigines die at rates significantly higher than non-Aborigines from several other categories of disease. Among these are:

• mental disorders (primarily alcohol and drug related conditions) which are the sixth and tenth leading causes of death for Aboriginal men and Aboriginal women and from which they die at rates about 10.3 and 5.5 times greater than non-Aboriginal men and women; and,
• diseases of the genitourinary system (particularly kidney disease) which are the seventh leading cause of death for Aboriginal men and the sixth for Aboriginal women and from which they die at rates about 8.6 and 16.9 time greater than among non-Aboriginal men and women.

Although not among the most common causes of death, Aboriginal men die from infectious and parasitic diseases at rates about 8.9 times those of non-Aboriginal men, and Aboriginal women about 7.5 times more frequently than non-Aboriginal women.

Mortality data provides only a partial picture of the health status of Aborigines. Examination of hospital morbidity data—while not comprehensive and affected by factors such as accessibility of hospitals and varying admission policies and practices—provides an extra dimension to the problem. In Western Australia and South Australia, Aboriginal hospital admission rates are up to three times greater than non-Aboriginal rates (Thomson & Honari 1988); and when hospitalized Aborigines remain there longer (Waddell & Dibley 1986).

While there is some commonality between Aboriginal mortality and morbidity patterns, there are important differences. Aborigines are between six and nine times more likely to be admitted to hospital than non-Aborigines for non-life threatening diseases of the skin and sub-cutaneous tissues and infectious and parasitic diseases (Thomson 1991). Although deaths from infectious disease have decreased in the past two decades, morbidity data indicates that burden of infectious disease among Aboriginal people remains unacceptably high. Importantly, while diseases of the circulatory system, are a major cause of mortality, they not among the major reasons for hospitalization of Aborigines. This indicates that much circulatory disease is not being detected and treated.

As with the general population, the largest proportion of Aboriginal health problems are treated outside hospitals or are not treated at all. Among these common problems respiratory tract infections, ear disease (a major cause of hearing impairment and consequent learning difficulties), diarrhoeal disease and (in some areas) sexually transmitted diseases are all more common among Aborigines.

Illness and disease are not randomly distributed within populations, and social factors are major determinants of ill health. This is most clearly demonstrated in the Black Report (Townsend & Davidson 1982) which showed clear linkages in Britain between levels of mortality and morbidity and social class. While there is no single Australian study as comprehensive as the Black Report, various studies point to the same conclusion (Blatch & Lawson 1984, Burnley & Batiyel 1985, Dobson et al 1980, Martin 1976, Taylor 1979).

Rather than explain Aboriginal ill health by reference to inherent 'racial' or even cultural characteristics (though the latter play some role) we believe it is due to the same structural factors which result in the poorer health status of working class people and indigenous minority groups in other countries. The causes of Aboriginal ill health are rooted in the political and economic structures of Australian society which have worked to exclude and marginalize Aboriginal people. These same structures now attempt, within a narrow range of action, to ameliorate the position of Aborigines but do little to radically transform it. Injustice is built into this system and the ill health of Aborigines is a direct consequence of that injustice.

Colonization of Aboriginal Australia

Prior to European colonization of Australia, Aborigines were hunter-gatherers living in small groups exploiting clearly defined territories. Ownership and use of land were validated in terms of kinship and religious knowledge and belief. Evidence from a number of sources (Flood 1989, Meehan 1982, Dunn 1968, Clark 1966), indicates that Aborigines lived relatively affluent lives. They expended less energy in meeting their subsistence needs and were generally healthier than working class people in Europe at the time of first colonization (Engels 1972). They had nutritious diets which, combined with the physical exercise required in the quest for food, contributed to their good health status. The small size of Aboriginal groups also afforded protection against epidemic diseases such as measles and smallpox which require large human host populations. The evidence suggests that the greatest threats to life were some diseases of infancy and trauma. The latter, along with various infectious and parasitic diseases accounted for the greatest part of the illnesses they faced.

Aboriginal explanations of serious illness and death were intimately bound up with their religious beliefs and were also a means of social control. To cope with illness, Aborigines developed a practical range of pharmaceutical and empirical medical practices known to all, as well as the specialist religious healing skills of Aboriginal healers (Cawte 1974, Elkin 1977, Gray D 1979).

Following British colonization in 1788, the Aboriginal way of life was irrevocably changed. Australia was first settled as a penal colony and to forestall potential territorial designs by the French. Initially, colonists appropriated land in the vicinity of Sydney to produce agricultural products to support the fledgling colony. However, the potential of the land to graze wool-producing sheep for Britain's rapidly industrializing economy was quickly recognized. This led to an expansion of the pastoral frontier which continued throughout the 19th and the early 20th centuries and was boosted by cattle grazing following the development of refrigerated shipping, which enabled the export of beef to Britain.

Seizure of Aboriginal land, its food sources and sacred sites and the Aboriginal resistance to this has been well documented (Elder 1988, Reynolds 1982). The effects of the violence this entailed, combined with the even greater impact of introduced diseases such as smallpox, measles, influenza and venereal diseases decimated the Aboriginal population. Estimates of the Aboriginal population at the time of the first British settlement, range from a low of 300 000 (Radcliffe-Brown 1930) to a high of 1.25 million (Butlin 1982). Whatever the number, this had been reduced to approximately 74 000 by 1930 (Smith 1980).

In the south of the continent where climatic conditions were more conducive to farming and grazing, settlement was more intensive and decimation of the Aboriginal population more complete. In these areas demand for labour for the expanding economy was met by the convict system and, following the gold rushes of the 1850s, by ex-diggers. Later, colonial and then Commonwealth Governments implemented comprehensive immigration policies aimed at increasing both the unskilled and skilled labour force. The southern remnant Aboriginal population, then, was largely irrelevant to the labour market. Despite this, a number of Aborigines did obtain some rudimentary vocational training but generally this was insufficient to enable them to take anything but low paid seasonal work such as farm labouring. Consequently, they and their dependents were forced to live in fringe camps on the outskirts of towns.

In the sparsely inhabited, less favourable environment of the north, pastoralists experienced a shortage of labour and were forced to make an accommodation with the Aborigines. In these areas Aboriginal men and women were employed as stockworkers and women as domestic servants. Despite being the backbone of the pastoral industry, Aborigines worked in conditions approaching serfdom. They were paid in kind—generally rations of tea, flour and sugar and occasional allocations of clothing and blankets— and did not have the opportunity to accumulate savings. Like those in the south, Aborigines on the stations lived in unsanitary camp conditions on the fringes of station homesteads. As late as the 1940s, conditions in station camps in the Northern Territory were so poor and took such a heavy toll on life that the Aboriginal work force was not even reproducing itself (Berndt & Berndt 1987). Furthermore, agreements were reached among station owners not to employ Aborigines from other stations, thus depriving Aborigines the opportunity to protest their conditions by seeking work elsewhere.

The desert regions of central and western Australia and Arnhem Land in the north were unsuited to the pastoral and farming activities which by the early twentieth century had become the mainstay of the Australian economy. In those areas Aborigines were disturbed to a lesser extent. However, drawn by the desire for western material goods and food, by the depopulation which made traditional life more difficult to sustain, and in some instances by their forced removal (as in the case of Pitjantjatjara speakers whose lands at Maralinga were appropriated for nuclear weapons testing), Aborigines were increasingly concentrated in large government or mission settlements. Living conditions in these settlements, like those in the fringe camps in the south or on pastoral stations, were generally poor and unsanitary (Middleton & Francis 1976). Although there were exceptions, Aborigines in these settlements received little training in skills leading to the development of independent means of support.

With their traditional lands appropriated, lacking education (Aborigines were generally either excluded or discouraged from attending schools until the 1950s in some parts of the country) and vocational training, Aborigines were either excluded from the labour market or given access to employment for such extremely low remuneration that they were barely able to meet their subsistence needs, let alone accumulate resources. Faced with overwhelming poverty, the health consequences were disastrous. An immediate result was malnutrition, particularly in children. This in turn lowered resistance to disease. Clean water for bathing and laundering of clothes and blankets was limited or absent. Lack of effective disposal systems led to the accumulation of human, animal and food wastes. Housing was rudimentary, often consisting of humpies and small shacks into which relatively large numbers of people were crowded. These factors interacted to produce a high burden of disease including influenza, pneumonia, diarrhoeal diseases, and a variety of parasitic diseases. These took a heavy toll and in the 1960s infant mortality rates of 150 or more per 100 000 live births were recorded—rates six times higher than among non-Aboriginal Australians (Moodie 1973).

While much of this disease was preventable, even when acquired it largely went untreated. Many Aborigines lived in areas where access to a medical practitioner was almost non-existent, and even in areas where medical care was available, few could afford either the cost of treatment or health insurance. Consequently, much minor disease developed into more serious conditions resulting in hospitalization or death.

Aborigines in contemporary Australian society

In a society oriented to the present, it is easy for Australians to ignore the injustices that Aborigines have suffered. It is only 65 years since the last major recorded massacre of Aborigines at Coniston in 1928 (Elder 1988), it is only a little over 40 years since curfews were imposed on Aboriginal entry into Perth (Biskup 1973), and it is only 26 years since the referendum which empowered the Commonwealth to count Aborigines as Australian citizens. These are all events which have occurred in the lifetime of living Aborigines.

Following the second world war, Aborigines made several significant protests about their position in Australian society. These began with the pastoral strike in the north-west in 1946. They continued with the 'freedom rides' through New South Wales, the Aboriginal walk-off Wave Hill Station in the Northern Territory in the 1960s and culminated with the establishment of the Aboriginal Tent Embassy in Canberra in 1972.

Towards the end of this period, conditions had actually worsened for many Aborigines in the pastoral regions of the country. In 1968 Aboriginal station workers were brought under the pastoral award which guaranteed them equal wages. The subsequent widespread expulsion of Aborigines from stations highlights the extent to which pastoral profitability was made possible only through the exploitation of Aboriginal labour. These expulsions led to further increases in fringe-dwelling populations in rural towns and to some extent fed the migration to the cities which began to gain momentum in the 1950s.

In the early 1970s the majority of Aborigines were poor, unemployed, uneducated (in the formal sense) and lived in sub-standard and inadequate housing. Fuelled by despair and boredom and facilitated by relaxation on the prohibition of the sale of alcohol to Aborigines, alcohol abuse became an increasing problem for some Aboriginal people. As public drunkenness remained a crime, this brought Aborigines into increasing contact with the police and exacerbated the discrimination they already suffered at the hands of the law (Eggleston 1976, Parker 1977).

The conditions of Aborigines were an embarrassment to Australia internationally when the Whitlam Labor Government was elected in 1972 and during its period in office it undertook a serious program of reform in Aboriginal affairs. Among these reforms were programs to improve educational opportunities for Aboriginal children, employment, housing and health programs. The most significant initiative, initiated by the Whitlam Government but implemented by the Fraser Government, was the granting of land rights to Aborigines in the Northern Territory. While these and subsequent programs have achieved some successes, they have been insufficient to transform the lives of Aborigines. This is made abundantly clear by the report of the Royal Commission into Aboriginal Deaths in Custody, which highlights the continuing injustices and inequalities faced by Aboriginal people (Johnson 1991).

There are several reasons for the failure of these programs. The first has to do with the amount of resources allocated. As we have pointed out elsewhere (Saggers & Gray 1991b), in 1986 the Aboriginal population totalled 227 645 and in 1986-87 Commonwealth spending on Aboriginal affairs was $542.5 million. Ignoring the fact that a significant proportion of this was consumed by administrative costs and salaries to non-Aborigines, per capita spending amounted to only $2383 for that year. By 1991-92 the Commonwealth claimed that this amount has been more than doubled. However in part this was creative accounting for in it included $204 million for the Community Development Employment Program, a scheme by which some Aboriginal communities agree to accept job search and other allowances (entitlements of all citizens) as a lump sum and pay community members to work. As can be seen these amounts are insufficient to bring about significant change in the economic position of Aborigines.

The Commonwealth's land rights program has been seriously compromised from the outset. Legislation relating to the Northern Territory only enabled Aborigines to lay claim to unalienated crown land—land that has been of largely marginal interest to non-Aborigines. Aborigines have been able to recover approximately 20% of land in the Northern Territory. However, much of it is economically unproductive except in terms of simple subsistence activities and, while it is important to Aborigines for cultural reasons, it is not likely to provide them with the resources to significantly alter their standard of living.

Similarly, the South Australian Government claims to have returned approximately 10% of the State's land area to Aborigines. This is inhospitable desert land returned to the Pitjantjatjara in the north-west. Again, it is largely unproductive in anything but subsistence terms. Elsewhere, Aboriginal gains in terms of land have been limited, and even opposed, as by the Burke Labor Government in Western Australia. The 1992 Mabo decision by the High Court recognizing 'native title' to unalienated crown land appears to open the way for Aborigines to lay claim more successfully to such land throughout Australia. However, in economic terms it is doubtful whether this either will produce widespread benefits to Aboriginal people.

While some successes have been achieved (improved infant mortality, for instance) other inequalities have either remained or worsened. In the early 1990s, unemployment rates for Aborigines have remained well in excess of 50% when the national rate is about 11%. In 1986 only 3% of Aborigines were earning more than $22 000 compared to 14% of other Australians. 53% of Aboriginal incomes derive from social security, compared to 11% for all

Australians (Thomson 1989). Aboriginal people are not simply poorer than other Australians. Their structural position makes it unlikely that the gulf separating them from non-Aborigines will decrease in any significant way. Recognition of these factors is essential to an understanding of the current health status of Aborigines.

Particularly in rural and remote areas Aborigines continue to live in poor quality housing. While new housing infrastructure has been provided to many communities, it has often been poorly designed, inappropriate for the needs of Aboriginal people and with little provision for maintenance. The housing situation is less acute in towns and cities but nevertheless constitutes a problem. Aboriginal families tend to be larger than non-Aboriginal families and this, combined with a shortage of housing, often leads to over-crowding and the breakdown of waste disposal systems, in turn leading to relatively high levels of infectious disease.

There has been a dramatic reduction in mortality due to infectious disease. This is due largely to medical interventions which, while preventing death, do nothing to address the causes of such disease. However, the number of people suffering from non-fatal illness remains relatively high.

Many Aboriginal people continue to experience poor nutrition, even though the incidence of clinically evident malnutrition has been reduced. Particularly for children, but for adults as well, 'convenience' foods which are high in fats and sugars have become a significant part of the diet. These are cheap, require little or no preparation and are attractive for people on low incomes. For many Aborigines, lifestyles have become increasingly sedentary due to decreased employment opportunities and lack of access to recreational facilities. This combined with poor nutrition appears to be a significant factor in the high levels of diabetes and heart disease found among Aborigines.

The abuse of alcohol and other substances also contributes to the high levels of Aboriginal ill health. Discussion of alcohol use among Aborigines is often coloured by prejudice. The stereotype of the drunken Aborigine is unfortunately one that is widely held. However, research from the Northern Territory (Watson et al 1988) found that there are larger proportions of non-drinkers among Aborigines than among non-Aborigines. Among those using alcohol, however, a larger proportion of Aborigines were found to drink at levels harmful to health. Alcohol abuse contributes to the high frequency of accidents and violence, to liver disease, and is associated with mental health problems among Aborigines.

Among Aborigines the proportion of people smoking tobacco is almost three times higher than among non-Aboriginal people (Guest et al 1992). Smoking contributes to the high frequency of heart disease and to carcinoma of the lung and high levels of respiratory disease among Aborigines. Given, the number of Aborigines currently smoking, it is likely that morbidity and mortality from these causes will actually increase in the coming years.

While not of the magnitude of alcohol and tobacco related problems, the abuse of other substances is a problem for Aboriginal communities. Petrol sniffing is of particular significance in the central desert areas and Arnhem Land (Brady 1992). In urban areas, reports of increasing amphetamine abuse among Aboriginal youths and glue sniffing among children are also of concern.

Studies from around the world have documented high levels of harm related to the abuse of alcohol and other substances among dispossessed indigenous populations such as native Americans (Heath 1983, May 1982) and Hawaiians (Alama & Whitney 1990). There are a variety of reasons for this, some positive and some negative. Among the positive factors are the effects of the substances themselves and the valued social contexts in which consumption takes place. Excessive use is also a response to lack of occupational or recreational alternatives, associated boredom, alienation from the wider society and despair at the situation in which people find themselves. Clearly, alcohol-related harm to the health of Aborigines cannot be understood apart from this broader social context.

Responses to Aboriginal ill health

Within the Australian health care system, primary medical care is largely provided by general practitioners in the private sector. Where there are no private general practitioner services, state health departments provide a service of last resort—usually through the outpatients departments of public hospitals or nursing posts. The hospital sector is mixed with services being provided by both state governments and the private sector. Within the health care system, public health services have been the poor relation. State public health authorities have traditionally had responsibility for the enforcement of legislation dealing with matters such as food and hygiene, the testing of pollution levels of various kinds, immunization against infectious diseases, health education, and infant, child and school health services.

While public health services generally have been provided at no direct cost, patients have usually had to pay directly for medical and hospital services, to insure against the need for such services, or to forego them altogether. Prior to the introduction of the first national health insurance scheme (Medibank) by the Whitlam Government, it was estimated that two million Australians out of a total of approximately 13 million were unable to afford private health insurance (Davis & George 1993). This included most Aborigines, only some of whom were able to obtain care from the public sector or through missions.

The introduction of a second national health insurance system (Medicare), like its fore-runner, has altered the basis for the financing of health care. However, it has done little to change the basis for the provision of health care. It is important to recognize this because it is within the framework of this structure that health care for Aborigines continues to be provided.

It is also important to recognize that this system itself has done little to improve the health of non-Aboriginal Australians. As McKinlay and McKinlay

(1977) have demonstrated for the United States, provision of health and medical services have made only a limited contribution to the reduction of mortality rates. The major decreases in mortality from diseases such as measles, tuberculosis, pneumonia and poliomyelitis all occurred before the development of vaccines or effective treatments against them. Among non-Aboriginal Australians, the major factor in reducing levels of mortality and morbidity has been improvement in the standard of living. Included in this are increased levels of personal income, the ability to purchase better quality housing, and the provision by governments of infrastructural items and services such as clean water supplies, sewerage systems and waste disposal services.

In the early 20th century, state governments conducted some small programs aimed primarily at preventing diseases which were introduced into the Aboriginal population, such as leprosy and venereal disease, from spreading back into the non-Aboriginal population. Apart from these there were no specific health programs for Aborigines. Mainstream health services whether in the private or public sector were largely too costly, inaccessible, or inappropriate to the needs of Aborigines (Saggers & Gray 1991b).

After the late 1960s, a plethora of reports documented the poor health status of Aborigines (Moodie & Pedersen 1971, Thomson & Merrifield 1988). Among the most important of these are the reports by the House of Representatives Standing Committee on Aboriginal Affairs (1979), the Royal Australian College of Ophthalmologists (1980), and the National Aboriginal Health Strategy Working Party (1989). These reports identify a common set of factors responsible for Aboriginal ill health. Among these are environmental conditions (including inadequate housing and infrastructure), poor nutrition, lack of knowledge about health and hygiene issues, and inappropriate health services. Importantly, however, although these reports allude to underlying economic factors, none makes a coherent set of recommendations which directly address these.

With respect to the provision of infrastructure, the Commonwealth Government has taken the leading role. Through the Aboriginal & Torres Strait Islander Commission (ATSIC) and its predecessor the Department of Aboriginal Affairs, the Commonwealth has channelled funds for housing directly to Aboriginal community organizations and to state and territory housing authorities. However, as indicated in the previous section of this paper, the effectiveness of its various programs has been limited by the resources made available, the inappropriateness of housing, insufficient allocations for maintenance, and by the inability of Aborigines themselves to afford to maintain this infrastructure.

As discussed above, provision of public health services is the responsibility of state government agencies. It is through these, often with Commonwealth funding support, that most efforts at the improvement of health services per se have been directed. However, the responses of these agencies has not been uniform. By-and-large the most common response has been to attempt to enhance existing mainstream public health programs such as immunization and health education or supplement them by the development of some Aboriginal specific programs, such as the Aboriginal Health Promotion Program in Western Australia. In Victoria, New South Wales and Western Australia, Aboriginal units have been established to assist in the formulation of health policy and or programs. However, it is only in South Australia that an Aboriginal unit was established by government to provide services directly to Aboriginal people.

An important initiative to deal with the inappropriateness of mainstream services has been the employment of Aboriginal health workers and Aboriginal hospital liaison officers. Doubtless, such workers have facilitated contact between Aboriginal people and government health services. However, their role is circumscribed. While they provide an Aboriginal face at the point of first contact with health services, they are constrained by the rules and structures of the organizations by which they are employed. Their ability to respond to Aboriginal people in culturally appropriate ways is limited and they are often placed in positions where they are caught between demands of their community and the health bureaucracy.

There are several problems with these strategies. First, they do not address the imbalance which exists in the Australian economy between the allocation of resources to treatment rather than to prevention of health problems. Through Medicare the Australian government exercises some control over the cost of particular medical services. However, such intervention is minimal. There are no existing arrangements which would allow government to redirect resources expended on treatment in the private sector to the provision of preventive services. While this fundamental imbalance exists, Aborigines, whose need for preventive services is greater, will continue to be more disadvantaged than the rest of the community.

Strategies to address the problems of Aboriginal ill health have also been largely uncoordinated. Despite a Commonwealth Government proposal in 1973 to develop a ten year plan to address Aboriginal ill health, no common goals and targets were established and there has been little agreement between Commonwealth and state/territory governments and Aboriginal people about what is to be done and the best means of achieving it. The National Aboriginal Health Strategy (NAHS) with its emphasis on tripartite cooperation is an attempt to deal with this. However, as of early 1993, problems with the development of coordinating mechanisms and differences in priorities have constrained the effectiveness of the tripartite forums and the Council of Aboriginal Health established as part of the NAHS.

As discussed previously, inadequate resource allocation is also a fundamental problem with strategies to address Aboriginal ill health. The working party established to report to the Joint Forum of Ministers for Health and Aboriginal Affairs on implementation of the NAHS, estimated that $2500 million alone was required to bring housing and infrastructure for Aboriginal people up to an appropriate standard. However, for its part the

Commonwealth allocated only $232 million over a period of five years to the NAHS with equal amounts expected to be contributed by the states/territories. Clearly this amount is insufficient to deal with the problem and is not being adequately supplemented by resources from other programs.

Aboriginal health programs that have been implemented by governments have focussed particularly on health promotion strategies. These are obviously necessary. However, in the absence of more fundamental changes which address Aboriginal poverty, living conditions and access to resources, their effect is severely circumscribed.

The other major problem with mainstream strategies to address Aboriginal ill health is that they have been only minimally responsive to Aboriginal demands for community control. As various writers have demonstrated (Gray & Saggers 1990, Mowbray 1986, Tonkinson & Howard 1990), there is a wide gap between the rhetoric associated with the policies of self-determination and/or self-management and the real life experience of these by Aboriginal people. As indicated above, prior to the 1970s, medical services were often not affordable or accessible to Aborigines and were certainly not responsive to the aspirations of Aboriginal people. The attempt by Aborigines in Redfern to deal with this problem led to one of the most important developments in Aboriginal health—the establishment of Aboriginal medical services (AMSs).

The Redfern Aboriginal Medical Service was established in 1971. The aim of the service was to provide a free, culturally appropriate medical service to Aborigines which was controlled by Aboriginal people themselves. The service was started on a shoestring budget with the assistance of non-Aboriginal health professionals (Briscoe 1974, Foley 1975). Since that time, the number of services has expanded and currently there is in excess of 60 Aboriginal community controlled health services. These services are funded from a variety of sources including Medicare rebates and direct government grants.

The Aboriginal medical services have aimed to make primary medical care available to the community. To facilitate this, services are provided free of direct charge to patients. To enable access, the AMS's are generally located in areas in which Aboriginal people are concentrated and for some patients transportation is sometimes provided. Like government run services, the AMSs employ Aboriginal health workers to visit patients in their homes. In rural and remote areas these workers often play an important role in the delivery of primary health care, while in the cities their roles emphasize the provision of preventive care and patient advocacy. While the initial emphasis by the AMSs was on the provision of primary medical care, many AMSs have expanded their role to include a variety of other services, including para-medical and specialist services as well as public health programs including nutrition and alcohol programs.

Conclusion

The poor health status of Aborigines has been clearly documented. Life expectancy is considerably less than that of non-Aborigines, they die at rates several times higher and carry a heavier burden of morbidity than non-Aborigines. Political and economic factors underlie the patterns of mortality and morbidity suffered by Aborigines and have conditioned the various responses to Aboriginal health. For much of the 19th and early part of the 20th centuries, Aborigines were seen as a 'dying race' marginal to Australian economic development. Consequently, other than the provision of piecemeal charity, little was done to alleviate health problems among them. When it became clear that Aborigines were not facing extinction, and the magnitude of the health problems they faced began to be documented, various attempts to deal with the problem were undertaken. However, these have been constrained by unwillingness to implement the political and economic changes necessary to improve the position of Aborigines in Australian society.

While broad social processes have shaped the health problems of Aborigines and the response of the wider society to them, it should not be imagined that Aborigines have been merely helpless pawns at the mercy of impersonal forces. Aboriginal people have resisted colonization, they have actively worked to improve their position within Australian society, and have developed their own responses to the health problems they face. That these efforts have not been sufficient to transform their situation says more about the magnitude of the forces arrayed against them than about their own tenacity.

REFERENCES

Alama K, Whitney S 1990 Ka wai kau o Meleka: water from America: the intoxication of the Hawai'ian people. Contemporary Drug Problems 17(2):161–194
Australian Institute of Health and Welfare 1992 Australia's health 1992: the third biennial report of the Australian Institute of Health and Welfare. Australian Government Publishing Service, Canberra
Berndt R M, Berndt C H 1987 The end of an era. Aboriginal Studies Press, Canberra
Biskup P 1973 Not slaves, not citizens. University of Queensland Press, St Lucia
Blatch J C, Lawson J S 1984 Predictors of health in two adjacent Australian communities. New South Wales, State Health Publication No (NMR) 84–003, Sydney
Brady M 1992 Heavy metal: the social meaning of petrol sniffing in Australia. Aboriginal Studies Press, Canberra
Briscoe G 1974 The Aboriginal medical service in Sydney. In: Hetzel B S et al (eds) Better health for Aborigines. University of Queensland Press, St Lucia
Burnley I, Batiyel M 1985 Indicators of changing mortality in Sydney and Adelaide: inequalities in wellbeing. In: Burnley I, Forrest J (eds) Living in cities. Allen & Unwin, Sydney
Butlin N G 1982 Close encounters of the worst kind: modelling Aboriginal depopulation and resource competition 1788–1850, working papers in economic history, no 8.

Australian National University Press, Canberra

Cawte J 1974 Medicine is the law: studies in the psychiatric anthropology of Australian tribal societies. Rigby, Adelaide

Clark M 1966 Sources of Australian history. Oxford University Press, London

Davis A, George J 1993 States of health: health and illness in Australia, 2nd edn. Harper & Row, Sydney

Dobson A J, et al 1980 Excess mortality in the Hunter region. Social Science and Medicine 14D:169–173

Dunn F L 1968 Epidemiological factors: health and disease in hunter-gatherers. In: Lee R B, DeVore I (eds) Man the hunter. Aldine, Chicago

Eggleston E 1976 Fear, favour or affection. Australian National University Press, Canberra

Elder B 1988 Blood on the wattle. Child, Sydney

Elkin A P 1977 Aboriginal men of high degree, 2nd edn. University of Queensland Press, St Lucia

Engels F 1972 (orig 1892) The condition of the working-class in England. Progress, Moscow

Flood J 1989 Archaeology of the dreamtime, 2nd edn. Collins, Sydney

Foley G F 1975 The history of the Aboriginal medical service: a study in bureaucratic obstruction. Identity 2(5):38–40

Gray A 1990 A matter of life and death: contemporary Aboriginal mortality, proceedings of a workshop of the national centre for epidemiology and population health held at Kioloa, New South Wales, 10–12 July 1989. Aboriginal Studies Press, Canberra

Gray D 1979 Traditional medicine on the Carnarvon Aboriginal reserve. In: Berndt R M, Berndt C H (eds) Aborigines of the west: their past and their present. University of Western Australia Press, Nedlands

Gray D, Saggers S 1990 Autonomy in Aboriginal education: a quest at Carnarvon. In: Tonkinson R, Howard M (eds) Going it alone? Prospects for Aboriginal autonomy. Aboriginal Studies Press, Canberra

Guest CS, et al 1992 Smoking in Aborigines and persons of European descent in southeastern Australia: prevalence and associations with food habits, body fat distribution and other cardiovascular risk factors. Australian Journal of Public Health 16(4):397–402

Heath D B 1983 Alcohol use among North American Indians: a cross-cultural survey of patterns and problems. In: Smart R G et al (eds) Research advances in alcohol and drug problems 7:343–396

House of Representatives Standing Committee on Aboriginal Affairs 1979 Aboriginal health. Australian Government Publishing Service, Canberra

Johnson E 1991 Royal commission into Aboriginal deaths in custody: national report. Australian Government Printing Service, Canberra

McKinlay J B, McKinlay S M 1977 The questionable contribution of medical measures to the decline of mortality in the United States in the twentieth century. Milbank Memorial Fund Quarterly 55(3):405–428

Martin G S 1976 Social/medical aspects of poverty in Australia: Australian government commission of inquiry into poverty. Australian Government Publishing Service, Canberra

May P A 1982 Substance abuse and American Indians: prevalence and susceptibility. International Journal of Addictions 17:1885–1209

Meehan B 1982 Shell bed to shell midden. Australian Institute of Aboriginal Studies, Canberra

Middleton M R, Francis S H 1976 Yuendumu and its children: life and health on an Aboriginal settlement. Australian Government Publishing Service, Canberra

Moodie P M 1973 Aboriginal health. ANU Press, Canberra

Moodie P M, Pedersen E B 1971 The health of Australian Aborigines: an annotated bibliography. Australian Government Printing Service, Canberra

Mowbray M 1986 State control or self-regulation? On the political economy of local government in remote Aboriginal townships. Australian Aboriginal Studies 2:31–39

National Aboriginal Health Strategy Working Party 1989 A national Aboriginal health strategy. Australian Government Printing Service, Canberra

Parker D 1977 Social agents as generators of crime. In: Berndt R M (ed) Aborigines and change: Australia in the 1970s. Australian Institute of Aboriginal Studies, Canberra

Radcliffe-Brown A R 1930 Former numbers and distribution of the Australian Aborigines. In: Official yearbook of the Commonwealth of Australia, No 23. Government Printer, Melbourne

Reynolds H 1982 The other side of the frontier. Penguin, Ringwood

Royal Australian College of Ophthalmologists 1980 National trachoma and eye health program. Royal Australian College of Ophthalmologists, Sydney

Saggers S, Gray D 1991a Aboriginal health and society: the traditional and contemporary Aboriginal struggle for better health. Allen & Unwin, Sydney

Saggers S, Gray D 1991b Policy and practice in Aboriginal health. In: Reid J, Trompf P (eds) The health of Aboriginal Australia. Harcourt Brace Jovanovich, Sydney

Smith L 1980 The Aboriginal population of Australia. Australian National University Press, Canberra

Taylor R 1979 Health and class in Australia. New Doctor 13:22–28

Thomson N 1991 A review of Aboriginal health status. In: Reid J, Trompf P (eds) The health of Aboriginal Australia. Harcourt, Brace, Jovanovich, Sydney

Thomson N, Honari M 1988 Aboriginal health: a case study. In: Australia's health: the first biennial report of the Australian Institute of Health. Australian Government Printing Service, Canberra

Thomson N, Merrifield P 1988 Aboriginal health: an annotated bibliography. Australian Institute of Aboriginal Studies and Australian Institute of Health, Canberra

Thomson N 1989 Aboriginal health: a socio-cultural perspective. In: Lupton G M, Najman J M (eds) Sociology of health and illness. University of Queensland Press, St Lucia

Tonkinson R, Howard M (eds) 1990 Going it alone? prospects for Aboriginal autonomy. Aboriginal Studies Press, Canberra

Townsend P, Davidson (eds) 1982 Inequalities in health: the Black report. Penguin, Harmondsworth

Veroni M, Rouse I, Gracey M 1992 Mortality in Western Australia 1983-1989: with particular reference to the Aboriginal population. Health Department of Western Australia, Perth

Waddell C, Dibley M 1986 The medicalization of Aboriginal children: a comparison of the lengths of hospital-stay of Aboriginal and non-Aboriginal children in WA and the NT. Australian Paediatric Journal 22:27–30

Watson C, Fleming J, Alexander K 1988 A survey of drug use patterns in Northern Territory Aboriginal communities: 1986–1987. Northern Territory Department of Health and Community Services Drug and Alcohol Bureau, Darwin

PART 2

Inequalities in care

Introduction

What exactly do we mean by 'care'? What constitutes just health care? By what means can we ensure that just care is part of health care practice? These are some of the questions which are addressed directly or indirectly by the chapters in this part.

Health care is often used simply to refer to medical care. With medical care, the focus is on individuals, on biology, on scientific understanding, on clinical intervention, and on cure. In order to be cured, patients must hand over control of their bodies to the medical expert. This clearly entails the disempowerment of the patient. Health care, on the other hand, is or should be about empowering those who are ill by actively involving them in the healing process.

At least 'in theory', caring entails concern for 'the whole person'. This has been the stated basis for nursing practice, but also for other 'allied health' professions such as physiotherapy and occupational therapy. The term health care has been used to refer to a particular set of institutional practices in which health workers or other designated persons partake in order to facilitate the physical, psychological, emotional, and social support of their patients or 'clients', who are deemed not able to take control of their own needs. It is significant that in formal health care settings the word 'client' is often used interchangeably with 'patient'. This implies that the individual has substantial control over their interactions with carers. Whether or not they actually do can be questioned.

Caring skills are assumed to encompass concern or empathy for the patient/client ('getting to know them' personally and understanding their socio-cultural and economic circumstances), the ability to offer emotional support (simply listening and being attentive to unexpressed worries) and to do things for them (for example, various kinds of body restoration and maintenance—monitoring 'vital signs', assistance with toileting, attending to dressings, and so on), and the commitment to protect and advance their interests (advocacy). However, because health care involves the patient/client handing over some control to others, they can be disempowered. The attempt to define (and thus treat) the patient/client as *more* than a body may simply mean the reinstatement of the patient's capacity to enter into the process of their own surveillance and control (May 1992:485–486). And the

137

implementation of a regime of care involving a broad range of skills and qualities that may not be fully and publically acknowledged, can also serve to disempower the carer.

It is inevitable that people will experience some loss of control in a health care system dominated by 'experts', and by doctors in particular. The privileging of the rational, scientific knowledge of 'experts' has led to the relative neglect of the patient/client's perspective and of the role of intuitive, emotional, and spiritual factors on health and well-being. The dominance of so-called biomedicine within mainstream health institutions, means that attention tends to be focussed on physiology, disease, and on the individual's physical needs rather than on their total well-being. Scientific and biomedical assumptions have profoundly influenced the practices of *all* health care professions in modern western societies. Thus even the bio-psycho-social model of nursing which seems self evidently to be a 'holistic' model is, in practice, strongly influenced by science and a biological understanding. This understanding dominates the other components of the model and fails to accommodate key aspects of experience, including the understanding of the lived experience of embodiment (Lawler 1991:37–38).

The importance of attending to psychological, emotional and social well-being as well as physical needs in healing has been emphasized in the literature on the sociology and anthropology of health and health care. This literature points to the significance of the individual's 'definition of the situation' to their experiences and understandings of illness and in their recovery. For example, patients bring personal and cultural meanings to their encounters with health workers and these meanings affect their expectations of care, responses to carers and subsequent compliance with treatment (Kleinman 1988). But since meanings are constantly negotiated during interactions, the carer obviously plays a key role in the patient's experience of illness and recovery. Carers can do much to put patients at ease and attend to their needs without at the same time disempowering them. This implies, among other things, attention to skills of communication; that is, interaction involving a genuine exchange of information. Patients who are fully informed of their condition and treatment are known to make a quicker recovery than those not so informed (Russell & Schofield 1986:205). There is evidence showing that where patients' emotional needs are met, they are less likely to use pain killers and are discharged from hospital earlier (Davis & George 1993:170). As Russell and Schofield put it, 'the interests of both sick people and health care workers would appear to be optimized by a situation in which the management of illness occurs in an atmosphere of participation—of activity and interaction—rather than of patient passivity and "expert" control' (1986:205). If the satisfaction experienced by health workers is associated with a successful therapeutic outcome, then it makes sense for health workers to give greater control to the patients/clients.

The impersonal bedside manner of many doctors that is often remarked upon is but the most obvious indicator of a widespread tendency to treat patients as objects without thoughts or feelings. That patients themselves expect that care will equate with mainly physical care is suggested by Lindsey Harrison and Elizabeth Cameron-Traub's study of patients' perspectives on nursing care (Ch. 9). Patients from a range of ethnic backgrounds were found to be reluctant to seek opportunities to talk with nurses about personal and emotional issues because this was deemed to be outside the bounds of what hospitals and health care are seen to be about. As the authors argue, this perception may in part reflect the still dominant image of nurses' role as handmaidens to doctors (nurses merely carry out the instructions of the doctors and provide physical care), but it also reflects the structural organization of hospitals which calls for patient compliance and allows nurses little time to talk to patients. The impersonality and anonymity of modern hospitals has led to widespread dissatisfaction and complaints by patients, as Davis and George (1993:170) report. And the increasing specialization of tasks, and tensions created by conflicts between the demands of superior professional staff, their own occupational priorities and the demands of bureaucratic accountability, have led to decreased work satisfaction and the high resignation rates of hospital staff, especially nurses (Davis & George 1993:168). Achievement of just care, therefore, suggests the need for changes in broader social structures and values, including those of bureaucracy which is based upon a highly inequitable distribution of power, and involves surveillance, secrecy, and an orientation towards 'cases' rather than people with particular needs and desires.

What the following chapters hightlight to varying degrees is the need in health care to consider the influence of such factors as class, gender, race, ethnic background, age, and existing mental and physical disability on individual experiences. The biomedical assumption that health is 'normally' a fixed, stable, condition, and requires caring strategies that seek to return health to some hypothetical norm of physical well-being, denies the complex interaction of a variety of factors influencing physical and mental well-being. It leads to a view that the content of care should be unvarying across different social groups. The chapters by Martha MacIntyre (Ch. 10) and by Varoe Legge and Mary Westbrook (Ch. 11) indicate that recent immigrants and people of non-Anglo-Australian origins have experiences and face problems that affect their health, their beliefs about illness, their perceptions of health carers, their behaviours and treatment preferences, and the quality of care they are likely to receive. For example, as MacIntyre points out, migrant women often come from countries which have very different health care systems which may influence their expectations and use of Australian health services. The generally positive assessment of Australian health services by El Salvadoran and Vietnamese women is reflected in their reluctance to criticize or complain about those aspects of health care with which they are dissatisfied. Moreover, problems with English language may lead them to avoid seeking medical treatment, and where treatment is had there may be breaches of human rights or medical ethics. Legge and Westbrook argue, on the basis of their survey, that there is an association, between both individualistic values and the degree of modernity in the communities' societies of origin, and their aged people's feelings of control of health outcomes, concealment of pain, and preference for privacy when ill. Both chapters suggest that health care workers can do much to improve care by familiarizing themselves with such issues and problems and with the cultures of the people for whom they care (for example, conventions about describing sickness), and by developing communication skills. But such changes must occur alongside more 'macro' institutional changes such as increased language learning facilities, the development of interpreter services, and the provision of appropriate materials informing people, in their own languages, on health issues and services.

The need for health workers to be sensitive to social difference and associated problems of poor communication applies to the dying patient no less than the patient recovering from illness. In Chapter 12, Allan Kellehear argues that there is a need for more frankness and clarity in telling the patient that he or she is going to die. The issue of professional power is again manifest in the reluctance of patients to question the doctor, who is believed to 'know best' and to have the only legitimate authority to decide how and how much to disclose to the dying person. What Kellehear's chapter reveals is the varieties of experience of dying and the way in which interpersonal relations both reflect and reinforce inequalities, often in surprising ways. For example, well-meaning parents and friends may offer forms of support such as greatly increased contact or cleaning or cooking without consultation which unwittingly undermine the autonomy or independence of the dying person.

That there has been an increased questioning of the dominance of medical knowledge and its implications for just health care is evidenced by the arguments appearing in many of these chapters (but especially those by Ann Daniel (Ch. 13), Kevin White (Ch. 14), Stephanie Short (Ch. 15), and Evan Willis and Jeanne Daly (Ch. 16)). As Daniel indicates, in health and medicine, people's trust in 'the system' depends on the belief in expert knowledge. But trust is contingent upon the public's belief that practitioners possess superior knowledge and skills and that they are working in the public interest. And it may be put in jeopardy when there are allegations of medifraud and 'over-servicing', or during disputes, such as in 1983–85 in New South Wales, which lead to public perceptions of irresponsibility. A number of the chapters start from the premise that to create a just health care system requires some historical insight into how the present one came into being, and in particular how medicine became dominant.

The dominance of medicine has, in large part, depended on the profession's ability to present the content of medical knowledge as existing outside of society; as being objective 'value-neutral' knowledge. But the neutrality of medical scientific knowledge is called into question by evidence such as that presented by Kevin White, which examines the historical struggles of medicine to privilege its definitions of what constitutes disease and the role of medical knowledge in the legitimation of European domination and the destruction of indigenous peoples. As White indicates, the argument that progress in biological sciences is responsible for the development of the medical profession is widely accepted by social scientists writing the history of medicine. But as his data show, the very content of medical knowledge has been socially constructed and can be seen as an outcome of medical struggles with the state to control health and health care, and control of the the hospital seems to have been crucial in this struggle. A significant point to note is that, even though it had been long known by sanitary engineers and health authorities that reductions of infant mortality could come about as a consequence of controls over environmental conditions (for example, housing and sanitation), the medical profession continued to promote its view that it was individual factors or 'the weather' that was the source of diseases. In both South Australia and New Zealand, White argues, the effect of the predominance of medical definitions of disease and mortality was to shift attention from social causes of infant mortality towards the individual mother and (in the latter country) the Maori culture.

As Stephanie Short indicates, sociologists have been centrally involved in the struggle to scrutinize and re-define the content of medical scientific knowledge. However, different traditions of thought within sociology have taken different positions on the question of the objectivity and universality of the content of medical knowledge. For instance, according to Short, while Talcott Parsons held 'an apparently contradictory theoretical position towards medical knowledge'; for other later theorists such as Michel Foucault the content of medical knowledge has been inextricably linked with the exercise of power throughout society. Short is concerned to draw out the implications of the various sociological perspectives for the way we understand how medical research can and should be conducted. She suggests that only 'critical' sociologists have challenged medicine's monopolistic position in medical research and have called for a democratizing of the health research process to include others, such as sociologists and health care consumers.

One of the legacies of medicine's struggles to assert its definitions of health and disease is the dominance of a hospital based, curative, 'high-tech' health system. And it is to issues associated with the priorities of and pressures within this system that the chapter by Evan Willis and Jeanne Daly is addressed. As Willis and Daly argue, the difficulties in generating policy regarding medical technologies go beyond purely technical considerations of 'what works'. If social justice considerations are to be incorporated in medical technology policy then issues of access to new technologies, evaluation of their effectiveness, and consideration of the diverse interests of various groups (patients, health professionals, manufacturers of the technologies, and the state) need to be taken into account. The case of sleep disorder centres, which they explore, illustrates the complexity of issues and the difficulty of balancing social justice against the interests of the different groups involved in the process of technological innovation.

In reaction to the 'expert' and bureaucratic control of health, including its dominance by high technology, many have looked to less formal care in 'the community'. The ideal of community based care has a strong democratic overtone which is difficult to resist. However, much of the pressure for community based care has arisen with the state which is intent on cutting costs associated with a burgeoning health budget during a period of fiscal restraint and has not involved a substantial redistribution of power to communities. That 'experts' and bureaucrats have remained essentially in control of health is borne out by both Julie Mulvany's chapter on the compulsory treatment of mentally ill people within the community (Ch. 17) and Rosemary Cant's chapter on mothers caring for children with significant physical disabilities at home (Ch. 18).

Mulvany describes the operation of mental health legislation in Victoria which provides for compulsory community based treatment. Community Treatment Orders (CTOs), which involve patients living in the community and being supervised by medical practitioners, are seen to reduce problems of relapse when patients who are released from hospital fail to continue taking their medication. The CTO involves the recipient attending a mental health clinic once a month to be given an injection of anti-psychotic medication by a psychiatric nurse, which is the only 'treatment' received. This provides a 'safety net' for staff who may feel compelled, because of diminishing hospital resources, to discharge patients after only a short admission but, as Mulvany indicates, it does not address the need for appropriate community resources such as housing. It also places the 'burden of care' on relatives, most of whom are women.

The last point provides the focus for Cant's chapter which describes the control which is exercised by health professionals and bureaucrats over mothers who care for physically disabled children at home. In rhetoric at least, social justice emphasizes that care be given in a way that allows those with disabilities to live as autonomously and independently as possible. But social justice considerations have tended not to be extended to caregivers. As Cant asks, 'how can we ensure that carers also have their needs for autonomy met? How can we ensure that whatever their age, gender or social position, carers have the same access to leisure and paid work, that those who do not meet the dependency needs of others are able to enjoy?' An important point raised in this chapter, and also elaborated elsewhere (see, for example, Baldock 1990), is the exploitation and regulation of women's unpaid work that accompanies 'de-institutionalization' of health care. It is simply assumed that women are willing and able to take major responsibility for care and, where children are involved, the ideology of motherhood provides a powerful mechanism of control.

Where a child is disabled, the regulatory mechanisms are strengthened and there is an increased threat to the autonomy of women at home carrying out care-giving work. Along with traditional medical authority, this threat derives from other 'experts' such as nurses, the therapists and social workers who stake a claim in the control in care giving in their attempts to professionalize. But it also comes from growing 'rationalism' or 'bureaucratization' with which professional power has become linked. As Cant puts it, together 'these strands of control are woven into a braid in the helping agencies of the state that binds women into a position of subordination to their "helpers"'. Drawing on data from her own Australian study, Cant describes how this control is experienced and resisted by some of these mothers. She suggests that similar controls exist for other care-giving work carried out in the home to those with, for instance, schizophrenia or dementia, those recovering from surgery or acute illness, and the frail elderly, and that this is becoming an increasingly important issue as governments try to contain costs through 'de-institutionalization'.

The question of exactly what is meant by the 'health consumer' has also been increasingly posed as governments attempt to re-structure health care along free market lines. And this question provides the focus for the final three chapters in this section, by Victoria Grace (Ch. 19), Liz Eckermann (Ch. 20), and Arthur O'Neill (Ch. 21), respectively. These chapters question, in particular, the applicability of the concept of the autonomous rational actor that is taken to underpin economic life. The very concept of 'health consumer' is explored by Victoria Grace on the basis of an analysis of the concept of health articulated by health promotion professionals in New Zealand. As Grace argues, the 'health care consumer' appears within the discourse of health marketing whether one is talking about medical care, preventive services or health promotion. But the notion that health care can be 'consumed' like any other commodity, which underlies health care reforms in New Zealand and elsewhere, has been questioned by health professionals and consumer groups alike. Drawing on the work of the French theorist Baudrillard, Grace indicates difficulties in defining a fixed identity for the 'health consumer' when the object of consumption in our contemporary society is not in fact a commodity, but a sign which has a shifting meaning. She indicates a lack of congruence between the 'health consumer' who is merely an artifact of the health marketing system and the 'health consumer' who strives for a more equitable, fair and empowering health care system.

Liz Eckermann takes a different approach to the question of what it means to be a health consumer in exploring opportunities for the exercise of individual and collective agency on the part of health care consumers. In particular, she is concerned with investigating what it means to be a health consumer as an embodied agent, especially a female one. In the study, which is part of an larger ongoing project on 'consumer knowledge, opinions, satisfactions and perceived choices in primary health care provision', women who attend a women's health centre were questioned on the degree to which they feel they have genuine choice and control over decision making in their use of primary health care. Although the sample was small, and the results are preliminary, it seems that women have an enormous amount of knowledge about the mainstream health system, the alternative services that are available and caring for their own bodies. It emerged that women are not necessarily passive consumers, and 'only use outside professional services when absolutely necessary and when their self-healing repetoire did not extend to a particular condition'. Eckermann acknowledges difficulties in translating women's unique approaches to consumption of health care into policy, but warns, 'assumptions about health as yet another market may mask the extent to which demand from health professionals themselves and senior bureaucrats, rather than demand from consumers, influences the supply of health services (both quantity and type of services)'.

Finally, O'Neill touches on issues of consumer choice in describing medical attempts to protect their control of the 'pain marketplace' from alternative healers. In the face of patients suffering persistent pain, and ineffective medicine, members of the medical profession have tended to either deny the physical basis for pain or to send the patient to someone more expert at discovery 'which can lead to a downward spiral of referrals'. Many alternative practitioners, however, 'not only believe what their patients say but also endorse patient beliefs about pain having a meaning'. Pain is seen as indicative of bodily malfunction; as having a real source; as something that can be remedied. Alternative practitioners represent themselves as offering a holistic approach to treatment and as using only natural methods. O'Neill shows, by reference to the cases of acupuncturists and chiropractors, how the medical profession has responded to the threat to its attempt to monopolize the pain marketplace; for example, by denigrating alternative theories and practices; by casting doubt on reports of successes; or by incorporating therapies such as spinal manipulation or acupuncture into conventional medical practice. The medical argument is that governments can cause injustice by permitting and endorsing practitioners whose activities are supposedly inherently dangerous. However, as O'Neill argues, 'the public interest' can also be invoked to justify the opposite position: by giving alternative practitioners proper training and practice regulations, this can make them safe.

What these chapters reveal collectively is that the content of care is both complex and ambiguous and does not simply equate with medical care. It comprises a vast array of practices and value judgements that may have unexpected and inequitable outcomes. The chapters, each in their own way, contribute to making visible these inequalities and to articulating the nature of changes required in developing a more just health care system.

REFERENCES

Baldock C V 1990 Volunteers in welfare. Allen & Unwin, Sydney
Davis A, George J 1993 States of health: health and illness in Australia, 2nd edn. Harper Educational, Pymble
Kleinman A 1988 The illness narratives: suffering, healing and the human condition. Basic Books, New York
Lawler J 1991 Behind the screens: nursing, somology, and the problem of the body. Churchill Livingstone, Melbourne

May C 1992 Nursing work, nurses' knowledge, and the subjectification of the patient. Sociology of Health and Illness. 14(4)473-487

Russell C, Schofield T 1986 Where it hurts: an introduction to sociology for health workers. Allen & Unwin, Sydney

9. Patients' perspectives on nursing in hospital

Lindsey Harrison   Elizabeth Cameron-Traub

This chapter reports research into the nursing needs and expectations of hospital patients from different ethnic backgrounds. We chose to research nursing needs and expectations, as distinct from medical needs, for a number of reasons. Nurses hold a pivotal position in the delivery of health care services for individuals in hospital (Bonawit 1989) and yet, compared to doctor/patient oriented research, comparatively little has been carried out in this area.

Australian hospital services have also had to come to terms with great ethnic diversity in their patient populations. Indeed, present government policies emphasize the need for the health care system to be responsive to people from ethnic minority backgrounds. Measures have been taken to improve interpreter services and visiting arrangements and to cater for dietary preferences and religious observances. These changes, which have occurred within the last decade, followed criticisms that, for some, access to services was inadequate and communication within health care institutions poor (Bates & Linder-Pelz 1990, Garrett & Lin 1990). Johnstone (1989) points out that the patient's right to appropriate or quality services is an ethical issue as well as a health issue.

Two other issues formed a backdrop to this research. One is the changing nature of the relationship between health care providers and consumers of health care and the other is changes in the health care system itself. At the same time as the patient population in Australia has been changing in composition, the model of professional dominance in western health care has been questioned, particularly by consumer groups which call for a more informed public, able to be involved in decisions about health and medical care (Bates & Linder-Pelz 1990). It is usually medical personnel who are the main targets of these critiques, but they obviously have implications for the traditional relationship between patients and all health care providers, including nurses.

Cost control in the health care system has also had a profound effect on the way care is organized in hospitals. Davis and George (1993:235) consider that the search for cost control demands greater visibility in the work that is done, its quantification and rationalization against other like tasks, and the measurement of input costs against output values. They discuss literature which describes the progressive substitution of efficiency in patient care as an end in itself, which, they suggest, runs counter to the humanistic philosophy of caring for the patient as a whole person. Some of these points will be pursued later in this chapter.

Given this background, it was decided to focus on patients for this research and to listen to their 'stories' about their perceptions of their nursing needs and expectations. By interviewing patients from different ethnic backgrounds, including Anglo-Celts, we hoped to explore a diversity of viewpoints. In this chapter, we can only present a small portion of the findings and have chosen to concentrate on a number of related themes. These have been grouped under two headings: 'the contract' and 'contradictions'. The first looks at the patients' perception of their role and of the nurses' role, part of the 'expectations' side of the research question. The second section explores some of the more complex aspects of the nurse/patient relationship, again only from the patients' perspective, particularly the apparently contradictory need for patients to talk about matters other than physical concerns, a need rarely satisfied in the hospital environment, and yet their desire to maintain privacy by revealing little about themselves to nurses. These aspects tended to be less fully articulated by the patients than their expectations of nurses and nursing care, but this is an important issue and will be a fruitful area for future research.

Before turning to the discussion of the chosen themes, which are illustrated with excerpts from the interviews, we describe the research method and the participants in more detail.

Method and participants

Twenty six people in three Sydney metropolitan hospitals participated. There were two criteria for inclusion in the study. One was that the patients spoke English. This of necessity excluded many recent migrants of non-English-speaking background. The other criterion was that they had been in hospital at least three days, but were shortly to be discharged, which meant they had recovered from the condition which led to their admission. The Nursing Unit Managers, to whom the research was explained once Ethics Committee clearance had been obtained, were relied upon for this information. We felt that three days was a minimum time for patients to have a significant experience of nursing care and to be exposed to a number of nurses. We also wanted to be certain that patients were well enough to be interviewed. At the same time, we wanted their experiences to be fresh and for this reason, as well as for practical considerations, the interviews were carried out in the hospitals rather than later in the patients' homes. It should be borne in mind, however, that the timing of the interviews, and conditions in which they took place, may well have influenced the stories that the patients told. They were giving their opinions at a particular stage in their hospitalization and their perceptions may have been different at an earlier stage when they were unwell, or at a later

Table 9.1 Participants in the study

	Anglo-Celtic patients	Ethnic minority patients
Sex	5 male/8 female	2 male/11 female
Age (mean in years)	53, range 28-79	48, range 26-68
Medical/surgical	5 medical/8 surgical	5 medical /8 surgical
Length of stay in hospital (mean in days)	9, range 3-23	11, range 4-34
Mean years in Australia	N/A	22, range 2-40

stage, after they went home and had had time to reflect on their experiences.

Thirteen of the participants were Anglo-Celtic, that is, they were born in Australia (predominantly) of British or Irish heritage, or were migrants from Britain or Ireland and all spoke English as their first language. The other 13 were from a wide variety of backgrounds, they were all born overseas, did not have British or Irish heritage and their first language was not English. Nine other languages were represented in all. These patients from ethnic minority groups had lived in Australia from between 2 and 40 years. Diagnoses were not sought, though many of the patients volunteered this information.

Each of the two groups of 13 participants in the study was similar in composition in terms of sex, age, time spent in hospital and type of present hospital experience (medical or surgical). This information is displayed in Table 9.1. Informed consent was obtained from each patient who was then interviewed for approximately thirty minutes. The interviews, which were audio taped, contained some structured questions but most were open ended to allow participants freedom to respond to the topic areas in their own way. The transcripts of the interviews were coded for dominant themes and counting was carried out where appropriate.

This was a non-random sample, which means that caution should be observed about generalizing the findings. Some of the interpretation is necessarily tentative given the small sample size and the 'one-off' nature of the interviews, which meant that questions could not be followed up with the participants during the analysis stage. However, this type of research has the capacity to reveal issues which larger surveys cannot, because it allows the participants to 'speak for themselves'. Situating the findings within the available literature also increases their utility and generalizability.

The contract

...I've always strived to be a model patient in the sense that I only ask for what I need and I'm always polite and co-operative and willing to do whatever the nurses want me to, and I expect in return that they are going to be everything that I want them to be.

This quote sums up the themes that are discussed in this section. It is taken from an interview with a 61-year-old Anglo-Celtic man born in Australia, but it captures in a very succinct way the views of most of our patient sample. We found that, no matter what their ethnic background, patients enter hospital with similar, strong expectations about the appropriate role and demeanour of the nurse, the appropriate role and demeanour of the patient and about the nature of the care they will receive.

The 'contract' of the heading refers to the fact that, from the patients' perspective, the patient/nurse relationship is a reciprocal one, with clear obligations on both sides, as the quote illustrates. These obligations were obviously not formally articulated by all patients , but their components are generally clear in the interviews. The patients considered that nurses were there to carry out the instructions of the doctors and to provide the physical care that allowed the patients to recover from their medical conditions. On the whole, patients expressed satisfaction with the physical care they received, especially when it was carried out in a cheerful manner. Any shortcomings in the standard of care tended to be blamed on the system, rather than the nurses. Nurses were also perceived to be constantly busy and to have no time to talk. For their part, patients were required by their perceptions of their role to co-operate by not 'bothering' the nurses, unless it was really necessary. Elements of passivity, compliance and acceptance in the patient role and trust in professional judgement were striking in patient discussion; patients did not see themselves as appropriate partners in decision making.

The similarity and strength of these patient viewpoints may well be the result of nursing images, such as angel of mercy (Cockerham 1986, Smith 1980) and doctor's handmaiden (Aroskar 1980, Donley & Flaherty 1990), which are so well established in popular western culture. Donley and Flaherty (1990) argue that these images, which are widely shared both within the health care professions and the public, present a number of disadvantages for the nursing profession. Newton (1980), however, considers that these images are maintained by the public desire to have nurses around to tend them when the need arises.

The patients in our sample perceived nursing care as being physical care alone, that is, care related to bodily functions and bodily comfort, rather than psychological, emotional or spiritual care. These latter aspects were either not seen as nursing functions at all or only as potential ones, taking second place to physical care and carried out if there was time, which, according to the patients, there rarely was. Nurses and patients conversed on general topics while physical care was carried out, but otherwise rarely communicated, a finding discussed in a later section.

The routine carrying out of physical care, especially that of monitoring vital signs, no matter that this often occurred at inconvenient times, provided reassurance for the patients that the nurses were doing their job, which included spotting when things might go wrong.

Woman, 43, Anglo-Celt, born in Australia: But yeah, they do the things that you really expect them to do, make you comfortable, take vital readings...As far as the care goes, I mean, they're always sticking thermometers, taking pulses, which is reassuring, because you figure...if they're keeping an eye on it, I must be all right.

Woman, 26, born in Armenia, 6 years in Australia: So the general things are cleaning and working good. They are not lazy. This I expected.

Woman, 79, Anglo-Celt, born in Australia: They take your blood pressure, your temperature and pulse and give out the medications and then they leave you...they put the light out...That's at half past five [in the morning]. We try and have a little sleep.

These views of patients are consistent with the idea that nursing work comprises 'housework', general nursing care, healing functions and tests and observations, as identified by Game and Pringle (1983). Overall, much nursing activity is related to the care of the body and bodily functions. This has been explored extensively by Lawler (1991). Newton (1980) argues that this view of the role of the nurse is functional in the health care setting and that there is little doubt that it corresponds to a real and essential need.

As long as there are prescribed treatments that patients cannot administer to themselves, as long as patients get so sick that they cannot attend to their own physical needs, the health care system will require the technically skilled person to administer medical treatment (Newton 1980:37).

Patients prized qualities of kindness and friendliness in nurses, their manner and having a smiling face, which was seen to be morale raising. Joking was frequently mentioned.

Woman, 28, Anglo-Celt, born in Australia: There was a nice nurse on last night, a male nurse. He was quite funny, he lighted us all up...It was good having him come in and joking around with us.

Woman, 50, born in Lebanon, 30 years in Australia: She [has] always got a smile on her face, make the patients laugh, make a joke with them and talk to them and make them happy.

Woman, 32, born in Syria, 13 years in Australia: The nurses they are really good. They make you laugh. They have got good sense of humour.

Woman, 44, born in Taiwan, 8 years in Australia: I needed the warmth...I needed the smile.

Man, 54, Anglo-Celt, born in United Kingdom: I mean, they are all cheerful you know. We joke with them...

Buckenham and McGrath (1983:40) quote one nurse's explanation of this joking relationship, 'if the patients are bored, you're there to make them laugh, if it's going to make them feel better'. Hence, the nurse showing kindness, friendliness and warmth was important to the patients and generally met with their approval. It may be seen as part of the creation of a therapeutic environment by the nurse involved and may be symbolic of the apparent equality between nurse and patient, which is also expressed in the use of first names. In contrast, when patients mentioned particular doctors, they used their title and surname. However, at least one patient had doubts about the meaning or implications of nursing cheerfulness.

Woman, 71, Anglo-Celt, born in Australia: And you know, some of them are really quite jolly and cheerful and everything, but they don't do as much for you as the ones that are not so, you know, and they're just sort of a bit, what will I say, they're a bit—fun is not the word I'm trying to use—you know, flighty.

Cockerham (1986) discusses how hospitalization may lead to acquiescence, submission to authority, enforced co-operation and depersonalized status. Patients learn their role through talking with and viewing the behaviour of other patients, as well as 'being explicitly taught and controlled in certain situations by hospital staff' (Bond & Bond 1986:197). In our research, the interviews revealed aspects of the patients' perceptions of their role in hospital and of the ways they responded to their nursing care environment. In terms of decision making, patients in our sample were quite clear that they had no say in their care and most accepted this. They did not know what their requirements were; professionals did.

Woman, 79, Anglo-Celt, born in Australia: Well, I didn't expect to have a say. See that's left to the doctors and then that's given to the sisters.

Woman, 28, Anglo-Celt, born in Australia: No, I don't think I had a say in the care, but I think they know what to do and I don't know what to do.

Woman, 43, Anglo-Celt, born in Australia: The routine of the hospital makes the decisions, I guess. Yeah, I guess you don't really have a say. You go along with the routine of things.

These statements were common to all patients, regardless of ethnic origin.

The extent to which patients could or should be involved, particularly in clinically related matters, raises ethical and technical issues. Thomas et al (1991) report that many patients would prefer to be involved in this area, however in the present study this was clearly not the case. Indeed, Silverman (1987:25) warns that it is important to avoid making the assumption that all patients want, or should want, to be partners in decision making.

Moreover, two thirds (18) of the patients in our sample did not believe that nurses made decisions about their nursing care. Patients considered that nurses were there to carry out the doctor's instructions, to the extent that 11 patients (41%) believed that doctors take the decisions about nursing care as well as medical care. What happened to them in a nursing sense, they considered to arise from their medical condition. Four patients (15%) thought 'the hospital' made the decisions and three (11%) had no idea.

The patients considered that the nurses were busy and that unless they had needs (and that meant physical needs), they would, or should, not 'bother' the nurses. As a consequence, our patient sample strongly associated having needs or making demands with receiving nursing care. Nurses were seen as being constantly busy, and this was attributed by most patients to staffing shortages and there being other sicker patients. The outcome was that the patients sought to co-operate with the nurses by making minimal demands on nursing time. It should be remembered, of course, that this group of patients was almost ready to go home and so they were largely able to care for themselves, although they had all experienced the need for more extensive nursing care at the beginning of their hospitalization.

Man, 61, Anglo-Celt, born in Australia: I suppose there's a bit of an inbuilt tendency not to want to worry the nurses.

Woman, 28, Anglo-Celt, born in Australia: You can see that they are always busy so, I mean, when you really do urgently need them OK, but if it's not that urgent you should be able to just hold back.

Woman, 79, Anglo-Celt, born in Australia: When I'm in hospital, I'm not a complainer. I think they work that hard and unless I've really got to ask them for something, I don't.

Woman, 63, born in Italy, 33 years in Australia: They always busy and I no want to waste the time, you see.

Woman, 32, born in Syria, 13 years in Australia: I don't like to disturb them. I hardly use the buzzer.

There was also clear recognition that the needs of others may take precedence over nurses' time and attention.

Woman, 38, born in Italy, 32 years in Australia: The thing is, you've got to understand that you're not the only sick person in here.

Woman, 50, born in Lebanon, 30 years in Australia: I don't need any help from the sisters because they can't. They've got [patient's name] over there and they've got another lady. They needing the sister more than I am.

Some patients did criticize the nursing care they received. Few failed to mention the frustrations of waiting to receive something (a pan, medication—always physical needs) for a considerable length of time, or their request being forgotten entirely. Only one patient, a 53-year-old Anglo-Celtic man, born in the United Kingdom, considered this to be 'slack' although he also felt the nurses were 'basically pretty good'. Generally, the patients explained away 'slack' incidents by blaming the hospital organization for the perceived heavy workload of the nurses.

Woman, 63, born in Italy, 33 years in Australia: You ring and they no coming very very soon. But I understand because they are busy. That's nothing. Or [they] forget something. But never mind.

These findings indicate the patients' sensitivity to what they see as the focus of the hospital system and to the role and function of both patients and nurses within that system. Clearly the patients in our sample see their role as co-operating with the nurses, given the demands made on them and their apparent responsibilities. Patients did not want to be seen as impeding nursing care in any way. Given that they defined nursing practice as the provision of care to meet the physical needs of patients, their expectations of nurses and nursing were tailored to be consistent with this definition.

However, although the patients appeared very certain about these issues of role, there were elements of confusion, and even some contradiction, in the interviews and these are explored in the following section.

Contradictions

Despite the patients' view of the nurses as kind, friendly, cheerful, joking, as well as competent in tending to physical needs, a number of patients appeared to acknowledge a gap in nursing care. Physical needs were met in hospital, but psychological, emotional or spiritual needs were not necessarily met. Perhaps the emphasis on physical care, the perception that nurses were busy and the atmosphere of superficial cheerfulness were sufficient to distance patients from nursing staff. In the interviews, nursing staff were seldom referred to by name. Partly, this may be explained by the social organization of hospital work, which involves shift work and the frequent rotation of nursing staff. This means that patients may not have an opportunity to get to know many of the nurses with whom they come into contact. The rare exceptions when nurses were named occurred when individuals were praised by patients, interestingly often because they engaged in 'talk' about other than general topics or physical care.

Woman, 34, born in Indonesia, 5 years in Australia: One day I feel so lonely, so lonely and this nurse she know me...and she came in and ask me, what's going on with you? Because she came in and she is really understanding type. I need somebody to talk. I feel so happy.

However, patients were reluctant to seek opportunities to talk with nurses, despite the fact that a number of them clearly wished to talk to someone, as indicated by the stories that patients told after the tape recorder was switched off (e.g. fears of onset of dementia, loneliness after the recent death of a husband, thoughts of dying from (curable) cancer rather than having treatment, etc).

One explanation is that patients often did not have close contact with nurses once they were able to look after their own physical needs. Patients who had no needs were left alone. This was accepted as appropriate by the patients because nurses were seen to be busy with other patients.

Man, 52, Anglo-Celt, born in Australia: I think, I mean, they've seen that I was all right, we've sort of left each other alone most of the time.

Woman, 71, Anglo-Celt, born in Australia: You're really left to yourself. Like I haven't seen anybody since I put the stockings on after I had a shower and a bit of a walk...But they're understaffed and running all the time, you know.

Man, 61, Anglo-Celt, born in Australia: Well, actually, if I make no demands, they do very little.

Few patients explicitly expressed a need to talk and, indeed, most denied that they had needs that were not satisfied. When asked whether they had talked to the nurses about their nursing needs, 20 (77%) said no, and only 6 (23%) said yes. These figures were similar for both groups (Anglo-Celts: 85% no, 15% yes; ethnic minority patients: 69% no and 31% yes). What they talked about turned out to be their physical requirements, for example, the need for medication or to be repositioned in bed. Patients were also asked if they would have liked to have talked to the nurses about anything, but were unable to for some reason. Again 21 (81%) felt they had no need to talk to the nurses, while only 5 (19%) would have liked to have talked to the nurses but did not or could not. The numbers were similar for each group (Anglo-Celts: 85% no, 15% yes; ethnic minority patients: 77% no, 23% yes). When asked what they would have liked to have talked to the nurses about, all five replied that they would have liked to have asked for more information about their medical condition.

However, despite these denials of the need for 'talk', some patients appeared to contradict this in other parts of their interviews.

Women, 43, Anglo-Celt, born in Australia: ...but I think maybe if they could have the time in their schedule to maybe just come round and sit beside the bed and have a little chat to someone and people might open up, rather than ask for it, you know. People don't always ask. But the nurses just don't have the time. There's not enough of them.

Woman, 63, born in Italy, 33 years in Australia: [What kinds of needs have you had?] To talk to somebody. Something like that.

Woman, 34, born in Indonesia, 5 years in Australia: I feel so lonely...I need somebody to talk.

Woman, 46, Anglo-Celt, born in Australia: Even though, on and off, I cry by myself and they don't take any notice.

Woman, 50, born in Lebanon, 30 years in Australia: I've been able to talk only when the nurses come talk to me. Otherwise, when the nurses they are not here, I haven't got any visitors and you don't talk and you don't say much.

In fact, analysis of the interviews revealed feelings of loneliness, social isolation and perhaps dejection. Why did patients not reveal their feelings to the nursing staff? Some of the potential reasons, the perception that nurses were busy and lack of continuing contact, were explored above. But other dominant themes apparent in the interviews suggest that patients preferred not to divulge personal information to the nurses and, indeed, beyond a superficial friendliness, attempted to maintain their privacy. Other research has indicated that some patients do not disclose information to nurses or other health professionals, because they are uncertain about the possible effects of self-disclosure, including how others may respond to them (Northouse & Northouse 1992).

Nursing care frequently involves intimate physical care carried out by strangers. This is accepted as necessary, unavoidable and potentially embarrassing. To endure this, the patients in our sample attempted to maintain distance and privacy. This was plainly not always possible in a physical sense, however it was possible to do so in respect to other areas of their lives. Even when it came to unavoidable physical care, some patients made strong statements about their usual independence in their lives outside the institution and their desire to be as independent as possible, as soon as possible. Others found elements of independent functioning in hospital. They may well be reflecting a core value of Australian society and certainly these statements were most frequently articulated by Anglo-Celts, but the sentiments of several of the patients born overseas, many of whom have lived for years in Australia, were very similar.

Man, 54, Anglo-Celt, born in Australia: I don't really like anyone looking after me at all, but, I mean, there are times you have to, absolutely have to.

Woman, 71, Anglo-Celt, born in Australia: Well, I'm typically a very independent person and basically, if I could do it myself, I would rather be doing it myself...But you know, I think it's traumatic to start with, you know, people sort of having to do things for you, which you have always done for yourself and you get used to that.

Woman, 26, born in Armenia, 6 years in Australia: I like to do everything myself, you know.

Women, 66, born in Latvia, 37 years in Australia: I went to the toilet myself...I sponge myself. By the time they are able to come to me, I had done the job myself...I've always been like that.

All patients were adamant that although nurses have a legitimate need to know about their patients' medical histories, they do not need to know about their background or lifestyle in order to nurse them, which, again, reflects the fact that nursing is seen overwhelmingly to be about physical care alone. However, the ethnic minority patients in the sample were likely to express the view that those who cannot speak English, and could not make their demands known, would have special needs, and that nurses would need to know more about where they come from. The question of how much was not explored. Ethnic minority patients who could speak English, on the other hand, and that included everyone we interviewed, could decide for themselves what to reveal about themselves to nurses. In view of their statements that there was nothing that they wanted to talk to the nurse about, and the 'busyness' of nurses, such divulgence of personal information was likely to be minimal.

Woman, 26, born in Armenia, 6 years in Australia: Why? I don't want them to know [about my background].

Woman, 34, born in Indonesia, 5 years in Australia: I mean, if I couldn't speak English, probably they should know a bit [about my background], because it's very hard communication without speak English. But if I know a bit about English, I mean I can talk by myself, to say myself without anybody. So really, it's not necessary.

Woman, 44, born in Taiwan, 8 years in Australia: [Do nurses need to know about your background?] I think no. We can converse easily. My English not very good, but I talk something, they understand.

These patients could tell staff what they wanted and why. In that respect ability to speak the appropriate language gave them some degree of control over their situation and, like their Anglo-Celt counterparts, they could also control the amount of information they divulged.

Conclusion

From the interviews discussed in this chapter, it is clear that some patients were placed in contradictory situations. Their needs in some areas were clearly in conflict with their strong expectations of the role and function of the nurses. Only physical needs were legitimate and merited nursing time. To fulfil their expectations of the patient role, they were unable to make demands or to express needs which they believed to be inappropriate, or peripheral to what they saw as the main concerns of the nurses. At the same time, they did not consider knowledge about themselves, other than medical knowledge, to be relevant to their nursing care and were guarded with personal information. The result was that worries remained hidden. Sometimes these were transitory worries such as loneliness in the hospital environment, which, though not trivial, would resolve themselves. Sometimes they were major concerns, which the patients would take with them when they were discharged.

It came as a surprise to us that the similarities between the views of patients who came from Anglo-Celtic backgrounds and those from ethnic minority backgrounds were far greater than the differences. This finding suggests that there are aspects of the delivery of care in the hospital setting which impact on the perceptions of patients regardless of their ethnic background.

It is easy to assume, on the one hand, that changes to hospital food catering departments, the provision of interpreters and similar services are all that is required to ensure quality care to those from ethnic minority backgrounds and that, on the other, Anglo-Celts are well provided for within the present health care system. However, this research suggests that the hospital environment supports and encourages a view of nurses and nursing which ignores significant needs and hence potentially disadvantages patients, no matter what their background. The search for cost control in the health care system may be a factor here, with efficiency in patient care becoming an end in itself. This, as Davis and George (1993) suggest, runs counter to the humanistic philosophy of caring for the patient as a whole person. This is an important area which impacts on the delivery of appropriate nursing care and needs further investigation.

REFERENCES

Aroskar M A 1980 The fractured image: the public stereotyping of nursing and the nurse.
    In: Spicker S F, Gadow S (eds) Nursing images and ideals. Springer, New York
Bates E, Linder-Pelz S 1990 Health care issues, 2nd edn. Allen & Unwin, Sydney

Bonawit V 1989 The image of the nurse: the community's perception and its implications for the profession. In: Gray G, Pratt R (eds) Issues in Australian nursing 2. Churchill Livingstone, Melbourne

Bond J, Bond S 1986 Sociology and health care. Churchill Livingstone Edinburgh

Buckenham J E, Mcgrath G 1983 The social reality of nursing. Adis Health Sciences Press, Sydney

Cockerham W C 1986 Medical sociology, 3rd edn. Prentice-Hall, Englewood Cliffs, New Jersey

Davis A, George J 1993 States of health; health and illness in Australia, 2nd edn. Harper Educational, Sydney

Donley R, Flaherty M J 1990 Strategies for changing nursing's image. In: McCloskey J C, Grace H K (eds) Current issues in nursing. C V Mosby, St Louis

Game A, Pringle R 1983 Gender at work. Allen & Unwin, Sydney

Garrett P, Lin V 1990 Ethnic health policy and service development. In: Reid J, Trompf P (eds) The health of immigrant Australia; a social perspective. Harcourt Brace Jovanovich, Sydney

Johnstone M J 1989 Bioethics; a nursing perspective. Harcourt Brace Jovanovich, Sydney

Lawler J 1991 Behind the screens: nursing, somology, and the problem of the body. Churchill Livingstone, Melbourne

Newton L 1980 A vindication of the gentle sister: comment on 'the fractured image'. In: Spicker S F, Gadow S (eds) Nursing: images and ideals. Springer, New York

Northouse P G, Northouse L L 1992 Health communication, 2nd edn. Appleton & Lange, Norwalk, Connecticut

Silverman D 1987 Communication and medical practice; social relations in the clinic. Sage Publications, London

Smith S 1980 Three models of the nurse-patient relationship. In: Spicker S F, Gadow S (eds) Nursing: images and ideals. Springer, New York

Thomas S A, Wearing A J, Bennett M J 1991 Clinical decision making for nurses and health professionals. Harcourt Brace Jovanovich, Sydney

10. Migrant women from El Salvador and Vietnam in Australian hospitals

Martha MacIntyre

Over the past decade there have been numerous studies of migrant health and a range of policy recommendations aimed at promoting access to health services.[1] The problem of access is necessarily broadly interpreted to include 'communication barriers, ethnocentric cultural practices, and alienating structures of service delivery' (Alcorso & Schofield 1991:ix). Research into the cultural and social variations in migrant women's experience provides insights into the diversity of factors that constrain migrant women in their use of health services.

In a recent study of migrant women's access to hospital services, we have looked at the needs of migrant women who have arrived in Melbourne over the past five years.[2]

In studying migrant women's access to the health services of public hospitals we have directed attention to the special problems faced by recent immigrants, specifically those who have come here as refugees from countries where their lives have been disrupted (or even threatened) by political upheavals. While many of the women who have come to Australia from countries such as Vietnam, Lebanon, El Salvador or the former Soviet Union did not come as refugees in the official sense, most left their countries to escape violence, or an intolerable level of insecurity. In the first few years a majority of them see themselves as exiles rather than voluntary immigrants, yet they are bureaucratically subsumed by the label 'Non-English Speaking Background' (NESB). The emphasis on language, and the definition of such people exclusively in terms of a negative capacity serves to further rob them of their political and cultural identities. Their status as recent immigrants provides another dimension, as they should also be viewed as part of Australian society—sharing with others the structural disadvantages of unemployment and poverty. The problems of migrant access to health services must therefore be explored in terms of the social, economic and cultural factors prevailing in the country of origin and those that are specific to the new situation.[3]

The importance of language, or the right to be understood

Migrant women and health workers almost invariably identify language as the greatest problem for recent immigrants. Often women avoid seeking medical care because of the problems of communication. Both migrant women and health service providers agree that communicating through an interpreter, however skilled, is never as satisfactory as direct conversation between the service provider and client who share language and culture. So that while the need for trained interpreters is acknowledged, it should be seen as an interim measure and not a substitute for English language courses that will enable women to speak for themselves. Migrant women are particularly disadvantaged by current government policies regarding access to language courses. Those funded by the State are restricted to newly arrived migrants, so that families usually place priority on men attending in order to learn sufficient English to seek employment. Women with young children are often unable to attend because of child care obligations.

Another way of dealing with language barriers is to employ professionals who are from the various ethnic groups served by a hospital or health service and to encourage bilingualism in the workplace. At present this is often ad hoc, so that people who speak a language other than English are called upon occasionally to interpret or translate. Often this is unsatisfactory for all concerned and reduces confidence in the service. In interviews many Salvadoran women expressed a preference for a particular hospital because there was a sympathetic Spanish-speaking social worker employed there. Her presence was viewed by women not simply as a resource, but as an affirmation of their culture and values. As many people who arrive as refugees are forced to work in menial jobs because of language difficulties or policies that do not allow recognition of foreign qualifications, the presence of professionals from their ethnic group carried with it intangible, but highly valued, symbolic significance. Vietnamese women spoke in glowing terms of nurses and midwives from their community and Salvadorans resented the fact that there were people who were unable to work in their professions because their qualifications were not recognized by the relevant Australian professional body.

Problems of communication are manifold. Almost every woman and health worker could produce a 'horror story' about a situation where there was no interpreter available. Sometimes this involves discomfort, embarrassment or confusion, but on occasions there are breaches of human rights or medical ethics.[4] Women have had major surgery without their informed consent, have been denied appropriate medical treatment and have had to divulge confidential information to people who just happened to be sitting in a waiting room or polishing the floor. The appropriate use of interpreters is best used as the first line solution to communication problems— but it is not a panacea for migrant women and their difficulties with language.

Cultural barriers

If you fall ill in your own country you usually know a variety of ways to seek medical assistance. If you are Australian you know that you can see a local general practitioner, or go to a public hospital, or call an ambulance. The range of choices, knowledge about required payments and rights of access are aspects of cultural awareness and practices that are taken for granted as 'the health system'. The problem for migrants, especially those who do not speak English, is that there is often a lack of fit between the system that prevailed in their country of origin and the Australian system. In some countries there is no private health care, in others the state funded system is minor and provides care only to the very poor. In some instances all health services are located in one institution, while in others there is a separation of dental, pharmacy and medical service provision. The complexities of the Australian system, and the extent to which it differs from other national systems are major factors that restrict access for migrants, especially those who have recently arrived.

Ethnocentrism, or the tendency to view one's own cultural premises and practices as 'normal' or 'natural' (and better than others) is not exclusively a characteristic of western societies. Most people grow up with some confidence in the view that their language is comprehensible and convenient; that their religious views are affirmed in the world around them and that the food they eat is nourishing and good to eat. But the ethnocentrism of the dominant group in a culturally diverse society is often oppressive in its demands for conformity, and blindness to the virtues of the diversity that are so often acclaimed. In the area of health care and medicine, the ethnocentrism that characterizes Australian services has to be viewed globally and locally.

The majority of women in our survey valued those aspects of western medicine that they were familiar with from their own countries. Immunization campaigns, family planning projects, and a range of disease prevention programs in countries such as Vietnam, El Salvador and Chile were mentioned in discussions. While many had come from rural areas where health services had been poor—none were absolutely ignorant of western medicine and many indicated resentment of the assumption that they were all 'ignorant peasants' who had never set foot in a hospital. Several women drew attention to the extensive medical tests they had undergone in order to emigrate and the fact that facilities for these existed in their countries of origin. Others who worked in the health services area stressed that 1986 census data revealed that migrant women were generally healthier than Australian women (see National Health Strategy 1993). Vietnamese and Salvadoran women suggested that their diets were healthier than Australians' and that they placed greater emphasis on self-management of illness through diet (and herbal cures) than Australians whom they believed were 'always running to doctors'. Their views are supported by Australian research (Powles &

Gifford 1990, Alcorso & Schofield 1990) which indicates that, '[i]deas of immigrants being generally disadvantaged in their health experience are poorly founded', and that 'the composition of diet [is] the chief influence on mortality differences', that show that immigrant advantage (Powles & Gifford 1990:102–3).

The majority of women interviewed indicated that they were generally pleased with hospital care they received in Australia and considered it superior to that of their country of origin. Some Vietnamese women described the lack of privacy in consultations, the poorly equipped health centres and the long waiting times at hospitals in Vietnam and insisted that they felt more confident in the well equipped, relatively luxurious surroundings of an Australian hospital. In a group discussion Salvadoran women stressed the disadvantages of giving birth in a crowded, understaffed Salvadoran maternity hospital and the advantages of being in a small ward with only one or two women in Australia. In short, many of the differences between hospital services in their native countries and those in Australia were ones that they were glad existed. Indeed, those who made negative comparisons almost always had access to private health care in their native country.

The development of culturally sensitive health services does not require that providers set about recreating modes of health care that reproduce facilities in the countries of origin of patients. Quite often women suggested that such changes would not be desirable. For example, those Salvadoran women who had been attended by qualified midwives in El Salvador, when questioned on the issue indicated preference for an obstetrician in Australia. Similarly, women who had successful homebirths in El Salvador preferred to deliver their babies in a modern Australian hospital rather than at home or in a birth centre within a hospital. They associated the domestic environment with higher risk and drew comfort from the equipment and clinical atmosphere of a delivery suite. Coming from a country where maternal and neonate morbidity and mortality is high, they valued the sterile atmosphere of a hospital and the visibility of equipment that could be used to diagnose potential problems or save life. While all affirmed that birth was 'natural', many had experiences which meant that they did not see nature as necessarily benign.

The generally positive assessment of Australian health services is reflected in a reluctance to criticize or complain about those aspects of hospital care that made women feel unhappy, uncomfortable, baffled or affronted. Women who have come from war torn countries, where public services have been disrupted, and where health care services had to absorb those who were injured in fighting, tend to accept that maternity services will be minimal. By comparison then, Australian health services are viewed as excellent. Moreover, refugee women often feel grateful and beholden to the Australian government for accepting them as immigrants, and this further inhibits criticism of its services. The reluctance to criticize is compounded further by the widely held view that public patients have only minimal rights and must accept what is offered without question. In group discussions most women affirmed their right of access but felt that this precluded choices about care within a hospital. Only those women who had participated in community based groups for migrant women or attended Community Health Centres where there were programs informing women on health issues had a clear view of their rights as patients in a hospital.

While general questions eliciting views on degrees of satisfaction produced mainly positive responses, more specific questions about actual experiences revealed a wide range of dissatisfaction. Numerous accounts of incidents of discrimination and failures of communication were reported.

Troubles with doctors

Of all people working in hospitals, doctors were those who were most often seen as obstructive, inflexible and insensitive to migrant women's needs. There are many reasons why this is predictable, as in all hospitals doctors are clearly those responsible for decisions about the woman's treatment, but negative reactions to doctors provide a way of interpreting problems of access that moves beyond lists of complaints about individuals.

Australian doctors are not so thoroughly trained as Chilean doctors. Here you have a little training in everything and you become a GP. In Chile every doctor is a specialist. If your child is sick you go to a paediatrician, if you are pregnant you go to a gynaecologist/obstetrician. You don't have to be referred, you just go! (Chilean woman, 35 years old)

I have no confidence in Australian doctors. They are not like doctors in El Salvador. There, they don't have to look for things in books, they listen to you and examine you and then they know what to prescribe. Here, every time I go to the doctor he has to look in a book, even to prescribe antibiotics! I think they do not study for as long as El Salvadoran doctors, they don't seem to know how to treat people. (El Salvadoran woman, 40 years old)

The comments of the Chilean and Salvadoran women above reveal the ways in which differing systems and styles of medical practice become the basis for a lack of confidence in Australian doctors. Some women had so little faith that they sought help from unregistered practitioners from their own community and then arranged for relatives to send pharmaceuticals from overseas, where they could be freely purchased.

These comments can be analysed in order to elucidate the nature of cultural differences in medical systems. They are two of many similar complaints offered by Latin American women. Cultural awareness education as part of medical training could readily overcome problems that sometimes result in women avoiding doctors because of fundamental ethnocentric misunderstandings.

El Salvador and Chile are countries where the training and practice of medicine has many things in common with those in Australia. Doctors work within what is usually called the 'western' system of medicine and the specialities are basically the same. Their prestige in society is based on factors such as highly competitive academic selection; expensive, lengthy education and a recognition of their work as a social good. Doctors have relatively high incomes and most come from middle class backgrounds. So the class and educational similarities are apparent to migrant women.

On the other hand, the fact that there is no direct equivalent of 'general practitioner' does mean that people who are accustomed to seeing specialists tend to suspect GPs of being 'jacks-of-all-trades, masters of none'. This suspicion is often confirmed when the GP fails to treat the woman in a way that is consistent with previous experience. For example, many drugs that are administered orally in Australia are given by injection in Latin America. 'Having an injection' is seen as the most appropriate and effective way of taking medicine. Moreover, the state systems of pharmaceutical control are quite different and access to drugs is almost unregulated in many countries. In practice then, any Salvadoran who has enough money can purchase pharmaceutical drugs and have them injected by a person who charges a small fee. As a result of this system people self-prescribe, are more familiar with the trade names of drugs and Latin American doctors probably suggest pharmaceutical treatments more often, recognizing that people will self-prescribe if they do not. Very few women had heard about problems of drug resistance and over-use of antibiotics and so interpreted a doctor's failure to prescribe antibiotics for all respiratory ailments as proof of his lack of training or knowledge in this area of medicine. Unaware of the strict and changing regulation of prescribed drugs in Australia, Latin American women perceive the doctor's consultation of the most recent MIMS catalogue (a catalogue of therapeutic prescription drugs) as further confirmation of his ignorance. While an Australian woman might see a doctor's referring to recent articles or textbooks as a reassuring action, suggesting to them that he is 'double-checking' a diagnosis or prescription, many of the women interviewed found it alarming.

Community based health education programs are the obvious places to provide information about the Australian system and explain cultural and practical differences to migrant women. Basic information that would enable migrants to understand that general practitioners in Australia are qualified both as 'physicians' and as 'surgeons', would alleviate fears and prevent differences being perceived as incompetence. But the interviews with migrant women suggest that Australian doctors need to be culturally sensitive and informed about the needs and expectations of migrants and areas where misunderstandings are likely to occur if changes are to be brought about in the spirit of multi-culturalism.

The ethnocentrism of the Australian medical profession and hospitals is a major problem in any policy development that attempts to be pluralistic. In its most extreme form it is expressed in refusals to call an interpreter to explain what the doctor considers a minor or routine procedure or bullying insistence that a woman comply with instructions—instances of such behaviour were given by several women. But more often responses of impatience, or disregard for the women's views, were seen by women as evidence of intolerance or racism that undermined their confidence in the doctor and made them feel humiliated and anxious.

> I speak good English and I understood everything the doctor said. But I felt weak and sick and had terrible pains after the birth. I felt cold and tired. When I told the doctor and asked for a hot water bottle he just said no and told me I could not feel cold because the room was very hot. He wanted me to walk around, but I was too tired. I would not go back to that hospital. The nurses were kind but the doctors never listened. (Vietnamese woman, 34 years old)

This woman's account of her dissatisfactions may not at first appear to be 'culturally different' from the sorts of complaints that many people make about medical treatment. A culturally sensitive interpretation would illuminate the fact that the woman's use of the English term 'cold' should not be seen as a simple reference to physical sensations of temperature. Rather, she is translating a Vietnamese term which in its cultural context conveys information about debilitating feelings of weakness, lassitude or even muscle pain. The refusal of a hot water bottle may have been because of a safety regulation in the hospital, but as no explanation was offered, the woman saw it as a dismissal of her perceived needs as well as a rejection of Vietnamese customary treatment of humoral imbalance.[5]

So, in thinking about the problem of access, we need to consider it from several perspectives. It is not sufficient to facilitate access simply by making it easier for women to receive medical care. Confidence in the system and the service providers is a critical factor. Indeed, in our study we found no cases of women whose language difficulties actually prevented them from getting to a hospital. Rather the problems of access were often presented in terms of a lack of confidence, that inhibited the woman from seeking health care after negative experiences. Women who had been embarrassed or humiliated avoided returning to a hospital for treatment.

Embarrassment, confusion and humiliation are more often the result of insensitive service delivery than simple inability to understand English. Many migrant women reported problems over mispronunciation of names, so that they missed their turn and were treated rudely by hospital staff who said that they had called them. Others were spoken to condescendingly when they asked for clarification of instructions that hospital staff considered routine, such as producing a urine sample or standing in a queue. People who lack confidence in their verbal communication skills are often very sensitive to non-verbal indications, so that facial expressions suggesting amusement or exasperation, or gestures of impatience or irritation are perceived as the major import of a response. Anxious to avoid hostile reactions or being seen as 'a problem', many women retreat into passivity as a defence against demeaning interactions.

Rather than seeing the 'communication barriers' simply as the women's language difficulties or lack of familiarity with the system, health service providers need to consider their own ignorance or lack of understanding as inhibiting or obstructing factors. The example of the Vietnamese woman who used the English term 'cold' meaning it to connote sensations of tiredness, weakness and humoral imbalance as well as the physical sensation of the body to low temperature, instances one sort of cultural insensitivity. The doctor did not know Vietnamese cultural conventions about describing illness and so failed to comprehend the woman's statement. This type of misunderstanding can be remedied in part if health service workers learn about the cultures of women who use the hospital, so that they can anticipate and respond to problems from an informed position. In the last instance however, there has to be a commitment to communication that is inspired not only by the desire for efficient service delivery, but by curiosity and imagination.

Too often, the barriers to communication take the form of inflexible ethnocentrism on the part of health workers. Sometimes this derives from racist attitudes towards people from different ethnic backgrounds, but very often it springs from indifference or failure of imagination. Repeatedly, Salvadoran and Vietnamese women expressed satisfaction with service delivery simply because they encountered one or two people who made every attempt to understand their needs and overcome their anxieties. They recounted with amusement and good humour the mimes and hand signals or line drawings that had been the last resort when words failed. A Salvadoran woman expressed her reason for travelling across the city to a particular hospital thus:

Well, whenever I think of the trouble of travelling I also remember how nice the sister was when I first went. She tried so hard and telephoned for an interpreter but there was nobody to help her. The only words I understood were 'please' and 'interpreter'. In the end she gave me a card with an appointment on Thursday but she looked so upset and I think she was telling me to 'Please come back on Thursday when the interpreter will be here.'—So I thought I should go, as she tried so hard to help me. I didn't want to disappoint her. (Salvadoran woman, 38 years old)

The idea of 'access' needs to incorporate the notion of continued utilization of a service. This is especially true with respect to women's health where preventive and follow-up care are important. Avoidance of regular screening for breast or cervical cancer and failure to return to a hospital for postnatal checks were attributed by the women to dissatisfaction with the service. In the main, such dissatisfaction derived from feelings of alienation because of negative experiences. In examining the stories and comments of migrant women several strategies present themselves as ways to solve problems of access. At one level there are the 'macro', institutional solutions which would mean increased language learning facilities for women, development of interpreter services, in-service training for health workers, and provision of written material informing women, in their own language, on health issues and services. At another level, much more consideration needs to be given to the development of communication skills of all health workers so that they pursue problems with a view to developing culturally sensitive solutions and responses. Extreme passivity, nervousness, hostility or obvious distress can be seen by the health worker as signals of a problem which needs to be explored. Curiosity, imagination and a willingness to accommodate difference (rather than seeing it as threatening or disruptive) are fundamental to the improvement of migrant women's access to health services. But whereas institutional change can be achieved by policy and procedural revision, the changes in attitude, personal interaction and awareness of cross-cultural variations require education and the development of flexibility and responsiveness among providers of health care. Migrant women make enormous cultural adjustments and changes as they adapt to their situation. By comparison, the cultural changes required of health providers are not nearly so dauntingly huge as is sometimes imagined. Moreover, the changes in the culture of health service provision that would enhance migrant access are those that encourage pluralism and flexibility that would benefit all Australians disadvantaged by the narrowness and institutional rigidity of current services.

NOTES

1. There are numerous studies of migrant health and the health needs of people from non-English speaking backgrounds. Published research by the National Health Strategy (1993), Alcorso and Schofield (1991), Reid and Trompf (1990) and Powles and Gifford (1990) provide a wide range of information, policy recommendations and insights into the problems of access for immigrant women.
2. Associate Professor Lorraine Dennerstein of The Key Centre for Women's Health and Dr Martha Macintyre undertook this research as a joint project.
3. In this paper I have refrained from giving detailed, tabulated data in the interest of brevity and accessibility. My concern is to raise issues and indicate broad findings. More detailed analysis of the study of Migrant Women's Access to Health Services in hospitals will be found in Macintyre and Dennerstein (forthcoming). The study into migrant women's access was funded by DILGEA and was a joint project of the Key Centre for Women's Health, University of Melbourne, the Mercy Hospital for Women in Melbourne, and the Sociology Department, La Trobe University. I thank Maria Robles, Rocio Amezquita, Ha Tranh Anh, Lan Vuong and Raffaela Lopez for their assistance in the research on which this paper draws.
4. While almost all surveys of migrant women's experience of health services generate anecdotal evidence, studies such as that by the Health Department Victoria (1991) and material referred to in Lee and Silburn [WICAG] (not dated) indicate that there are serious problems in the areas of informed consent and patients' rights.
5. The belief that physical well-being depends on a person actively maintaining the balance of those elements that make up the body is found in many cultures (see Parsons 1990:113). The idea of distinct, complementary elements in Chinese medicine is referred to as yin/yang opposition. Vietnamese culture draws on Chinese traditions to a great extent and the yin/yang relationship is central to ideas of health as a harmonious state and illness as a manifestation of imbalance.

REFERENCES

Alcorso C, Schofield T 1991 The national non-English speaking background women's health strategy. Australian Government Publishing Service, Canberra

Health Department Victoria 1991 Health services and ethnic communities: report of the ministerial taskforce on ethnic health. Health Department Victoria, Melbourne

Lee S, Silburn K n.d. An analysis of the existing literature on informed consent in relation to obstetrics and gynaecology and women of non-English speaking background. Women's Informed Consent Action Group and Women's Health Service for the West

National Health Strategy 1993 Issues Paper No 6 Removing cultural and language barriers to health

Parsons, C 1990 Cross-cultural issues in health care. In: Reid J and Trompf P (eds) The health of immigrant Australia: a social perspective. Harcourt Brace Jovanovich, Sydney

Powles J, Gifford S 1990 How healthy are Australia's immigrants? In: Reid J, Trompf P (eds) The health of immigrant Australia: a social perspective. Harcourt Brace Jovanovich, Sydney

Reid J, Trompf P (eds) 1990 The health of immigrant Australia: a social perspective. Harcourt Brace Jovanovich, Sydney

11. Ethnicity, illness and aged people

Varoe Legge   Mary T. Westbrook

Australia, in common with all other developed countries, has an ageing population. In addition Australia has one of the most culturally diverse populations in the world. People over the age of 65 years accounted for 11.1% of the population in 1990. This figure is expected to reach 12.3% by 2001, 17.6% in 2021 and 21.5% by the year 2031 (Rowland 1991). In 1990 immigrants to Australia represented 23% of the population, of whom 22.5% were born in the United Kingdom or Ireland, 30.2% elsewhere in Europe and 21.5% in Asia and the Middle East (Australian Bureau of Statistics 1992, National Population Council 1991). The people from non-English speaking backgrounds (NESB) are primarily the result of the large migration inflow which commenced at the end of World War II, augmented by aged family members arriving under family reunion provisions. The majority of the ethnic aged migrated while young or in early middle age. They have lived in Australia for many decades and they are eligible for all the available social service benefits. The important, though considerably smaller, segment of the NESB aged who migrated to rejoin their already established children are eligible for all social service benefits, housing and medical services, however the aged pension is obtainable only after 10 years' residence unless a special benefit is obtained.

The rapid changes which are taking place in the composition of Australia's aged population are evident when the statistics from 1981 to 2001 are examined. In 1981 the largest numbers of NESB born overseas came from Italy, Poland, the Netherlands, Germany, Greece, Yugoslavia, the USSR/Ukraine, the Baltic States, Hungary, India, Malta, China, Egypt, Austria and Czechoslovakia. This order changes when the ranking criterion used is the proportions of the birthplace groups who are aged. The Australian Institute of Multicultural Affairs (AIMA 1983) used 1981 census data to show that 44% of people from the Baltic area were over 60 years old followed by the Ukraine/USSR (43%), Poland (36%), Hungary (27%), China (22%) and Czechoslovakia (20%). Table 11.1 shows the rapidity at which selected migrant groups are ageing.

Many of these national groups are composites of a number of different peoples whose language, religion and history differ. In addition their reasons

Table 11.1 Projected percentage changes in age groups from 1991 to 2001 of Australian residents born overseas and in selected countries.

Age group	Overseas	Country of birth			
		Germany	Greece	Italy	Baltic states
40–59	74.6	24.8	−6.4	−25.4	−69.9
60–64	105.8	129.4	445.7	129.2	−33.7
65–69	104.8	164.2	406.4	165.4	−43.6
70–74	105.2	334.8	361.8	204.6	−14.9
75 +	147.0	340.5	356.9	210.9	153.1

Source: AIMA 1983

for migrating and their experiences in their countries of origin, were extremely diverse. The countries from which they came also had very different educational systems, levels of economic development and political systems. As a result generalizations about immigrants' values, needs and attitudes should be treated with extreme caution. In addition to the pre-migration factors there are those associated with post migration experiences. The attitude of the Australian government was strongly assimilationist in the early post World War II period. Migrants were expected to accept the values and behaviours of the host society. This attitude gradually changed to an integrationist position. In the 1980s multiculturalism was recognized by all Australian governments as the official policy. Economic circumstances at the time of arrival also changed. During the long post war boom immigrants were fully employed although usually in blue collar, heavy labouring work. Major economic recessions however occurred in the 1970s, 1980s and 1990s, and newcomers have experienced high levels of unemployment. As a result of these two factors migrants vary considerably in their post-migration experiences. The above changes have been documented in both governmental review enquiries and academic writing and as a result a number of initiatives have been instituted which are designed to improve migrants' access to services and to sensitize professionals who are involved in the delivery of such services.

English language fluency is one of the crucial factors in being able to access services and in communication between professionals and clients. Lack of English language competence is also an indicator of the extent to which a person, or group of people, is likely to retain the values of their country of origin as they existed at the time of migration. Despite the differences mentioned above, for all NESB immigrant groups in Australia three generalizations can be made: older people are less likely to be fluent in English than are younger people, women are less likely to speak English than are men and the fewer the years of schooling in the country of origin the greater the likelihood that the person will not use English at home or in conversation. It follows, therefore, that aged women with few educational skills are the group most at risk of inadequate support and inappropriate professional and medical treatment. They are also the group most likely to have retained the values and behaviours of their youth.

The issue of ethnic differences in behaviour when ill is an important one in a multicultural society where increasing numbers of patients and practitioners come from non-Anglo backgrounds. The aim of the survey reported in this chapter was to compare the illness behaviour of aged people in six Australian communities, five ethnic and the mainstream Anglo community whose values can be considered to dominate the provision of health services.

The five ethnic communities in the survey were the Chinese, German, Greek, Italian and Arabic speaking. These communities were chosen because they are particularly large and/or significantly different in their values from the core Anglo Australian community. They represent some of the oldest and newest immigrant groups, the most highly educated and the least educated, ones whose members arrived as displaced people and refugees and others whose members have been involved in a well established chain migration program.

The major migration period for people from Germany was the 1950s. Their educational profile is similar to that of the host society, although slightly higher percentages are in the professional and administrative categories. They have been highly exogamous (marrying outside the community) and geographically disbursed (Jupp 1988). Only 7% of aged Germans do not use English at home (Pensabene & Kabala 1986). People of Chinese origin are the most recent and currently the largest of the immigrant groups. There was a small well-established Chinese community which had been in Australia for many generations. The present flow of Chinese immigrants commenced in the early 1970s and it has not yet peaked. The group therefore has a low median age, however as family reunion has been comparatively easily obtainable, a large number of parents have arrived. The younger generations have high English language ability and educational standards considerably higher than those existing in the host society (Jupp 1988). Australians of Chinese ancestry have been attracted to the health professions; they are proportionally strongly over represented as medical practitioners and nurses. Few of the parent generation speak English, nor is their educational level high. The older generation is almost exclusively endogamous, (marrying within the group) the younger generation is not.

The Greek and Arabic speaking communities differ again; endogamous, with poor English language skills and educational achievement, they tend to be geographically concentrated. However the high point of Greek migration took place several decades before that of the Arabic speaking group. As a result 23% of the Greek community is over 55 years old as against only 11–12% of the Arabic speaking community. Sixty per cent of aged Greeks do not speak English well or do not speak it at all. This figure can be further divided into 49% of men and 72% of women who either do not speak English well or at all (Bureau of Immigration Research 1990). This pattern has reduced the likelihood of cultural transmissions and it has been argued that the values of the aged are similar to those of their country of origin as they existed at the time of migration (Storer 1985). Although the possibility of cultural change existed through continued chain migration, in actuality both the Greek and Italian communities are experiencing a reverse flow as aged people remigrate rather than have younger members arriving in Australia (Birrell 1990).

Italian migration to Australia commenced prior to World War II. Many rural areas, especially those in fruit growing and irrigation areas attracted comparatively large Italian communities. During World War II a number of prisoners of war arrived many of whom stayed in Australia and acted as anchors in an active family reunion program. Despite the length of time in Australia, the Italian community maintained strong links with their families in Italy, and it has also maintained a considerable degree of geographic concentration. Spouses were sought in Italy when suitable Italo-Australians were not available. It was possible to live in Australia without learning English, and, as most of the immigrants were from village society, language and values were slow to change.

Illness behaviour

People from different cultures vary in their beliefs about the causes of illness, in their behaviour when ill and in their expectations as to how illness should be treated (Helman 1986). Cultural differences in illness behaviour have been well documented in anthropological literature (Harwood 1981, Kleinman 1980). However, relatively little research has examined the effect of cultural factors on illness behaviour within western societies. Zola's (1966) classic study showed variations in illness behaviour between Jewish, Italian, Irish and Anglo Americans. The groups differed in their descriptions of similar symptoms and the effects of illness on their daily lives and personal relationships. In Australia, Westbrook et al (1993) found that in many ethnic communities people with a wide range of disabling and chronic health conditions were more stigmatized and more likely to be excluded from social roles than were Anglo Australians who had disabilities.

Health practitioners' beliefs regarding appropriate sick role behaviours and their professional assessment of symptoms are unconsciously located within their cultural backgrounds. Payer (1988) argued that physicians in Germany, France, England and America not only describe but diagnose conditions differently. Workshops conducted by, and for, interpreters in the New South Wales Department of Health provided evidence of the extent to which culture influences illness behaviour. The interpreters also discussed the difficulties resulting from the imposition of Anglo Australian values by health professionals (Legge 1981, 1982). Davitz and Davitz (1980) surveyed nurses from 13 countries and reported significant cultural differences in their perceptions of patients' pain and suffering. For instance English nurses inferred that patients were experiencing the least amount of physical pain and these nurses occupied the ninth rank in their estimation of patients' psychological distress. Health practitioners tend to approve of, and treat more benignly, those patients whose illness behaviour resembles that of the practitioner's culture. The Davitzes reported that American nurses were highly approving of Asian patients' more stoical behaviour when in pain. Surveys of staff in Sydney nursing homes found that staff experienced more tension when caring for NESB residents than Anglo residents (Westbrook & Legge 1990a,b). However the patterns of tension associated with nursing Greek, Italian and Chinese residents differed significantly. For example, the major tension that nurses reported when caring for Greek and Italian patients occurred when patients were experiencing pain. Greek patients' behaviour toward staff, particularly in regard to touching staff, caused problems. Even though Chinese patients had poorer English speaking skills and had been in Australia for fewer years than the other two groups, nurses reported experiencing less tension in caring for them. This was due to Chinese patients' illness behaviour meshing more comfortably with staff values. While NESB residents in nursing homes experience difficulties in interacting with Anglo staff, Anglo residents encounter difficulties with NESB nursing and domestic staff due to differences in language and attitudes (Westbrook & Legge 1991).

Survey of illness behaviour

Method

A questionnaire was devised to measure community attitudes towards ageing and health care. Respondents were asked to answer the questions 'in terms of your experiences with the Australian (respondent's) community'. The question which examined illness behaviour had the following instructions: 'People differ in their beliefs as to how you should act when you are sick. Do you think the typical older person in the Australian (respondent's) community would agree or disagree with each of the following statements?' The question consisted of the 18 items. Seven were concerned with beliefs about illness (see Table 11.2), five covered treatment preferences (see Table 11.3) and six investigated attitudes toward health practitioners (see Table 11.4). Four optional answers were provided for each item, viz. strongly agree, agree, disagree and strongly disagree.

The questionnaire was completed by 371 health workers from the six communities, viz. Anglo (72), Arabic (54), Chinese (69), German (32), Greek (62) and Italian (82). To be included in one of the community samples a respondent had to identify him or herself as a member of that ethnic community and to have some involvement in providing health care to community members. Health workers were chosen as subjects because they were seen as community representatives competent to report on both the cultural and health care issues being investigated.

Female health workers made up 67% of the total group and predominated in all samples except the Arabic speaking, of which they comprised 45% of subjects. The average age of the respondents was 42 years. The percentages of the samples who were born in Australia were Arabic (6%), Chinese (4%), German (0%), Greek (37%), Italian (33%) and Anglo Australians (82%). The average age at arrival in the country of members of the NESB groups born overseas ranged from 19 years (Greeks) to 27 years (Germans and Chinese). Only 2% of the ethnic respondents had a parent who was born in Australia.

The survey was conducted in Sydney. The NESB samples were recruited by consulting lists of ethnic health practitioners and contacting ethnic health, welfare and social organizations to request names of health workers. Anglo Australian respondents were contacted via community health centres. Initially respondents were contacted by phone and asked if they would participate in the survey. Questionnaires were then mailed to the respondents who returned them anonymously. The return rates from the various communities was as follows: Anglo (72%), Arabic (51%), Chinese (69%), Greek (61%), German (60%) and Italian (80%). Chi square analyses were performed to examine whether there were significant differences in community attitudes.

Results

The results of the chi square analyses (see Table 11.2) revealed significant community differences in six of the seven illness beliefs investigated.

Table 11.2 Results of chi square analyses comparing illness beliefs of the aged in six Australian communities

Community endorsement[1]							χ^2
Arabic	Chinese	German	Greek	Italian	Anglo	Total	(df 5)
When you feel pain you should conceal your distress							
22(43%)	39(57%)	15(48%)	21(34%)	23(29%)	40(56%)	160(44%)	17.92**
When you are sick you should try to regain your independence as soon as possible							
36(67%)	58(84%)	32(100%)	44(72%)	49(61%)	67(93%)	286(78%)	37.99***
If you take proper care of yourself (e.g. good diet, exercise) you will ensure that you remain healthy							
41(77%)	67(97%)	31(97%)	45(75%)	53(65%)	57(79%)	294(80%)	30.37***
There's not much you can do to protect yourself from ill health							
27(51%)	24(35%)	6(19%)	26(43%)	32(40%)	20(28%)	135(37%)	12.84*
Not much can be done to alleviate the health problems of the aged							
25(46%)	35(52%)	15(47%)	28(46%)	44(56%)	32(44%)	179(49%)	2.63
When you feel sick it is usual to tell people all about your symptoms							
45(83%)	58(84%)	14(45%)	51(84%)	67(83%)	39(55%)	274(75%)	39.60***
When you are ill you like to have lots of visitors							
48(89%)	43(62%)	9(29%)	44(72%)	49(61%)	27(38%)	220(60%)	49.44***

* p <.05, ** p <.01, *** p <.001

[1] Numbers and percentages of respondents who strongly agreed or agreed

All groups, with the exception of the Chinese, were less in favour than were the Anglo Australians of concealing distress when in pain. The Anglo and German communities believed more strongly than the other communities that sick people should try and regain their independence as soon as possible. German and Anglo Australians wanted fewer visitors when ill and considered it less appropriate to tell other people about their symptoms. Relative to the Italians, Arabs and Greeks, the Chinese, German and Anglo Australians considered that people can exert control over their health; 97% of the Chinese and German respondents endorsed the importance of factors such as diet and exercise whereas only 65% of the Italians did so. The Arabic speaking group was the most fatalistic concerning their health; over half of the group said that aged people believe there is little they can do to protect themselves from ill health whereas 28% or less of the Anglo and German aged were said to hold this view. However the communities reported similar beliefs regarding what can be done to alleviate health problems that occur; 49% of the total group believed that not much can be done for the aged. Overall this set of findings indicated a marked similarity in the illness beliefs of older German and Anglo Australians. The Chinese also resembled the Anglo aged in their preferences for concealing pain, regaining independence and attempting to maintain health.

Significant community differences were found regarding four of the five attitudes toward medical treatment (see Table 11.3). The Greek and Anglo aged were believed to be less likely than the aged in other communities to criticize modern medicine for being too interventionist. All NESB communities were described as being more in favour of traditional remedies than were Anglo Australians. For example, 87% of Chinese and 76% of Arabic respondents reported that aged people believed that traditional

Table 11.3 Results of chi square analyses comparing treatment preferences of the aged in six Australian communities

	Community endorsement[1]						χ^2
Arabic	Chinese	German	Greek	Italian	Anglo	Total	(df 5)
Modern medicine is too interventionist(e.g. too much surgery)							
38(73%)	52(75%)	19(63%)	30(52%)	52(63%)	40(57%)	231(64%)	10.96*
Traditional and home remedies work better than modern medicine							
24(44%)	40(58%)	11(34%)	20(33%)	29(37%)	20(28%)	144(39%)	16.13**
Home or traditional remedies should be tried before seeking medical advice							
41(76%)	60(87%)	17(55%)	30(49%)	50(62%)	32(44%)	230(63%)	37.19***
Injections are more effective than oral medicine							
41(77%)	54(78%)	19(61%)	33(59%)	66(81%)	26(37%)	239(66%)	44.22***
When you are ill you feel safer being cared for in hospital							
33(64%)	46(67%)	27(84%)	43(71%)	55(67%)	43(61%)	247(67%)	6.35

* p <.05, ** p <.01, *** p <.001
[1] Numbers and percentages of respondents who strongly agreed or agreed

Table 11.4 Results of chi square analyses comparing the attitudes regarding health practitioners of the aged in six Australian communities

Community endorsement[1]							χ^2
Arabic	Chinese	German	Greek	Italian	Anglo	Total	(df 5)
Doctors should explain the diagnosis to the patient							
47(90%)	64(93%)	32(100%)	52(85%)	67(84%)	60(85%)	322(88%)	8.87
Doctors should give the diagnosis to the family rather than the patient							
25(48%)	26(39%)	5(16%)	24(41%)	39(49%)	9(13%)	128(35%)	32.95***
Doctors know what is best for patients							
44(83%)	54(78%)	22(69%)	41(67%)	48(60%)	42(58%)	251(68%)	14.37**
Doctors should discuss the treatment options with their patients							
48(89%)	65(94%)	32(100%)	58(95%)	73(90%)	64(89%)	340(92%)	6.16
Doctors are inclined to give patients too much medication							
31(60%)	39(57%)	25(78%)	36(59%)	57(70%)	57(79%)	245(67%)	13.20*
Patients should be cared for by nurses and therapists of the same sex as themselves							
43(81%)	33(48%)	8(25%)	30(49%)	46(57%)	37(51%)	197(54%)	28.55***

* p <.05, ** p <.01, *** p <.001
[1] Numbers and percentages of respondents who strongly agreed or agreed.

remedies should be tried before seeking medical advice compared to 44% of Anglo Australians. Moreover, 58% of Chinese and 44% of Arab respondents said that older community members believed that such remedies worked better than modern medicine whereas only 28% of the Anglo aged were reported to do so. All communities had much greater faith in the efficacy of injections over oral medication than did Anglo Australians. No significant differences were found in community preferences for being hospitalized when ill. Overall the findings revealed that the treatment preferences of aged people in NESB communities were described as differing significantly from those of Anglo Australians. Once again Germans' attitudes were seen as similar to those of the core culture as were those of the Greeks.

Community attitudes toward health practitioners were found to vary significantly regarding four of the six issues investigated (see Table 11.4). While the communities were similar in their strong belief that doctors should explain the diagnosis to the patient and discuss treatment options, the Anglo and German aged were significantly less likely than those in the other communities to consider that doctors should give the diagnosis to the family rather than the patient. The communities differed significantly in the faith they had in their doctors' views. The Arabic speaking and Chinese aged were most likely to believe that doctors know what is best while Anglo Australians were the group least likely to agree with this statement. The majority of respondents in all samples considered that older community members thought that doctors over prescribe, but this view was most strongly endorsed by Germans, Anglo Australians and Italians. There were significant differences in aged people's preferences that they be cared for by nurses and therapists of the same sex as themselves. Arabs gave the strongest endorsement to this item and Germans the least. Overall these results indicated that the aged in NESB communities differed from the Anglo aged in having greater faith in doctors' knowledge and prescribing patterns. There were also marked differences in the preferred method of communication of diagnoses and some differences in attitudes regarding the appropriate sex of those caring for the sick. Again the Germans exhibited similar attitudes to the Anglo aged. The Italians' attitudes were also similar to those of Anglo Australians except for a strong preference that diagnoses be communicated to the family rather than to the patient. Arabic attitudes deviated most from those of the core culture.

Discussion

When considering the sickness behaviour of the frail aged, it is seldom the case that the enormous cultural diversity of the Australian population is fully appreciated. The results of the survey demonstrate that illness beliefs, behaviours and treatment preferences spread across a very wide range, with those of aged people from Germany being closest to those of Anglo Australians. While these results were not unexpected, given the composition of the various migrating groups, they have not previously been sufficiently analysed in relation to health, health professionals and the health delivery system.

Modernization theorists have postulated a connection between the ascribed roles of traditional societies and the achieved roles of industrialized societies and the values held in such societies. Traditional roles are associated with particularistic ascriptive values and community based relationships, whereas in industrialized society roles are more likely to be individualistic, competitive and based on rational, scientific values. The results of our survey indicate that medical sociology needs to incorporate an understanding of the values which underlie sickness behaviour in a society such as Australia, which is composed of people from many different cultures whose degree of modernity differs widely.

The responses to the questionnaire indicated there is an association between both individualistic values and the degree of modernity in the communities' societies of origin, and their aged people's feelings of control of health outcomes, concealment of pain, and preference for privacy when ill. When assessing attitudes to medicine, people from societies with strong medical traditions, e.g. Chinese and Arabic, were more likely to see modern medicine as too interventionist and to endorse traditional remedies. The Anglo Australians were the only community which did not view oral medicine as less effective than injections. Despite these differences, respondents from all six communities endorsed the view that sick people feel safer in hospital. There were considerable differences in community preferences regarding the communication of diagnoses. Almost all Anglo Australians and Germans considered that the patient should be told, whereas less than half the Italian and Arabic respondents considered that the patient should be told. There was however strong endorsement by all communities that the doctor should explain the diagnosis to, and discuss treatment options with, the patient.

For health professionals and for service providers the research has considerable implications regarding the design of interventions and the education of health professionals. For the community respondents themselves, the study may be useful in understanding and explaining aspects of service delivery and the attitudes of health professionals. In the past, cultural differences in illness behaviour received little attention in education programs for health practitioners, but an increasing number of training institutions now incorporate elements of multicultural studies in their curricula in order to sensitize health workers to the importance of culture in the definition and description of, and reactions to illness. However the task of understanding cultural variations in a society which comprises over one hundred different groups is clearly impossible. Furthermore what Fitzgerald (1992) describes as the 'cookbook' approach of compiling lists of illness beliefs and behaviours assumes that the information applies to all people in a community and ignores the diversity within communities. The aged, the young, first and second generation members of a community and those who have received tertiary education particularly in the health sciences, will all vary in their beliefs about and reactions to illness. The 'cookbook' approach can lead to stereotyping when knowledge about a community's beliefs are overgeneralized and patients' individual characteristics are ignored. Our research has shown that Anglo Australian health practitioners are becoming more sensitized to the dangers of stereotyping. Some react to discussion of cultural differences in illness behaviour by arguing that a client's ethnicity is irrelevant; an ethnic patient needs to be treated with 'tender loving care' as an individual (Legge & Westbrook 1989, Westbrook et al 1991). Such an approach may lead to ethnocentric misinterpretation of patients' behaviour and to the provision of care that is meant to be, but is not, interpreted by the client as either tender or loving.

Health practitioners require a flexible approach. Turner (1990) has suggested a tripartite diagnostic paradigm which takes account of clients' biology, culture and individuality. It asks, 'How is this client like all human beings? How is this client like some human beings? How is this client like no other human being?' (Turner 1990:16). In answering the second question Fitzgerald (1992) suggests that health practitioners expand their knowledge of the ethnic communities from which their clients are drawn but that they also develop an interviewing style that elicits culturally relevant information from patients. She suggests the use of Kleinman et al's (1978) protocol which asks patients questions such as: What do you think has caused your problems? Why do you think it started when it did? What are the chief problems your sickness (injury) has caused you? Pfifferling (1981) proposed a similar 'cultural status exam' which includes questions such as: What do you think is wrong, out of balance or causing your problems? What do you think will help to clear up your problem? Apart from me who, or what, else do you think can help you get better?

The present survey has examined a relatively small sample of illness behaviours. Furthermore it has sampled health practitioners from ethnic communities rather than aged people themselves. Research is needed to investigate both a wider range of illness beliefs and treatment preferences and a more representative sample of community respondents. Overall the results reveal the wide range of attitudes toward health and health care that exist among aged people in Australian communities. Appreciation of such differences is essential in the provision of quality health care and successful public health programs.

REFERENCES

Australian Bureau of Statistics 1992 Social indicators. Australian Bureau of Statistics, Canberra

Australian Institute of Multicultural Studies 1983 Papers on the ethnic aged. Australian Institute of Multicultural Affairs, Melbourne

Birrell R 1990 The chains that bind: family reunions migration to Australia in the 1980s. Australian Government Publishing Service, Canberra

Bureau of Immigration Research 1990 Community profiles. Australian Government Publishing Service, Canberra

Davitz L J, Davitz J R 1980 Nurses' responses to patients' suffering. Springer, New York

Fitzgerald M H 1992 Multicultural clinical interactions. Journal of Rehabilitation 58(2):38–42

Harwood A 1981 Ethnicity and medical care. Harvard University Press, Cambridge

Helman C 1986 Culture, health and illness. Wright, Bristol

Jupp J (ed) 1988 The Australian people: an encyclopaedia of the nation, its people and their origins. Angus & Robertson, Sydney

Kleinman A 1980 Patients and healers in the context of culture: an explanation of the borderland between anthropology, medicine and psychiatry. University of California, Berkeley

Kleinman A, Eisenberg L, Good B 1978 Culture, illness and care: clinical lessons from anthropologic and cross-cultural research. Annals of Internal Medicine 88:251–258

Legge V 1981 Migrants and health. Cumberland College of Health Sciences, Sydney

Legge V 1982 Disability in cultural context. Cumberland College of Health Sciences, Sydney

Legge V, Westbrook M T 1989 Provisions made for ethnic patients in nursing homes. Australian Journal on Ageing 8(4):7–14

National Population Council Population Issues Committee 1991 Population issues and Australia's future. Australian Government Publishing Service, Canberra

Payer L 1988 Medicine and culture: varieties of treatment in the United States, England, West Germany and France. Gollantz, New York

Pensabene T, Kabala M 1986 Conduct and findings of the survey of aged migrants. In: Australian Institute of Multicultural Affairs: community and institutional care for aged migrants in Australia. Australian Institute of Multicultural Affairs, Melbourne

Pfifferling J H 1981 A cultural prescription for mediocentrism. In: Eisenberg L, Kleinman A (eds) The relevance of social science for medicine. Reidel, Dordrecht

Rowland D T 1991 Ageing in Australia. Longman Cheshire, Melbourne

Storer D (ed) 1985 Ethnic family values in Australia. Prentice-Hall, Sydney

Turner F J 1990 Social work practice and theory: a transcultural resource for health care. Social Science and Medicine 31:13–17

Westbrook M T, Legge V 1990a Ethnic residents in nursing homes: a staff perspective. Australian Social Work 43(3):15–26

Westbrook M T, Legge V 1990b Staff perceptions of caring for Italian, Greek and Chinese
nursing home residents. Australian Journal on Ageing 9(3):22–26
Westbrook M T, Legge V 1991 Life in a mainstream nursing home: a survey of Chinese,
Greek and Anglo Australians. Australian Journal on Ageing 10(4):11–16
Westbrook M T, Legge V, Pennay M 1993 Attitudes toward disabilities in a multicultural
society. Social Science and Medicine 36:615–623
Westbrook M T, Skropeta C M, Legge V 1991 Ethnic clients in diversional therapy
programs. Australian Occupational Therapy Journal 38:251–258
Zola I K 1966 Culture and symptoms: an analysis of patients' presenting complaints.
American Sociological Review 31:615–630

12. The social inequality of dying

Allan Kellehear

What lessons about social inequality can be learned through a study of human dying behaviour? Sociological studies of conscious dying behaviour have seldom explored this question. It is more common to find studies that link social status (e.g. age, occupation, religious affiliation) to people's treatment of the comatose (Sudnow 1967; Simpson 1976) or already dead (Prior 1989).

So in this chapter, I shall revisit my own earlier sociological study of dying (reported in Kellehear & Fook 1989, and Kellehear 1990) and offer some reflections and observations through the prism of social inequality. That study discussed the findings of interviews with 100 terminally ill cancer sufferers with less than 12 months to live. My task was to connect their beliefs and behaviour to the broader cultural and historical influences of modern Australian society.

As I look back to that study, several interesting observations emerge around the general question of social inequality. These observations do not exhaust every aspect of the problem of inequality but they are sufficient to illustrate two of the most important dimensions of it. These may be described as the structural and the interpersonal dimensions of the experience of inequality. By structural dimension, I refer to the disempowered patterns of social fortune and treatment associated with broad group characteristics such as age, ethnicity or gender. These are indirectly associated with any social study of cancer. Most discussions in health sociology textbooks focus on this indirect experience of inequality. They attempt to show how health in Australia is very much determined by group membership. Whom and how these groups live influences the likelihood of their health, illness or death, although the members of that group may not *consciously* be aware of this inequality. On the other hand, there are much fewer discussions about the interpersonal dimension of inequality. When I refer to an interpersonal dimension of inequality, I mean the experience of inequality which comes to people directly and consciously through their day to day encounters with other people. Through examples from the study of dying, it is easy to see that dying can be seen to both reflect *and* create problems of social inequality. I will begin, as other writers do, by discussing how dying reflects structural inequalities in the wider society. But then I will move to a discussion of how interpersonal inequalities are created by the circumstance of dying itself.

The aim of focussing on both structural and interpersonal dimensions of dying behaviour is to reunite the impersonal and personal elements of inequality. I will demonstrate that a sociological study of inequality is not simply about historical and political forces as abstract as 'white settlement' or the social conventions surrounding the 'sick role'. Inequality is also mediated and felt in social encounters by people who experience these encounters as highly personal and individual. And yet focussing on these personal experiences can revise some of our views about patterns of social inequality just as surely as a focus on solely structural issues. Some of these important insights are summarized at the end of the chapter.

The structural experience of inequality

One of the first observations that one makes about cancer, particularly the solid tumour variety (e.g. bowel, breast, lung cancers) is that it is a disease of modern affluence. The mean age of respondents in my study was 59 years of age. This highlights the fact that cancer is a degenerative disease, in other words, a disease associated with ageing. This fact is of only recent origins.

In the Middle Ages in Europe the life expectancy of the typical peasant worker was in the twenties. The bourgeois and aristocracy who experienced better housing, food and daily work conditions could expect, on average, to live into their forties. In this context, low life expectancy was only partially due to high infant mortality. The spread of better housing, food and work conditions to all social classes after the Industrial Revolution, and particularly after the First World War, meant that life expectancy rose sharply only this century for most Anglo-Europeans around the world. Before this century, high infant mortality, infectious diseases, accidents and war took a great toll on average life expectancy. When living conditions improved, most people were able to grow old and then, of course, they began to experience the diseases of old age: rheumatic illnesses, cancers, and diseases of the circulatory system (e.g. heart attacks, strokes etc). In an ironic way, cancer can be seen as a status symbol for any population who has successfully managed to get most of its members to grow old. In Australia therefore, one might imagine that this applies to all of our people. But this is not true.

In the sample of one hundred terminally ill cancer respondents in my study *Dying of Cancer* (Kellehear 1990) there was not one Australian Aborigine. This does not mean that Aborigines do not develop the disease nor does it mean that the sampling procedure undertaken by the study was exceptionally unusual. The sample of the study represented most of the people defined by doctors as terminally ill over a period of fifteen months. In that time, and in the places where the study was conducted, no Aborigines were met. There are several reasons for this experience. First, most Aborigines live in rural areas (Kellehear 1988) so there are significantly fewer Aborigines in ratio to white people in the cities. This is particularly the case in Newcastle, where the major part of the sample was drawn. This means only a larger sample over a longer time would procure Aboriginal respondents. Secondly, Aboriginal people tend to use Aboriginal health personnel and services if and when these are available in their area, thereby further reducing the prospect of meeting Aborigines in services used mainly by whites. But in epidemiological terms, that is, in terms of the pattern of illness and death across Australia's population, cancer affects marginally fewer of Australian Aborigines. One possible reason for this is simply that the average Australian Aborigine doesn't live long enough to develop the illness at the same rates as their white counterparts.

The average life expectancy of Australian Aborigines is some 15–20 years less than for non-Aboriginal populations in Australia. Saggers and Gray (1991:102) estimate that for Aborigines in rural New South Wales, this life expectancy is as low as 51 for males and 59 for females. Other illnesses significantly shorten the life expectancy of Australian Aborigines. Aboriginal deaths due to respiratory illness are almost three times higher than for whites. Indeed Lincoln and others (1987) report that the mortality rate from infectious disease is 90 times the average in Queensland alone. The structural aspects of cancer, that is, who develops it and at what rates, show us on first inspection that as a disease it occurs disproportionately among the old, being the leading cause of death among Australians (Castles 1992). But the absence of Aborigines in my study *Dying of Cancer* highlights the epidemiological plight of another sector of Australian society. The lesser rates of cancer for Aborigines does not highlight a better lifestyle, or more successful strategies of prevention, but is tragically only the further consequence of a lifestyle of poverty and marginality characteristic of life as an Aborigine in Australia.

Another structural observation one may make about inequality and dying of cancer is about gender differences. When working in a Sydney hospice (a place where some dying people spend their remaining time in round-the-clock nursing care) I noticed that most of the residents were women. Indeed the high proportion of women in hospice care is quite common. This is an interesting phenomenon given that cancer rates are generally higher for men (Castles 1992:11). What are the possible reasons then, for the apparent disproportionate number of women in hospices?

To begin with, according to the Australian Institute of Health and Welfare (1992) men have a shorter life expectancy than women from birth and across the lifespan generally. Twice as many working age men (25–64 yrs) compared to women die and three times as many young adult men (15–24 yrs). So although the rates of cancer are higher in men, there are fewer men than women at the older age groups expected to develop cancer. However, this factor alone must explain very little of the problem. More relevant is the probability issue of who, of an average pool of men and women, will die first and in that case be cared for by the other. If men are more likely to die earlier than women, then it is likely that very many women will not have their male spouses around to care for them. In a single income nuclear family this would lead to a higher proportion of women than men being the subject of institutional care, e.g. hospices and nursing homes. The interesting conclusion one may draw from this is that, although cancer affects marginally more men, it is women who are more likely to experience institutionalization because of it.

Finally, when discussing the practical issue of preparing for death with people who are dying, two further structural factors emerge. First, the wealthier the dying person then the more likely that this person will make preparations, and many of them. People in the higher social classes will engage lawyers and accountants to help them make financial plans. These are also the people most likely to have insurance policies, or superannuation funds or property and shareholding folios. The more educated and wealthy respondents will have thought more about forward planning and the problem of dependents. In that case of course, they are also the people more likely to have wills, to have made or discussed their own funeral plans and to have discussed arrangements for organ or body donations to medical institutions.

Poorer people more commonly do not have wills or when they make them (usually after they learn of their fatal illness) this may be the major preparation. Financial planning for these people may also be rather simpler. Common are the 'special' bank accounts with one or two thousand dollars set aside as 'untouchable' and for 'emergency' purposes only. Often these funds will be earmarked for funeral costs.

As one would expect, people who have wealth need preparation for its satisfactory disposal and dissemination in the advent of their own death. But also those who are most active in making arrangements for the security and welfare of dependents are those most likely to be able to afford them. The issue of affordability is not, however, confined to the issue of social class. There is also a tendency for men rather than women to favour legal and financial preparations for death. Furthermore, more women seem to favour 'willing' of personal items, particularly between dying mothers and their surviving daughters. The fact that most of the women in my study were older women, and that many of these had been life long 'home-makers', perhaps meant that the role of being a 'personal provider' continued even when dying. The men in the study, on the other hand, continued to see their caring role in material terms of banking, superannuation, will making, the purchase of prepaid funeral plans and so on.

In summary then, the structural features of dying of cancer in Australian society demonstrate that people die very much in the way that they have lived. In social terms this means that people's lives are rarely altered by them in radical ways which contradict the usual social positions and expectations they have had as men or women, wealthy or poor, young or old. Furthermore, the fact that more or less of one group is represented in various treatment centres points to patterns of health and illness as diverse as the epidemiology of Aboriginal health or the people most likely to become personal carers of the elderly or terminally ill. Often people's private thoughts on life change when they are confronted by the prospect of their own death. Just as frequently friends and relatives alter their behaviour to the dying person, commonly, it must be added, in helpful and positive ways. But overall it is unusual to meet people who desire, or who actually attempt, to change their social life in major ways. Most people continue, for better or worse, 'till death do them part', to live out their remaining time within the well known and safe orbit of their usual circles of work, church and family.

However, although the broad parameters of work, church and family rarely alter for the dying person, the usual expectation and exchanges with those people do often alter. Not all of these altered relationships change for the better, and in these ways the interpersonal experience of dying can actually create, rather then simply reflect, an experience of social inequality.

The interpersonal experience of inequality

In theory, there are many ways that a person may become aware that they are dying without actually being directly told by a medical practitioner. Among those ways which emerged in my book *Dying of Cancer* were the mental association of the word 'cancer' with death; the observation of recurrence of dramatic symptoms (e.g. the return of severe pain, bleeding or lumps); observing the nervousness of their own doctors; looking one's symptoms up in a medical textbook; talking or experience with others with similar symptoms who had subsequently died; and finally, of course, overhearing about one's dismal prospects from the conversations of others. However, despite this diversity of sources, only 26% of people in the study learned in these ways that they would die from their current illness; 47% of those interviewed had no idea that their illness was terminal until told by their doctor, while a further 27% had suspicions but depended on their doctors for confirmation. If these figures are anything to judge by then, over 70% of dying cancer sufferers depend on their doctors to inform them of the gravity of the prognosis.

The survey literature in this area indicates that, at least since 1950, people overwhelmingly favour being told by their doctors whether their disease is fatal. The problem here has been that similar surveys of medical practitioners during this period have not favoured disclosure (Kellehear 1990: 79–80). The desire to prepare oneself and one's friends and family for one's own death has consistently been behind the 'need to know'. The fear held by some doctors of 'unnecessarily upsetting patients', of hysterical reactions and mental disorders, or the misplaced and non-empirical belief that 'most patients' know anyway, has meant decades of poor or absent communication on this important matter.

Since the 1980s, more doctors are beginning to disclose prognosis to the terminally ill (Veatch & Tai 1980), but the experience is complex. Younger doctors are more likely to be frank then older ones, and hospital based medical practitioners tend to be more willing in this area than the commonly older general practitioner (Bates 1979). Furthermore, there is some debate about what constitutes 'telling the patient'. Asking for an explanation and receiving an adequate one are distinctly separate issues. Some medical explanations are so cryptic and laden with jargon that many people simply do not understand. This communication difficulty revolves around the deeper problem of the inequality of professional relationships. For the terminally ill, who are sometimes fearful or anxious, the traditional view of doctors as all knowing and capable looms large, fuelled by personal hope and inadequate medical knowledge. In this unsure and unwell state, the ill person's desire to be more rather than less co-operative frequently rises, while the competing desire to question the doctor slips easily away.

The reluctance by both patient and doctor to alter the social rules in the game of 'compliant patient and medical authority' leads to frequent problems (see Kellehear & Fook 1989). In *Dying of Cancer*, one person learned of their prospects by overhearing a conversation between hospital wardsmen. Kearl (1989: 386) cites a 12-year-old boy who learnt on TV the reason for a visit to him by a local baseball star. In the program, the boy learnt that he had been suffering from cancer for the last three years and had less than a couple of months to live. These are not the appropriate ways to learn about these matters, but they will continue as long as ordinary people believe 'doctor knows best' and that it is up to professionals to decide how and how much to disclose to the dying person. In this way, dying can become an interpersonal experience of social inequality.

Of course, awareness of dying is not the only problem that dying persons may encounter with their doctors. The lack of medical knowledge, or informed consultation about medical matters, can also lead to an inability to choose treatment strategies which suit. Because it is the doctor who has both the knowledge and experience here, it is the doctor who has the ultimate control over how much or how little he or she will share with the patient. And yet the patient is dependent on the quality of this information to make decisions about the treatments which will significantly determine the quality of remaining life left.

The issue of professional authority in medicine is given greater historical and sociological discussion by Willis (1989). But from the experience and point of view of the dying person, the problem of inequality is a problem concerning lack of control. In medical encounters, this is a lack of control over information. This in turn, interferes with the usual desire to maintain personal autonomy particularly as regards decision making about the future. But this lack of control is not simply confined to encounters with professionals, although of course, this is a central concern of the sociological literature. Family and friends can contribute to the experience of inequality in surprising, but not entirely unexpected, ways.

The social reaction of friends and relatives toward the dying person is generally unchanged or, if changed, then usually this reaction is more positive. In general, people rally to help, support and maintain their relationship. But negative experiences do occur and positive experiences sometimes have negative consequences. For the moment I will focus on 14 of the 100 people interviewed whose social experiences suggest an interesting and often overlooked experience of inequality for the dying.

As adults, most people collect around them a group of friends with whom they share some common interests and values. With respect to parents, most people have developed, through mutual effort, a kind of friendship which manages to transcend the child-parent politics of their earlier years. Those who have not enjoyed this achievement have, instead, developed strategies that allow each to enjoy each other's company on regular occasions, but not so often as to threaten the independence of the now adult sons or daughters. For some dying persons, the experience of terminal cancer overturns these gains and strategies. Well meaning parents return, often insisting on greatly increased access, or occasionally, even moving in to their adult offsprings' houses. Friends, on the other hand, whom one formerly enjoyed meeting once a week, are suddenly seen two or three times daily. And spouses take on extra duties (e.g. cooking or cleaning) and sometimes extra roles (e.g. driving the kiddies to school) that the dying person formerly performed and perhaps with not a little satisfaction.

The problem, from the point of view of the dying person, is that most of these changes are well motivated. The dying person is classified by parents, friends and spouse as ill, and they react by relieving the burden of daily activities for 'the sick' one. In this process, the communication rules have altered from comparatively equal social relations to a set of exchanges which are based on 'the helpers' and 'the needy'. In this case, the needy dying person is rarely consulted. When consultation takes place it can be enthusiastically pursued by the well for the purpose of taking control over from the ill. Agreements are not checked or adjusted to the cycles of cancer illness.

People with cancer, particularly those who are receiving chemo- or radiotherapy treatments, commonly experience days of prolonged tiredness, nausea, pain and/or diarrhoea. But on other days, they can be up and about and feeling generally well. It is on these good days that the dying person feels the loss of control over some cherished and even some trivial activities and roles. The interpersonal politics of goodwill and intention so often prevent the dying from complaining or complaining too strongly for fear of appearing ungrateful. The sick role is not a set of equal expectations and exchanges. The sick are helped and they must desire to get well, but they never direct the help offered to them on a day to day basis. At home this control transfers to parents, friends and spouse. That transfer of power further contributes to an interpersonal experience of social inequality for the dying in their own homes and work places.

A casual inspection of the interpersonal experience of inequality for the dying yields several important insights. Many students of sociology have looked to events or circumstances of maltreatment and stigma to identify problems of social inequality. But we can see in the experience of inequality in professional settings that unequal social status does not equate with maltreatment or stigma. Yet the disadvantages can be just as real in their consequences. The disadvantages which accrue to the compliant dying patient is lack of access to information flow and control. The dying patient's status in the health care system is often so low that they are sometimes referred to by professionals as disease systems (e.g. the melanoma in ward F) or social stereotypes (e.g. the whinger in the Maling Wing). The circumstances of dying, in common with the circumstances of serious illness, can lead to the problem of depersonalization. This means that so often decisions are made (or not made) without consultation, and information withheld or obscured for the convenience of the more powerful professional.

And if this were not serious enough as a problem for the dying person, other problems can arise from equally well meaning family and friends. Inequality of social relations can result in positive, caring responses to the dying. However intimacy, as the social opposite of depersonalization, can lead to a politics of care which fails to consult, to respect, or even notice former boundaries of privacy and autonomy. And finally, a single style of social response can be inadequate to a disease which creates multiple and changeable health consequences for the dying person.

In these two interpersonal examples the fundamental problem of inequality is an inability of the dying person, because of social or professional conventions, to obtain a share in making the rules which affect him or her. Often referred to as the problem of participation (Turner 1986), this type of deprivation has been traditionally discussed and identified with large scale political institutions and movements. However, studying the problem of social inequality through measures of wealth (Social Justice Collective 1991) or theories of industrial society and social stratification (Giddens 1986) can sometimes obscure the fact that inequality is a way of seeing and relating to other people in day to day encounters. It is true that group membership can attract hardship and negative labelling simply by virtue of that membership (as we have seen in our earlier discussion of Australian Aborigines). But inequality viewed solely in these terms overstates the group specific side of social inequality. The fact of the matter is that inequality can happen to anyone. If circumstances or associations alter sufficiently to encourage other people to believe that you are somehow less than capable of full participation and independence, you will become a prime candidate for unequal social treatment.

Summary and conclusions

Reflections on the inequality of dying demonstrate several social issues. First, people die very much as they have lived. Not only do their activities reflect the usual inequalities of their daily social positions and respective lifestyle but the likelihood of developing types of fatal illness is also linked to these. Second, unequal treatment does not always mean frank maltreatment and stigma.

Despite popular myth and clinical opinion to the contrary, the dying are not an especially stigmatized group. And yet disadvantage can come to them through inappropriate beliefs about illnesses such as cancer. People often decide too early, and then demonstrate a reluctance to revise, what terminal illness means for a dying person in practical day to day terms. Such care, and it often expresses itself as care as we have seen, privileges too highly the professional and lay need to act. This anxious need to act can lead to according a lower priority to the social value of daily listening and learning from someone whose social circumstances have altered dramatically.

Third, the problem of social inequality, as one of the central concerns of sociology, is not simply about identifying which groups experience discrimination. That is only one part of the critical story of social inequality. Just as importantly, the study of the inequality of dying demonstrates that unequal social relations often result from perceptions by others of personal and social inadequacy. In this respect, we are all at risk. It is this diagnosis then, taken by so many, and so rashly, of others, which lies at the heart of the universal problem of social inequality.

REFERENCES

Australian Institute of Health & Welfare 1992 Australia's health 1992. Australian Government Publishing Service, Canberra
Bates E 1979 Decision making in critical illness. Australian & New Zealand Journal of Sociology 15:45–54
Castles I 1992 Causes of death, Australia, 1991. Australian Bureau of Statistics, Canberra
Giddens A 1986 Sociology: a brief but critical introduction. Macmillan, London
Kearl M 1989 Endings: a sociology of death and dying. Oxford, New York
Kellehear A 1988 Country health: another side of the rural crisis. Regional Journal of Social Issues 21:1–8
Kellehear A 1990 Dying of cancer: the final year of life. Harwood Academic Publishers, London
Kellehear A, Fook J 1989 Sociological factors in death denial by the terminally ill. In Sheppard J.H.(ed) Advances in behavioural medicine, vol 6, pp 527–537
Lincoln R A, Najman J M, Wilson P R, Matis C E 1988 Mortality rates in 14 Queensland reserve communities. Medical Journal of Australia, April:357–360
Prior L 1989 The social organisation of death. Macmillan, London
Saggers C, Gray D 1991 Aboriginal health and society. Allen & Unwin, Sydney
Simpson M A 1976 Brought in dead. Omega 7:243–248
Social Justice Collective 1991 Inequality in Australia: slicing the cake. William Heinemann, Melbourne
Sudnow D 1967 Passing on: the social organisation of dying. Prentice-Hall, New Jersey
Turner B 1986 Equality. Tavistock, London
Veatch R M, Tai E 1980 Talking about death: patterns of lay and professional change. In: Fox R (ed) The social meaning of death. The Annals of the American Academy of Political and Social Science 447:29–45
Willis E 1989 Medical dominance, 2nd edn. Allen & Unwin, Sydney

13. Medicine, state and people: a failure of trust?

Ann E. Daniel

This government has destroyed trust. We're in a sort of partnership with the government, state and federal, to get health care to the people. Now the partnership's breaking down; we can't trust them any more.

It was 1984 and I was interviewing antagonists on both sides of a battle between state and profession over control of medical services in New South Wales. That story was told in a book published in 1990, a book which was primarily concerned with professions and the strategies they employ to maintain command of their sphere of practice (Daniel 1990). Since writing about the long-running strife between medical practitioners, their associations and learned colleges, on the one hand, and the politicians and bureaucrats who run the health service organisations on the other, I have had more time to reflect on the key issues. It seems to me that much of the trouble arose when trust broke down, when the trust between those who provided and those who managed and administered that provision of health services in public hospitals was worn down; trust disappeared, suspicion was rife and a fierce enmity set in.

Trust between patient and practitioner has long been assumed as integral to that relationship and it was feared that the doctors' political troubles were putting it at risk. Trust between state and profession has, however, always been hesitant and, indeed, distrust had already become endemic in all quarters. In the health systems, trust eroded, and everywhere effective relations between health professionals and the politicians and administrators running the health system wore down. The dissipation of trust between medical profession and health bureaucracies apparent in Australian during the early 1980s was also evident in the relation between nurses and health administrators later in that decade. The industrial action of nurses in hospitals throughout the country was at once symptomatic and exacerbating of misunderstanding and trust within the public hospital system.

Trust is widely stressed as integral to the therapeutic relation between patient and health practitioner—what Giddens (1990:84–88) terms 'facework' commitments. Related to this person-to-person trust is the more generalized concept of system trust, in this case a professional 'expert system'. Issues of trust are addressed frequently in theory of and research on professions. Often forgotten, however, is the requirement for trust between those practising in

191

the health field and the agencies providing the infrastructure and, to a greater or less extent, the payment for those services. This latter sphere of trust lies at a more generalized level between social and cultural institutions (in this case between profession and state in its administrative capacity). An exploration of this area underlines the point that the efficacy, efficiency and equity, beloved of social planners, are predicated on relations of trust, and where trust fails social justice is endangered. Justice is predicated on the dependability and responsibility of those endowed with authority.

This chapter first examines the concepts of trust and confidence and related notions of distrust, risk and danger. An exposition of a sociological concept, like trust, can readily become abstruse and abstracted unless it is aptly illustrated. To leaven the theory I will refer to incidents drawn from empirical research in the field of medicine and health to promote mental digestion.

The second section of the chapter will examine the bases of trust in medical practice. Trust rests on the certified, trained competence and integrity of the profession inculcated by professional discipline. Beyond the guarantee held out by a profession and underwritten by state registration, lies the protective encirclement of law. But, while the presence of law buttresses trust, it is invoked only when trust fails. Implicit in patient-practitioner relationships is the interplay of trust and distrust which rest on confidence in the competence and integrity of the practice of scientific medicine. The appeal to discipline as the basis for trust and the procedures for instilling discipline (in the body of the organization as well as of practitioner), rather than the formal procedures of law, are the concerns of this section.

The third section returns to questions of system trust, but this time trust between medical profession (as clinical service provider) and federal and state governments (as managers of health services). Profession and government are necessarily in partnership and the rhetoric of both institutions extols the importance of partnership. But without trust partnerships founder. Medicine and state in many countries constitute a very troubled partnership; the Australian case is instructive.

The notion of trust

Trust in its most general application has been examined by a number of contemporary sociologists, whose reviews of its workings have particular application to our concern with professional practice. Some of these social thinkers write quite abstractly of the concept of trust; others ground their expositions in particular settings, like family, business, politics. In drawing on these theoretical discussions I shall relate issues of trust to our specific concerns in the sphere of health and medicine.

In an original and generative essay Niklas Luhmann relates trust to the exigencies of human existence and to strategies for coping with the hazards and difficulties of that existence. He begins his long essay by claiming 'trust, in the broadest sense of confidence in one's expectations, is a basic fact of social life' and continues by proposing that the necessity for trust stipulates the starting point for the derivation of rules of proper conduct (1979:4). It is this understanding of trust which makes its contemplation an excellent beginning for an inquiry into the proper, ethical conduct of medical practice and the responsible provision of health services to all the people. As the world grows more complex, trust serves to reduce complexity and allow action. Without some measure of trust we dare not do anything; we would not get up in the morning! Trust is not further defined but rather taken as a fact of life and the mode, par excellence, for reducing the complexity of life, particularly the intricate complexities of modern life: 'the social dimension of human existence in both its aspects—added complexity and new possibilities for the absorption of complexity—increases the potential for complexity and thus extends the human world' (Luhmann 1979:7). Trust, in this highly abstract essay, is integral to the formation of expectations which permit generalization over time and over a plurality of subjects and objects. So trust provides the grounds on which we act.

Trust is learned through experience, but distrust is equally learned—'Familiarity is the precondition for trust as well as distrust' (Luhmann 1979:19) and this condition arises in experience, in contemplation of things past. Trust assumes that persons or things relied on in the past may continue to be relied on. It goes beyond the information available and defines the future and what might be expected. Familiarity and trust are complementary ways of dealing with complexity and carry the past into the future. As one's world becomes more complex, more unpredictable, trust serves to diminish the complexity and provides the emotional stability for considered action. Yet, trust is precarious. Distrust arises when the threshold of trust is over-reached. The person distrusted at first reacts with forbearance and then shifts to caution and eventually resentment.

Distrust tends to be endorsed and reinforced in social interaction and is taken by the one who is distrusted as an exemption from the moral obligations which were initially acknowledged—and so distrust becomes 'a self-fulfilling prophecy'. If one continually encounters distrust or suspicion, the intention to be trustworthy can be readily set aside—the practitioner who experiences public or sustained distrust can more readily become a rogue and not to be trusted. (The connections with labelling theory can be seen.) Either trust or distrust can establish the mind-set which interprets events and transforms doubt into conviction. For instance, if I distrust the competence of male practitioners in the field of women's health, I will tend to mistrust the course of action recommended by the male doctor I inadvertently visit. I may query the evidence supporting his diagnoses, prognoses and therapies and he, in turn, may despair of securing my confidence and finish the consultation by angrily justifying my suspicions about his lack of understanding. Distrust may, however, be obviated by a system which patently punishes self-exemption from obligations of compassion, care and competence.

Luhmann argues for the rationality of trust on the basis of its function of increasing the potential of a system to deal with complexity and secure time to achieve distant effects. In health and medicine 'system trust' depends on a belief in expert knowledge and counts on explicit processes for the reduction of complexity and the function of the system's own internal controls. Trust in a practitioner's superior knowledge and skills prepares a person to wait patiently till therapy alleviates or cures a distressing condition. While a system of high complexity, like medicine and health care, operates on trust, it can, at the same time, engender distrust (the risks may be high or the disappointments many). Within such a system, trust is institutionalized in supervisory arrangements which respect the differentiation of areas of trust and depersonalize potential mutual hostility of distrust. For instance, in the example of the woman who distrusted male practitioners working in the field of women's health, if her confidence had been predicated on a generalized trust in the system of medical science, the identity of a particular practitioner would have been irrelevant. The medical profession, while not neglecting the doctor-patient relation, is constantly concerned about its image and the high standing of medical science generally. Audacious or premature claims for medical advances put its reputation for dependability at risk.

Giddens (1990:83–88) explains the distinction between the more abstract trust of systems and the specificities of personal trust. Modern institutions, he claims, are deeply bound up with the mechanisms of trust in abstract systems. Such systems are negotiated at access points by 'facework' commitments with individual practitioners or through 'faceless commitments' with the knowledge held in the system. The 'facework' commitments with medical or nursing practitioner depend heavily on her or his trustworthiness. The strong emphasis traditionally placed on the moral character, the calm dependability, the apparent knowledgability and skill of nurse or doctor, is oriented to engendering and bolstering trust. 'Faceless commitments', on the other hand, are generalized to confidence in a knowledge system, like medical science, which is similarly sensitive to imputations cast on its reliability and integrity.

Law, Luhmann reminds us, can limit uncertainties and so allow trust a milieu for its flourishing. But law, legislation and regulation, does not obviate the need for trust; rather it patrols the fields of risk and danger to intervene if the trusted systems should fail the expectations of trust. In the fields of health and medical practice, the law provides a safeguard, or at least a remedy, in the case of negligence, incompetence or wrongdoing. In this way legislation which defines the limits to acceptable conduct pushes back distrust. 'Trust and law must largely operate *independently* of one another, be connected only through the *general conditions which make them possible, and, when the need arises,* be capable of mutual co-ordination with reference to individual problems of some significance' (his emphasis; Luhmann 1979:35).

Trust in Luhmann's account is not undifferentiated, but rather specific to activities or functions of either systems or individuals. They are trusted in specific respects and within set limits. Trust is learned—through family, schooling, everyday discourse. So when the news media trumpet another medical marvel, trust in medical science is enhanced; conversely a chronicle of ignorance or fraud will promote distrust. Allegations of medifraud and 'over-servicing' promote suspicion and cynicism towards the profession generally and can readily be carried into the doctor-patient relation.

Trust deals with the unpredictability of complexity by accepting an internal order with its own problematic for the more complex external order with its perilous problematic. For example, the peril of disease and personal disintegration can be dispelled by medical diagnosis, therapy and prognosis. Anxiety subsides even when 'the worst' becomes known and a plan of action is put forward to cope with the troubles or difficulties ahead. Trust is about securing simplification so that the fearful unknown can be knowable and hence controllable.

Bernard Barber in *The Logic and Limits of Trust* (1983) grounds this somewhat abstract analysis in particular contexts in business, government, science, professions—and draws on empirical research to elucidate the nature of trust. In relating trust to professions, Barber claims that it is integrally tied to the powerful knowledge, considerable autonomy, and high level of legal and moral obligation and responsibility which professions espouse. Taken together these afford grounds for trustworthiness, but if one or other is called into question confidence is eroded. Powerful knowledge is dangerous and, as Gouldner (1971:486–488) had warned, power must be held in check by a strong sense of humanity and responsibility—an issue taken up in the next section on discipline. Barber perceives a diminishing of public trust because science and technology is seen to be fraught with danger, because a better educated public grows more critical and because demands for personal autonomy restrict the concession of authority to science.

Trust legitimates authority and so can control and sustain authority. If the doctor is distrusted her authority is undermined. Trust in professions is limited by perceptions of the extent and adequacy of knowledge, the effectiveness of practice and the responsibility for public and individual welfare with which practice is carried out.

The paradox of trust is that other forms of social control, which reduce the unpredictability and the unmanageability of the complexities of life, both substitute and bolster trust:

the greater authority and power generated by our changing social system and the greater knowledge and competence throughout the population demand higher levels of trustworthiness from all citizens (Barber 1983:170).

Barber poses but does not answer the question, how is trustworthiness to be ensured? The answer might be by wisdom and vigilance. During the doctors' disputes in Australia in 1983-85, widespread concern was voiced in the councils of the profession about public perceptions of irresponsibility. Emergency systems were set up to recall visiting specialists, who had protested by formally resigning their hospital posts, to treat emergency patients in the public hospitals. The hospitals, which had little interest in sustaining 'striking doctors' credibility', refused to call on the visiting specialists and managed a holding operation for the critically ill. The withdrawal of medical labour (whether by resignation or strike) stopped short of children's hospitals and children's wards in public hospitals—that would have been widely viewed as a complete betrayal of trust.

Luhmann had perceived trust as integral to all social relations, but especially required in large measure to cope with the complexity of modern life. Other writers have argued that the division of labour (seen by many, who follow Durkheim, as being the major force of modernity) necessitates an ever increasing level of trust. Rueschemeyer (1986) had linked trust to the power of expert groups grounded in the structure of the division of labour. Horobin more explicitly ties the necessity for trust to the division of labour and emergence of experts and follows Simmel who claimed 'modern life is based to a larger extent than is usually realised upon faith in the honesty of the other' (quoted in Horobin 1983:102). Giddens takes these insights further and finds, along with other developments of modernity ('time-space distantiation', 'disembedding', 'symbolic tokens' like money), the establishment of expert systems which depend for their authority on the concession of trust. Trust, Giddens had earlier argued, is 'the foundation of a tension-management system' in personality formation (1984:54). And in the construction of society, trust is essential to the authority, control and operation of expert systems.

Trust presupposes awareness of risk. Giddens stipulates that trust is 'confidence in the reliability of a person or system regarding a set of outcomes or events where that confidence expresses a faith in the probity or love of another, or in the correctness of abstract principles (technical knowledge)' (1990:34). Trust/confidence is socially created, it arises where there is uncertainty and where there is recognition of risk and it generates a sense of security despite risk. 'The nature of modern institutions is deeply bound up with the mechanisms of trust in abstract systems, especially trust in expert systems' (Giddens 1990:83). Such systems are negotiated at 'access points' by 'facework' commitments with individuals and 'faceless commitments' with the knowledge held in the system. Situations which require such trust are commonplace in the health system—a person undergoing an operation will know of, and will have been warned of, the dangers of the procedure; such a person submits because she, or he, has confidence both in the skill and care of surgeon and anaesthetist (each will normally have introduced themselves to the patient) and in the science of surgery and anaesthetics which have developed this operation. The 'access point' in this example is hospital or doctor's surgery, the patient meets and makes arrangements with the specialists ('facework commitment') and these negotiations occur in the context of a confidence in the integrity and capacity of medical science ('faceless commitments').

Trust, in Giddens' account, is necessary for 'ontological security' and psychological well-being and development: the opposite of trust is not distrust or the more emotion-laden mistrust, but angst or dread, i.e. persistent existential anxiety—those who cannot trust suffer the most acute anxiety and distress. 'Trust and risk, opportunity and danger—these polar, paradoxical features of modernity permeate all aspects of day-to-day life once more reflecting an extraordinary interpolation of the local and the global' (1990:148). Most people are pragmatic and simply accept abstract systems which impinge on them, but they may react with alarm to perceived inconsistencies in expert knowledge and then lose trust. Controversies in medicine generate alarm. For example, arguments about the reliability of diagnostic tests diminish trust in medical science. Publicity disclosing the latitude for error in cancer detection techniques, such as mammograms or cervical smear tests, has prompted dismay and distrust in diagnostic medicine generally.

Sociologists, whose work focuses more explicitly on occupations and professions, find that the concession of trust increases with the degree of expertise claimed and demonstrated in the work of a profession. (This trend is integral to the more general phenomenon of the division of labour). John Goldthorpe holds that trust is an inherent dimension of the work of 'the service class', that prestigious set of senior managers and professionals prominent in contemporary society. Their work necessarily involves an important measure of trust because of the authority, albeit delegated authority, wielded by senior managers or because of the authority, based on specialist knowledge and expertise, assumed by professionals (1982:168). A moment's reflection can remind us that if one can trust no one with a task the only alternative is to do it oneself—and in large work organizations and complex societies like ours that is simply impossible. The problem is a familiar one. In professional practice the requisite degree of autonomy and discretion is conceded on the basis of trust in the authenticity of expert knowledge fostered within the profession and, at a secondary level, on acceptance of claims for the integrity and good intentions of the practitioner.

In conditions of risk or complexity, engagement of professional services is predicated on trust. Without some measure of trust the relationship, with its inherent dependency, cannot be sustained. Knowledge, technique and dependability diminish the risk of the contingencies faced and the reliability of these is underpinned by the discipline of profession and the regulation of law. Trust is a hazardous business and, despite its demonstrated necessity, it is only given where there are grounds for believing it will be respected.

Discipline

In relation to systems, trust is reinforced by both perception of effective self-regulation and confidence in the external surveillance of law—the discipline of profession and the law of society acting in concert. This goes to what Dietrich Rueschemeyer calls the central sociological issue in the study of professions, 'the social control of expert systems, its different institutional forms and their structural conditions' (1983:54–55). The differentials of power and the exigencies of experience can call forth distrust which looks for explicit controls to ensure trustworthiness. Trust in professions is limited by perceptions of the extent and adequacy of knowledge, of the effectiveness of practice and of the responsibility for public and individual welfare.

While trust, necessary for any level of co-operative activity, is so salient in client-professional relationships and is integral to modern institutions utilizing expert systems, discipline, in the several meanings of that word, is critical to professions. The term implies the field of esoteric knowledge, the mental and moral training for its application, the definition of standards and the imposition of sanctions where those definitions are transgressed. Discipline, understood as abstract or scientific knowledge, rigorous preliminary training and continuing commitment to high standards of expertise, is crucial to sociological interpretations of professions. A number of writers of both conservative and radical persuasion have pointed to the growing authority and prominence of professions (and intellectuals generally) in contemporary society (Bell 1973, Konrad & Szelenyi 1979, Gouldner 1979, Clegg et al 1986, Rueschemeyer 1986, Daniel 1990).

So pervasive is the ideology put around by contemporary professions, several writers, including those identified above, maintain that the 'professional ideal' exerts a hegemonic force in social and economic arrangements. In a most detailed social history Harold Perkin (1989) demonstrates the ascendancy of professions exploiting ever expanding resources of abstract and technical knowledge as a form of 'property' and shows the extent of the influence of professional ideologies such that society itself endorses professional values and the educated and trained workforces are intent on a professionalizing project. 'The professional ideal, based on trained expertise and selection by merit, differed from the other three [aristocratic, entrepreneurial, collectivist ideals] in emphasizing human capital rather than passive or active property, highly skilled and differentiated labour rather than simple labour theory of value, and selection by merit defined as trained and certified expertise' (1989:4). Professions claimed to provide services of high expertise, beyond the grasp of the uninitiated and hence not readily evaluated and having to be taken on trust (Perkin 1989:16).

Discipline is implicit in all of these analyses, and discipline, or rather the perception of discipline, is the basis for trust in a profession. A professional is given access to our secrets—secret fears or guilty secrets—when we require help; some professionals, particularly medical practitioners, may take extreme liberties with our bodies (consider any surgical procedure). This is permitted because they are trusted to know and do good for us; the reasons for this trust lie with the discipline of the profession in which they are registered and which they are certified as fit to practise. The strength of disciplinary practices underwrite the trust required in professional—client (in our case 'doctor-patient') relations.

The concept of discipline has been extensively investigated by Michel Foucault, who links it to the constitution of institutions—initially as the correlate of 'punish' in his account of the prison. Foucault moved on from *Discipline and Punish* (1977) to an analysis of the links between power and knowledge that were, in one guise or another, to hold his attention to the end—'the constant articulation of power on knowledge and of knowledge on power' such that 'the exercise of power itself creates and causes to emerge new objects of knowledge and accumulates new bodies of information' (Foucault 1980:51). Knowledge and power are integrated with one another—the exercise of power requires knowledge and knowledge engenders power. Foucault explicates the forms of mediation between power and knowledge in the two lectures of January 1976. Here he outlined the question which directs his later research—'what rules of right are implemented by the relations of power in the production of discourses of truth?' (1980:93) His preliminary answer—'power never ceases its interrogation, its inquisition, its registration of truth: it institutionalizes, professionalizes and rewards its pursuit' (1980:93)—is a fine portrayal of the professionalizing project.

In a number of his writings, Foucault pursues the notion of sovereignty as a traditional power conceded and limited (limited in that sovereignty exceeded to the point of oppression strikes its limit and provokes a reaction which denies its legitimacy and threatens its existence). The theory of sovereignty he traces as the ideology of law and as the organizing principle of major legal codes. Foucault, however, postulates other modes of domination lying outside the legal form of sovereignty and these he identifies as disciplinary power. His demonstrations showed disciplinary power to be gathering persuasiveness rather more than the sovereign power expressed in the laws of the state. Our contemporary society he pictures as one of normalization where power is exercised simultaneously through the traditional law concerned with rights and duties and through techniques to which the disciplines give rise such that 'the procedures of normalization come to be ever more constantly engaged in the colonization of those of law' (Foucault 1980:107). His exemplar of this force for normalization is found in medical science and its extensions where the ascent of power is tied to scientific knowledge and the disciplinary normalization of the learned college. Illustrating Foucault's account is the viewpoint on proper medical practice currently held by the law. Medical practitioners are, of course, subject to the law; but in matters of medical practice, standards of competence, care and responsibility, their conduct is judged according to the standards set by the profession. A long line of judgements in most common law countries (those based on the English law system like Australia, Canada, the United States) have held that it is the profession which judges what are acceptable standards.

It is this sense of discipline which is important for control within professions—disciplines and all the effects of power and knowledge that are linked to them. Foucault elicits through some painstaking analyses of historical events the working of discipline oriented both to generating and sustaining knowledge and to controlling the practices of knowledge.

Implicit in this perspective on the disciplinary practices of professions is a sense of danger. I would argue that professions are at some pains to reassure that their practice is both informed and conscientious—that their work is 'good'. Gouldner had emphasized the human predeliction for imputing goodness to power that impinges closely on personal life as 'a general condition of all permitted social worlds' (1971:486). It can be claimed, as Shils does, that the authority of professions is charismatic on account of their closeness to 'the centres...those positions which mediate man's relationship to the order of existence—spiritual forces, cosmic powers, values and norms—which legitimates or withholds legitimation from the earthly powers or which dominates earthly existence' (1968:107). Passages like this recall the religious origins of professions and suggest the significance of rituals, symbols, language in the creation of a professional ethos. And it calls up the issue of risk, and the invocation of medicine particularly in moments of personal danger. Hence the salience of trust and ontological security, which Giddens and Luhmann postulate as essential for sanity.

The great civilizing process of transition to system trust gives humanity a stable attitude towards what is contingent in a complex world, make it possible to live with the realization that everything could be otherwise (Luhmann 1979:58).

Discipline in professions

The discipline of a profession typically begins with the university education and continues into the technical training of hospital, courtroom, worksite. There are many accounts of the inculcation of professional discipline, of which the outstanding exemplar is the classic phenomenological study of medical students by Becker, Geer, Strauss and Everett C Hughes (1961). In Australia the longitudinal research by Anderson and Western (Anderson & Western 1967, Anderson et al 1973, Western & Anderson 1968) follows four cohorts of students (engineering, law, medicine, teaching) from their early university studies into mid-career and middle life. The medical students are still drilled in lecture hall, tested for their command of medical information and then set to the long hours of 'walking the wards' (the traditional apprenticeship of physician or surgeon). The 'pre-clinical' years require concentrated study and frequent submission to examination. Clinical training occurs under surveillance and continuing assessment. Students, whose education is constantly regulated and monitored, progress together towards the common identity of 'doctor' and develop a sense of commitment and collegiality, which outsiders readily dub an elitist esprit de corps. The compulsory hospital internship and residency instil a loyalty to the team and regard for the rules governing practice. In the course of researching the battles involving the medical profession, I was frequently reminded by practitioners taking different sides in those disputes of the importance of the teaching hospital in the training years and subsequently. An older practitioner of firmly socialist views agreed with his more conservative colleagues:

It is impossible to underestimate the importance of the hospital and the way doctors work in hospitals; you are working with each other in life-threatening situations, your work is interconnected in so many ways, you are meeting often and unpredictably over your work, you must cooperate, you must trust each other. This makes for a solidarity which people outside hospitals and medicine may find baffling. Medical solidarity is forged in the hospital during training and reinforced every time you come back into it. There is no way anyone could hold out against colleagues, lest for the rest of your professional life you are a marked person (quoted in Daniel 1990:84).

Randall Collins points out that 'all education is a ritual in a certain formal sense' (1990:38). Collins draws on the notion of the 'sacred' in elite education creating a bond among the acolytes in the 'sacred realm'. The aspiring professionals participate so intensively that they come to identify themselves with the subject of the curriculum. After the formal education and the clinical (practical) training, medical practitioners assume their place in the collegiate of their fellows, an association characterized by the solidarity of shared experiences, expectations, values, goals—not unlike that solidarity which Durkheim termed the mechanical solidarity of strongly cohesive, homogenous, simple societies.

In some earlier writing I have argued that the authority of any profession is secured by a variety of strategies. These are directed to securing a monopoly of relevant knowledge and expertise and, by collaborating with the state, to ensuring the exclusion of those whose knowledge is not certified, whose practices have not been disciplined in the regulatory, approved manner (Daniel 1990:62–64). Evan Willis, whose focus is on health and medicine in Australia, had pointed to the strategies of subordination, limitation and exclusion which produced medical dominance (Willis 1989). Paul Starr's long story of medical sovereignty in the United States told of the dependence of peoples on medical science and the legitimacy secured by scientific knowledge and technique which together engendered the modern authority of medicine as profession (Starr 1982). The authority of medicine he describes as 'cultural authority', based on the persuasion of expertise and distinguished from political authority, based on law and regulation—a distinction reminiscent of Foucault's differentiation of the power of the sovereignty of law and that of pervasive discipline of normalizing practices.

Professional standards of practice rest on control over admission to training, quality control of standards of competence and ethics instilled by that training and ongoing surveillance of the maintenance of high moral and standards. Michael Bayliss (1989) in *Professional Ethics* describes the surveillance of character and competence of practitioners and catalogues the penalties imposed for violation of prevailing standards; these range from the informal sanctions of blame, ostracism and boycott to the more formal reprimands, fines, exclusion from professional college or association, revocation of licence to practise; and, beyond the authority of profession, the law's investigation of malpractice and determination of damages, criminal penalty or imprisonment.

Professional bodies in the economically developed nations are firmly involved in setting, maintaining and patrolling standards and have become more concerned with their obligations for regulation and surveillance. Prevailing practice in the Organization of Economic Community Development (OECD) countries concedes to the medical profession's official bodies the regulation and determination of clinical and professional matters of which they are held to be the best judges. In common law countries, the courts have deviated little from the principle of the medical profession's primacy in determining what is proper and improper professional conduct and what is misconduct. The judgements of Australian state courts have maintained this view, although in practice matters before the court can frequently appear as a contest of experts.

In Australia, Medical Registration Boards, composed largely but not exclusively of medical practitioners, are responsible under state legislation for setting, maintaining and monitoring standards, for receiving and investigating complaints and for assisting and funding the tribunals which hear complaints. The constitution of the NSW Medical Tribunal exemplifies the interdependence of profession and state, where the presiding judicial officer and the lay person sitting on the tribunal are government appointed, and the two medical practitioners are appointed by the Board. In the case of disagreement the state appointed judicial officer, however, has a further casting vote. In Australia, the recipient of most complaints about medical practice is a specialist unit within the state health department. The officers of these units investigate and prosecute cases before tribunals and professional standards committees. Beyond the professional conduct tribunals, persons who believe they have been injured may have recourse to common law and state legislation and seek damages or bring action alleging gross negligence or criminal offences. While the law serves to bolster the rationality of trust, resort to the law occurs when trust is gone.

This outline of discipline and disciplinary practices in medicine is necessarily schematic and fragmentary. A sustained and detailed excursion into the many theoretical and practical issues involved appears in Joseph Jacob's path breaking book on *Doctors and Rules* (1988). Readers who wish to follow up some of the matters raised in this section will find Jacob's work instructive and challenging.

Profession and state

This chapter has been concerned to elucidate the nature of trust immanent in all co-operative relationships and essential in most of the activities that fill our lives. Distrust is not its opposite, but a moderating, a diminishing of the primary basis of trust. The complete disappearance of trust predicates outright conflict—a state of 'war'.

The prolonged doctors' dispute of 1983–85, when the profession was locked in battle with state and federal governments, was preceded by the erosion of trust and an accompanying rise in suspicion and antagonism. Professions grow strong in relations of interdependency with the state, and medicine in Australia and elsewhere had gained authority and influence as the state provided the conditions for its certified monopoly of medical science and practice. (For fuller accounts of this process in various countries see Freidson 1970, 1986, Starr 1982, Rueschemeyer 1983, 1986, Derber 1982, Willis 1989, Crichton 1990, Daniel 1990) In the years after World War II governments in many countries had sought to ensure public provision of health services. The United Kingdom led in this development, a story told by Rudolf Klein. He points out, among other things, that the British Labour government consulted continuously with the British Medical Association on every aspect of the planned National Health Service and secured through negotiation and compromise the profession's co-operation with its free health care for the British people (Klein 1983:1–28). Governments in other countries were not so skilful.

The twenty years before the introduction of Medibank by the Whitlam government in Australia in 1975 were punctuated by skirmishes with the medical profession's representative associations. Labor policy was much feared because of a perception of ill-concealed intentions to 'nationalize medicine'. Some doctors became paranoid about Labor policy and most were distrustful. Nonetheless the worst fears failed to materialize. Medibank was established and eventually secured broad based support from most of the profession which profited from the extension of the market for medical services. But, Medibank was dismantled in a piecemeal fashion during the years of the conservative Fraser government. Then, in 1983 Labor came to power with a mandate to implement again a national health scheme. The new system, Medicare, was erected in the same year, but it built in ancillary provisions which medical practitioners interpreted as whittling away the conditions under which they practised in public hospitals. The earlier suspicions about Labor's intention to 'nationalize' medicine and put all health services on a salaried basis re-surfaced. That story I told in some detail (Daniel 1990). The relevant point to note at this juncture is the failure of trust to which the opening passage of this chapter alluded.

There was no consultation between the government and the profession, so medical practitioners feared the worst. There had been earlier intimations in published policy speeches of the desirability of a salaried medical workforce. Changes in hospital contracts with visiting medical officers were unilaterally ordered. The basis of the partnership between profession and government to deliver health services to all Australians was being eroded. The conflict spread throughout the nation. In the hospitals visiting specialists withdrew their services; salaried specialists prepared to withdraw their services in sympathy and meantime refused any duties usually taken by those who had resigned; hospital based medical services wound down; only emergency care and paediatric care services were sustained. The evening news carried reports from 'the front'; media commentators orchestrated debates and confrontations; spokespersons for trades unions, community organizations and interest groups of all persuasions had their say; bureaucrats entered the public arena; a premier declared 'I will change the law' and Parliament legislated to ban those who resigned from appointment to any hospital for seven years; and Parliament was recalled a month later to repeal the inflammatory act. Months went by and negotiations swung back and forth. Suspicion was everywhere rife, but it was vague and amorphous; it did not always identify 'the enemy'. The solidarity of the profession held despite some cracks along structural divisions and cleavages along politico-cultural lines. Trust was at a premium within the profession; and there was no trust to create links between profession and government.

Trust for the future?

Those times are gone and some healing of the deep wounds has occurred. Consultation about proposed changes is now mandatory. Health Ministers are better at conciliation (and one suspects that skills in diplomacy count in their appointment). But the partnership between profession and government in Australia is still riven with mutual suspicions, and trust grows very slowly.

Questions of trust in the future provision of health services cut across many parties involved. Is trust between public and politicians possible? Democratic ideals prompt us to believe it should be. Is trust between bureaucrat and professional possible? Sociologists have discerned the common class origins of bureaucrats and professionals, their shared educational profiles, similar lifestyles and life chances, and have suggested that these social and cultural bonds should promote understanding and co-operation. Work cited earlier in this chapter (Goldthorpe 1982, Goldthorpe et al 1980, Derber 1982, Clegg et al 1986, Rueschemeyer 1986) and the Australian research of Broom and Jones and their associates (1980) point to bureaucrats and professionals' shared social situation which should foster an effective partnership. But at work they live in different worlds, and a great pledge of trust is needed before they can be persuaded into cooperation on the project of ensuring a just and equitable health service adequate to the needs of everyone.

REFERENCES

Anderson D S, Western J S 1967 Notes on a study of professionalisation. Australian and New Zealand Journal of Sociology 3:67–71
Anderson D S, Western J S, Boreham P 1973 Conservatism in recruits to professions. Australian and New Zealand Journal of Sociology 9, 3:42–45
Barber B 1983 The logic and limits of trust. Longman, London
Bayliss M D 1989 Professional ethics, 2nd edn. Wadsworth, Belmont, California

Becker H S, Geer B, Hughes E C, Strauss A 1961 The boys in white: student culture in medical school. University of Chicago Press, Chicago

Bell D 1973 The coming of post-industrial society. Basic Books, New York

Broom L, Jones F L, McDonnell P, Williams T 1980 The inheritance of inequality. Routledge & Kegan Paul, London

Clegg S, Boreham P, Dow G 1986 Class, politics and the economy. Routledge, London

Collins R. 1990 Market closure and the conflict theory of the professions. In: Burrage M, Torsendahl R (eds) Professions in theory and history: rethinking the study of the profession. Sage, London

Crichton A 1990 Slowly taking control? Australian governments and health care provision 1788–1988. Allen & Unwin, Sydney

Daniel A 1990 Medicine and the state: professional autonomy and public accountability. Allen & Unwin, Sydney

Derber C (ed) 1982 Professionals as workers: mental labour in advanced capitalism. G K Hall, Boston

Freidson E 1970 Professional dominance: the social structure of medical care. Atherton Press, New York

Freidson E 1986 Professional powers: a study of the institutionalization of formal knowledge. University of Chicago Press, Chicago

Foucault M 1977 Discipline and punish. Penguin, Harmondsworth

Foucault M 1980 (edited by C.Gordon) Power/knowledge. Harvester Press, Brighton

Giddens A 1990 The consequences of modernity. Polity Press, Cambridge

Goldthorpe J H 1982 On the service class, its formation and future. In: Giddens A, Mackenzie G (eds) Social class and the division of labour: essays in honour of Eily Neustadt. Cambridge University Press, Cambridge

Goldthorpe J H et al 1980 Social mobility and class structure in modern Britain. Oxford University Press, London

Gouldner A W 1971 The coming crisis of western sociology. Heinemann, London

Gouldner A W 1979 The future of the intellectuals and the rise of the new class. Macmillan, London

Horobin G 1983 Professional mystery: the maintenance of charisma in general medical practice. In: Dingwall R, Lewis P (eds) The sociology of the professions. St Martin's Press, New York

Jacob J M 1988 Doctors and rules: a sociology of professional values. Routledge, London

Klein R 1983 The politics of the national health service. Longman, London

Konrad G, Szelenyi I 1979 Intellectuals on the road to class power. Harcourt Brace and Jovanovich, London

Luhmann N 1979 Trust. John Wiley, London

Perkin H 1989 The rise of professional pociety: England since 1880. Routledge, New York

Rueschemeyer D 1983 Professional autonomy and the social control of expertise. In: Dingwall R, Lewis P (eds) The sociology of the professions: lawyers, doctors and others. St Martin's Press, New York

Rueschemeyer D 1986 Power and the division of labour. Polity Press, Cambridge

Sax S 1990 Health care choices and the public purse. Allen & Unwin, Sydney

Shils E A 1968 Deference. In: Jackson J A (ed) Social stratification. Cambridge University Press, London

Starr P 1982 The social transformation of American medicine. Beacon Press, New York

Western J S, Anderson D S 1968 Education and professional socialisation. Australian and New Zealand Journal of Sociology 4:91–106

Willis E 1989 Medical dominance: the division of labour in Australian health care, 2nd edn. Allen & Unwin, Sydney

14. Nineteenth century medicine, science and values

Kevin White

To construct a just health system it is necessary to have some idea of how the current one came into being. There is a commonsense understanding of how modern medicine has developed since the 19th century. In the first place, it is thought that the state gave the profession its status and right to practice because it self evidently served the purposes of life (Larson 1977). In other words because medicine deals with life and death it was granted a privileged place in the occupational structure of society by the government. Second, it is presumed that the way in which the medical profession explained disease was unproblematic. The assumption is that medicine developed on the basis of scientific theories which were unquestioningly welcomed by the general public. Third, following from this, modern medicine is seen as the outcome of science, with little or nothing to do with politics and values. Last, modern medicine is thought of as an unqualified boon to those indigenous peoples whose countries were colonized in the 19th century.

This chapter will challenge these assumptions. It examines the dispute over the control of the Adelaide Hospital in 1896 showing that the profession was involved in a deeply political struggle with the government of the day over the control of the hospital and its resources. The government, in brief, was not prepared to give the profession free reign over public resources and wanted to keep control of the hospital. In examining debates on the causes of infant mortality I will show how the profession's perspective on it was challenged by other social groups. It will be seen that medicine adopted a highly individualistic perspective, pointing to individual lifestyle factors, while other groups in the society pointed to environmental conditions, such as slums and the living conditions of the people. In all, what is demonstrated is that the development of the medical profession is the outcome of political debate and social struggle over what constitutes disease, what causes it, and how it should be treated. Thus the development of modern medicine, its links with the state, and its knowledge base are all the outcome of social processes. I will also refer to the New Zealand case. In this it will be shown that Western medicine can be analysed as an ideology of domination which contributed to the destruction of indigenous peoples and their cultures of healing. At the very least medicine depoliticized the destruction of indigenous cultures by explaining their dissolution in biological terms. Furthermore

207

medicine, because of its identification with science and rationality legitimated European domination (MacLeod & Lewis 1988).

The lesson to be learnt from these case studies is that the organization of medicine and what constitutes a just health care system is the product of social struggles. In this struggle competing groups generate alternative pictures of both nature and society. There is a struggle over the role of scientific knowledge in understanding and explaining sickness and disease; over the contribution of social factors to sickness and disease; over the role of the individual's own behaviour in the cause of disease; and over access to state resources. It will be suggested that the reason for the success of modern medicine relates to its congruence with the social structure of capitalist society. By adopting a scientific view of the origins of sickness, medicine depoliticized the social environment as a cause of disease. By focusing on the individual it located the problem of disease in the individual rather than in the organization of society (Labish 1985, Ringen 1979).

This chapter will show that the way in which medicine developed at the turn of the century was affected by the social and political situation of the time. In pursuing this argument the chapter adopts a historical sociology and it is important to explain the distinctiveness of this approach (see Stedman-Jones 1976, Hicks 1982, Shortt 1981).

A historical sociology of medicine

The way in which we understand medicine to have developed has large implications for how we go about establishing a just health system. If we think that medicine evolves out of the natural sciences, on the basis of biological discoveries, then we also tend to think that the contents of medical knowledge exist outside of society. Medical knowledge in this perspective is objective, scientific and value free. This approach can, for convenience, be called the positivist approach.

A positivist approach to the social history of medicine, and to history in general, sees historical data as self-evident information to be analysed by the historian. The data are self-evident in that the past consists of a series of stepping stones which lead inevitably to the present. The present, more advanced state of society can be traced backwards, through great institutions, great ideas, and great men whose contributions to our welfare are seen as self-evident. The present is seen as the inevitable outcome of the historical progress towards truth, enlightenment and the better society.

This approach to the history of medicine sees medicine's development as the inevitable unfolding of human rationality, driven by the logic of scientific discovery. Technological and scientific changes are seen as the motor of Western societies. Analysis such as this—which might be called the technological determinist—tends to describe medical phenomena and developments isolated from other social factors; it sees medicine as a science and focuses on its achievements rather than its failures; and emphasizes great men and institutions (Youngson 1979). By viewing medicine as a natural science we can fail to see that medical thought and organization are as much the product of social and political factors as any other human endeavour (Grob 1977, Veith 1980).

A sociological approach argues that historical data do not just exist 'out there' for us to go and find. We have to know what it is in the past that we are looking for, that is what is relevant to us today, before we can go and find it. In other words, for those who adopt this approach, history itself is constructed by us in the present to serve present needs and interests. Indeed those who adopt this approach are highly critical of those historians who see the past as a series of self evident 'facts'. They argue that to see the past like this is to give a sense of the inevitableness of the present; it is to leave out much of history. The focus on parliaments, constitutions, and ideas leaves out 'the common people' and obscures the contradictoriness of history: historical materials do not lead inevitably to our present but could have taken many different turns (Hobsbawm 1971).

It is against this background that we can study the early development of the medical profession in South Australia. By adopting a historical sociology approach, the intent is to conduct the research in such a way that the debates over the role of organized medicine are made evident. It does not set out to show how 19th century developments led progressively to the 20th century. Rather the research seeks to illustrate the ways in which what counts as medicine is the outcome of political events.

Knowledge and the medical profession in the 19th century

The argument that progress in the biological sciences is responsible for the development of the medical profession is widely accepted by social scientists writing the history of medicine. One study of the rise of the medical profession in Australia locates the development of the medical profession in technological change and in the structure of its knowledge base: 'The source of the profession's power was its control over a body of systematic knowledge relating to medicine' (Pesabene 1980). But it was not this straight forward.

Conflict between the medical profession and the government over the control of the hospital was endemic throughout the 19th century. To help us explore the dynamics of the development of the profession, we need to be clear that taking over the hospital was critical to its development. The benefits which accrued to the medical profession in controlling the hospital were immense and can be briefly summarized.

Appointment as an honorary to a hospital connected the practitioner to the wealthy patron of the hospital (in the English case), or to the state-provided resources in the Australian case. Once in the hospital this honorary position gave the practitioners independence from and, through the control of medical committees, dominance over hospital processes. Additionally, gaining control of admissions procedures allowed an increase in status of the profession since it could now accept only those cases that were curable or short term (Waddington 1973). It thus appeared that the practice of medicine was improving people's survival rates when in fact the profession was only taking treatable cases. In terms of intraprofessional developments, the location of the medical educational system in the hospital allowed consultant physicians and surgeons to control the whole profession and paramedics, while the prevention of private practice of junior doctors in the hospital protected the incomes of the consultant (Parry & Parry 1976).

Thus a lot was to be gained in taking over the hospital and it is not surprising that it was the site of enormous political struggle. In South Australia it resulted in the dismissal of the Colonial Surgeon (1839), the resignation of the honorary staff (1841), the dismissal of the matron (1866), the dismissal of the board of management (1896) and, associated with this, the resignation of the honorary staff (1896–1901). Each of these disputes alerts us to the social and political nature of the development of the medical profession, but it is the last that is of concern here.

In the 19th century the medical profession was not as highly regarded as it now is. The demands of the medical profession to have a monopoly over medical practice were seen more as the self interested actions of a trade union than as the acts of a professional group. As a member of parliament put it: 'the points at issue are the right of the representatives of the people to control public institutions supported by public funds...No union however influential can be allowed to usurp the functions of government' (Holder 1896).

As part of the ongoing battle between the profession and the government the medical staff at the Adelaide Hospital resigned in 1896. Following this Dr Allan Campbell tabled a motion in parliament calling for a Royal Commission into the management of the hospital. He proposed that the commission be comprised of a judge of the Supreme Court and two medical practitioners— one nominated by the government and the other by the medical profession (South Australian Parliamentary Debates 1896, Nov. 11, 341). The Chief Secretary responded furiously:

What right had the Medical Association to be represented on any Board of Enquiry into the management of the hospital? Were they to become an estate of the realm that they were to be considered and to appoint Judges in a matter of public interest of this sort? (South Australian Parliamentary Debates 1896, Nov. 11, 342).

The government was not going to allow the profession free control of the hospital. The government staffed the hospital with its own employees and then proceeded to advertise overseas for staff—since the British Medical Association had boycotted the hospital. It appointed Dr Leith Napier and Dr Ramsay Smith. Both men were highly qualified practitioners in their fields. But the local members of the profession wanted to discredit them by attacking their qualifications without calling into question the profession's general claim to a knowledge base. Extensive debate was carried out in the parliament, in an environment of mutual hostility between the medical members and the lay members.

The claims of medicine to be a science were still doubted by many prominent people. The Chief Secretary in South Australia's parliament, J. H. Gordon, in a debate on the hospital pointed out:

If he [the Chief Secretary] told some of the stories of that kind which doctors had told him, many of the public would perhaps turn in despair to faith healers. The science of medicine was empirical and mistakes were unavoidable. As the miner often did not know what was at the end of his pick neither did the doctor often know what was at the end of his knife (South Australian Parliamentary Debates 1896, Dec. 12, 429).

It was against this background that the profession and its spokesmen (there were no women), in attempting to take control of the hospital from the government, sought to discredit the qualifications of the two overseas doctors. A number of strategies were open to them. At the most general level it could be argued that no two people, no matter how competent, could replace a whole hospital staff:

What was the use of bringing two men from England to do what a staff of specialists had always done?...in the advanced state of science in medicine and surgery it was necessary to have specialists. No one man could do the work of the specialists in medicine and surgery (South Australian Parliamentary Debates 1896, July 8, 120).

In mounting this argument the profession was on its strongest ground. It left outside of the discussion the specific qualifications of the two doctors and did not raise general questions about the relationship between medical qualifications and medical practice. Nevertheless, given the uncertain status of the profession and the fact that the qualification of its leading parliamentary spokesman, Dr Campbell, was in homeopathy, it was difficult to prevent broader issues from arising. The strategy that the profession adopted was to emphasize its clinical skills rather than the technical achievements that the award of degrees reflected. Thus as one of its spokesmen put it:

A great deal had been said about the great quantity of degrees that the present doctors had got [Drs Napier and Smith]. He [the spokesman] was told by a well educated gentleman that it was not such a difficult matter to get those degrees, and that he had some himself. He placed more reliance upon the results of a man's practice and its extent than on the number of books he had written or of degrees he had got. A man might write well, and take degrees, and not be a practical man at all (South Australian Parliamentary Debates 1896, Dec. 9, 465).

Dr Campbell took this argument even further. He recognized the need for professional training but only a minimal one. As Dr Campbell described his own qualification in homeopathy, it was 'a nominal qualification for the practice of medicine'. He continued:

He esteemed a qualification very highly, but he never esteemed it beyond the measure that it simply enabled him to practise as a medical man. They would generally find that those who laid greatest stress upon qualifications were not always the most competent...These repeated references to degrees of qualification

were simply childish. The whole thing lay with a man's right hand and brain'
(South Australian Parliamentary Debates, 1896, Dec. 9, 467).

Thus to the profession the role of qualifications was problematic. They could not be over-emphasized because they would generate schism within the profession, given that some leading members of the profession did not have orthodox qualifications. In the particular case of Drs Napier and Smith, their qualifications had to be undermined, but not at the cost of the profession's integrity. Thus we see the profession trying to find a way to maintain its claim to a scientific base, but simultaneously suggesting that technical training and knowledge were not the essential characteristic of a medical practitioner. Emphasis was placed on the idea of medicine as an art—as an interpretive skill. This strategy was not peculiar to South Australian doctors. Studies in England (Lawrence 1985) and in France (Jamous & Pelloille 1970) have revealed similar strategies. The issue was not just the specific problem presented to the South Australian medical profession by Drs Napier and Smith. It was that if the developing profession emphasized the technical aspects of its development then it was open to the challenge that its work was really only a more sophisticated form of manual labour. It had to counter this challenge by emphasizing the interpretive aspects of its practice. It was not enough just to have technical knowledge—one had to know how to understand it. It is from the resolution of this dilemma about the profession's knowledge base that the claim that medicine is both an art and a science developed.

While the medical profession in South Australia was busy trying to defend itself from government employment and attempting to take control of the hospital, it also had another battle to fight. Medical knowledge and explanations of disease were being contested by other social groups as shown in the following case-study.

The causes of infant mortality

In the ten year period ending in 1875 South Australia recorded the highest infant mortality rate of any colony in Australia, 157 deaths per 1000 live births. Of the deaths registered, only 1708 specify a cause of death: 34% were caused by diarrhoea and dysentery (or from another perspective impure food and water); 5% were recorded as dying of privation (Hayter 1878–79). If we examine the statistics for children under 5 in the year 1876, of the 1345 deaths recorded, 731 were registered as being due to zymotic disease (the 19th century word for infectious disease). That is, 54% of all childhood deaths in that year were due to environmentally mediated infectious diseases. The second (1875) *Report of the Central Board of Health* expressed its understanding of the causes of infant mortality quite bluntly:

The causes which lead to this high rate of mortality among children are well known and may shortly be stated as consisting of neglect, or ignorance of sanitary matters, the use of impure water, overcrowding in houses, often imperfectly constructed, badly drained and inefficiently ventilated, to which may be added carelessness in the administration of nutrition during the hot months of the year.

However when the literature produced by the medical profession is examined quite a different explanation is found. When we turn to the contemporary medical literature, we find the following reasons given for these high rates: temperature, humidity, barometric pressure, and the direction of the wind. To quote from the clearest example of this approach, Dr Sylvannus Magarey set out to

compare the variations in the death rate with the variations of the temperature, rainfall, barometric pressure, evaporation and humidity during the years 1873–77 (Magarey 1878–79).

He concluded that 'the rate of mortality depends to a very large extent upon the height of the thermometer', but that rainfall had no connection with mortality rates (Margarey 1878–79).

In focusing on the weather (an uncontrollable event) medical practitioners effectively precluded reference to social conditions affecting health (which are potentially controllable). As late as 1890 an Adelaide doctor could claim that 'there is no overcrowding, no noxious trades or injurious occupations, no destitutions or privations of any kind' (Borthwick 1890). If this was indeed the case then there are few factors other than the weather which can be confidently identified as a source of disease.

Dr Joseph Verco was convinced as to the significance of the weather. But after an exhausting 40 pages of tables and graphs comparing infant mortality and meteorological indices, admitted that while the seasons must play some part in mortality rates, he could come to no conclusion as to what it was (Verco 1878–79).

Even when a disparity in social conditions was recognized, they were not seen as a sufficient cause of disease, and indeed were even asserted to have no special significance. Dr Magarey acknowledged that the highest infant mortality rates existed in the most overcrowded, poorly drained and polluted parts of Adelaide, yet concluded: 'I believe that time will show that bad drainage is not so efficient a cause [of infant death] as heat' (Magarey 1878–79). Indeed, he criticized a Dr McCarthy of Victoria, who 'in a singularly weak way ascribed this excess to careless dieting, improper clothing and impure air' (Margarey 1878–79).

Other commentators were less concerned to point to the weather and more concerned to point to its interaction with social conditions. To the extent that disease and temperature correlated, it was due to inappropriate social custom (Stephens 1839). In 1849, Stephens had pointed out that disease was due less to the hot summer, than to the importing from England of inappropriate housing and clothing fashions. As he put it:

Rigid custom binds men down to a certain class of domestic arrangements, and they condemn the climate when they ought to confess their own want of perception (Stephens 1849).

Magarey's writings on the relationship between heat and mortality were the most explicit in denying social factors. What of other medical authors? Some of them did point to social actions that would mitigate or exacerbate infant mortality during the hot months. Dr Handyside Duncan suggested that infant mortality was the consequence of the 'mismanagment and imprudence' of weaning children in the hot summer months (Duncan 1850). But he took care to exclude the medical profession from any culpability. As the minutes of the Adelaide Children's Hospital recorded in 1876: 'There can be little doubt that our exceptionally high rate of infant mortality is more largely attributable to unskilful nursing than any lack of medical ability' (quoted in Trained Nurses Centenary Committee 1938, 69). Dr Campbell in a pamphlet called *How To Manage a Baby* (1878) identified mothers as the cause of infant mortality. He argued that those babies who died in the summer months did so because they had not been breast fed:

> You may not have every comfort at your command that the rich man's baby has. It may be that your baby does not very regularly get its daily bath, or it is not waited on with the attentive care that a special nurse would give it, or even does not sleep in the cosiest cot in the world. Deprived of all this it will survive but it will not survive if you depart entirely from the order of nature with its food (Campbell 1878).

Here we have an expression of the medical view of the world. Social phenomena are excluded entirely and all problems are reduced to the level of the individual. This becomes even clearer when we look at the solutions offered for the problem of high infant death rates by medical practitioners. There is no reference to housing or to social conditions. Magarey and Campbell both called upon philanthropists to step forward and perform a community service. As Magarey said:

> it is to be hoped that...benevolent persons will cause large, well ventilated, cool resorts to be built in this city to which babies might be taken during the heat of the day. The place might be made attractive with fountains and flowers etc (1878–79).

Can we, albeit briefly, evaluate the claims of the medical practitioners that disease was caused either by individual behaviour or the weather? One way to do this is to examine the incidence of death before and after the introduction of deep drainage—a public health initiative—in 1884 (Jamieson 1887–88). In the ten years prior to 1884 the average annual death rate in Adelaide was 21.38 per 1000. In 1885 it had dropped to 14.34 per 1000. If we break this figure down, into causes of death dependent on the contamination of the water supply by sewage, the following picture emerges. Between 1882–4 typhoid was responsible for 4.8% of deaths; between 1885–6 it dropped to 3.17%. Similarly, diarrhoeal diseases were responsible for 10.44% of deaths between 1882–84, but only 7.37% in 1885–86. While the validity of these figures was debated at the time (Whittell 1887–88) the general thrust of them was accepted: that the introduction of deep drainage had a remarkable effect on the health indices of the population—especially those which depend for their existence on unsanitary conditions: typhoid and gastrointestinal disease.

Thus reductions in mortality and morbidity came about as a consequence of controls over the disposal of waste, over the quality of foodstuffs and protection of the water supply (McKeown 1979).

In New Zealand concerns were also expressed in relation to the infant mortality rate. As in South Australia, the individual mother was blamed for causing the death of the infant. When account is taken of the social circumstances of the mother and child, the effect is to attack Maori culture. Here is a Dr Mason addressing the New Zealand House of Representatives in 1903:

> More than half our Maori die before they are four...and one is not surprised to find this state of affairs when inquiry is made into the infant life of the Maori. The marvel is that more do not die. Lucky is the infant who has a mother's breast...A host of diseases snatch away lives of infants who would have been saved if the mothers were more enlightened as to how to feed their babies (New Zealand 1903).

In Dr Mason's view, it is not only the mother's failure to feed the children, but also Maori culture itself which kills the children:

> The Maori hui [meeting] and prolonged tangis [feasts] are no doubt great curses and are to blame in great measure for infant mortality...these useless huis and tangis ought all to be abolished. It is no wonder that the infant mortality is great when we have these little mites taken into badly ventilated, overcrowded, smoke filled whares [rooms], their meals given to them at irregular hours, their clothes too scanty to keep them warm (New Zealand 1903).

In a situation where a subordinate ethnic culture exists, western medicine attacks and undermines the culture's lifestyles and social organization.

We can see from the above evidence the way in which medical knowledge is located within a political, ethnic and economic environment. The examples show the way in which the developing profession sets out to present itself as scientific—through developing correlations between temperature and infant mortality and implying a causal relationship between them. We can also see the way in which it shifts the blame for the problem onto subordinate groups such as nurses or mothers, or in the New Zealand case, the Maori. Lastly, in its appeals to individual philanthropists, medicine deflects attention away from the need to undertake changes to the economy or the urban environment. We can see too how this knowledge was contested by other groups who located the cause of infant mortality in the social arena—pointing to the outmoded English customs, to the deprivations of urban slums, and to hunger.

Conclusion

This chapter has argued that medical science is the outcome of power struggles between groups in society. It is not the result of the disinterested development of science. The case studies have shown how medical knowledge was contested, how in South Australia the profession had to fight with the state to gain control of the hospital, and how in South Australia and New Zealand other groups disputed its accounts of the causes of infant mortality. The fact that medical concepts became dominant can be explained as a consequence of their fit with the requirements of a capitalist society. The sanitary engineers recognized that it was the environment that needed to be monitored and cleaned up if society was to stay healthy. From this perspective scientific medicine had very little part to play in the improvement of the people's health, or in the understanding of what caused disease (Waitzkin 1981). However the sanitationist's approach did not fit with the political or economic climate of the time. With its focus on the group rather than the individual and its implications for state intervention, it was rejected. Modern medicine, with the aura of the physical sciences, focusing on the individual and denying the need for collective action to prevent disease, was more congruent with 19th century capitalism. In colonial societies such as New Zealand medical knowledge was shaped in such a way as to facilitate the undermining of the indigenous culture. It acted as an ideology legitimating this destruction by being presented as being an impartial and scientific knowledge (Arnold 1988).

In pursuing the development of a just health system we must keep the lessons of a historical sociology of health in mind. We must remember that medical knowledge is as much a social product as it is a product of the natural sciences. Further we must reject the individualism of modern medicine: we must focus on the social, cultural, political and economic structures that shape a health system if we are to produce a just health system. Developing a medicine that has this focus is the outcome of politics and values, not nature and science.

REFERENCES

Arnold D 1988 Imperial medicine and indigenous societies. Manchester University Press, Manchester
Borthwick T 1890 A contribution to the demography of South Australia. Bailliere Tindall & Cox, London
Campbell A 1878 How to manage a baby: a lecture delivered at the City Mission Hall 6th June. South Australian Public Library, Adelaide, p 6
Duncan H 1850 The colony of South Australia. T & W Boone, London, p 27
Grob G 1977 The social history of medicine and disease in America. Journal of Social History 10(1):391–409
Hayter H H 1878–79 Infantile mortality in South Australia. Transactions and Proceedings Philosophical Society of South Australia, vol XI, Adelaide
Hicks N 1982 Medical history and the history of medicine. In: Osborne G, Mandle W (eds) New history—studying Australia today. George Allen & Unwin, Sydney
Hobsbawn E 1971 From social history to the history of society. Daedalus 100(1):20–45
Holder F W 1896 The Adelaide Hospital dispute: the case for the government. South Australian Public Library, Adelaide, p 16
Jamieson J 1887-88 The deep drainage of Adelaide and its influence on the death rate. Royal Society of South Australia Transactions and Proceedings, vol XI, Adelaide
Jamous H, Pelloile B 1970 Professions or self perpetuating systems: changes in the French

university hospital system. In: Jackson J (ed) Professions and professionalisation. Cambridge University Press, Cambridge

Labish A 1985 Doctors, workers and the scientific cosmology of the industrial world. Journal of Contemporary History 20(4):599–615

Larson M 1977 The rise of professionalism. University of California Press, Berkeley, p 23

Lawrence C 1985 Incommunicable knowledge: science technology and the clinical art in Britain 1850–1914. Journal of Contemporary History 20(4):503–521

Magarey S 1878–79 Our climate and infantile mortality. Transactions and Proceedings, Philosophical Society of Adelaide vol II, Adelaide

McKeown T 1979 The role of medicine. Basil Blackwell, London

MacLeod R, Lewis M 1988 Disease medicine and empire. Routledge, London

New Zealand 1903 Journal of the House of Representatives. Government Printer, Wellington

Parry N, Parry J 1976 The rise of the medical profession. Croom Helm, London, pp 136–143

Pensabene T 1980 The rise of the medical profession in Victoria. Australian National University, Canberra, p 159

Ringen K 1979 Edwin Chadwick, the market ideology and sanitary reform: on the nature of the 19th century public health movement. International Journal of Health Services 9(1):107–21

Shortt S 1981 Clinical practice and the social history of medicine. Bulletin of the History of Medicine 55(3):533–542

Shortt S 1983 Physicians science and status: issues in the professionalisation of Anglo-American medicine in the nineteenth century. Medical History 27(1):51–68

South Australian Parliamentary Debates 1884–1896. South Australian Government Printer, Adelaide

South Australian Parliamentary Papers 1875 Second report of central board of health. South Australian Government Printer, Adelaide

Stedman-Jones G 1976 From historical sociology to theoretical history. British Journal of Sociology 27(3):295–305

Stephens J 1839 The land of promise. Smith Elder, London, p 44

Stephens J 1849 Sanitary reform: its general aspect and local importance. Register, Adelaide, p 2

Trained Nurses Centenary Committee 1938 Nursing in South Australia: the first one hundred years. Children's Hospital, Adelaide

Veith I 1980 Changing concepts of health care: an historian's view. Western Journal of Medicine 133(1):532–538

Verco J 1878–79 The South Australian statistics of consumption. Transactions and Proceedings, Philosophical Society, vol. II, Adelaide

Waddington I 1973 The role of the hospital in the development of modern medicine: a sociological analysis. Sociology 7(1):211–224

Waitzkin H 1981 The social origins of illness: a neglected history. International Journal of Health Services 11(1):77–103

Whittell H 1887–88 On the effect of deep drainage on the rate of mortality in Adelaide and suburbs. Royal Society of South Australia Transactions and Proceedings, vol XI, Adelaide

Youngson A J 1979 The scientific revolution in Victorian medicine. Croom Helm, London

15. Towards the democratization of health research

Stephanie D. Short

This chapter aims to provide a theoretical framework for analysis of sociological research on medical knowledge. It will explain why the critique of positivism (belief in the exclusive value of natural scientific knowledge) is central to a contemporary sociology of medical knowledge. The chapter also aims to draw out the implications various sociological perspectives have for the way we understand how medical research can and should be conducted. In doing so it is responding to the challenge posed by postmodernist theory which posits that there is no single truth within complex and diverse post-industrial societies such as Australia (Wickham 1990). Does this mean that anything goes; that, we can be no more certain about the knowledge of a medical practitioner than that of a relative or herbalist? Can we be no more certain that information in medical texts or journals is true, than say information in a self-help newsletter or a women's magazine?

Over the last four decades health sociologists have addressed concerns about the relative certainty of medical knowledge in numerous ways. As theoretical development in the sub-discipline of health sociology has developed in parallel with developments in the parent discipline we can discern several distinctive approaches or schools of thought within the sociology of medical knowledge. The four main theoretical developments that have contributed to our sociological understanding about medical knowledge will be analysed. The starting point for this analysis is the work of Talcott Parsons. We turn then to insights that can be drawn from the phenomenological work of Eliot Freidson and from the work of the most influential post-modernist in this field, Michel Foucault, before reflecting on a nascent critical sociology of medical knowledge. The chapter further contends that a critical sociology informed by postmodernist insights has important implications for more just health research.

Parsons' structural-functionalist perspective

Our journey into sociological thinking about medical knowledge begins with the theorist often referred to as the 'founding father of medical sociology', Talcott Parsons. Parsons' work was fundamental to the shaping of grand sociological theory in the 1950s and 1960s, particularly in the United States of America. His work was also crucial in drawing sociologists' attention to medical practice as a subject for empirical investigation and theoretical enquiry.

Parsons developed a structural-functionalist account of society, and of the structure and function of the institutions, such as the family, organized religion and medicine, within society. In this account, or perspective, society was likened to a living organism, in which each part contributes to the functioning of the whole. In this organic metaphor, Parsons viewed the doctor-patient relationship as a complementary role structure in which doctor and patient are engaged in a common task. In Parsons' (1951:432) now famous chapter on medicine as a social institution in *The Social System*, we note that

Modern medical practice is organised about the application of scientific knowledge to the problems of illness and health, to the control of 'disease'.

In Parsons' view of this complementary role structure, patients are obliged to seek medical advice and to follow doctors' orders, because the medical profession has a monopoly on scientific medical knowledge. The doctor knows better.

Parsons viewed the content of medical science as self-evident and unsuitable for sociological analysis. He shared the assumptions of 'medical positivism' in that he assumed that medical knowledge was objective and universal, and beyond the influence of society. He viewed medical practice as '...part of the general institutionalization of scientific investigation and the application of science to practical problems' (Parsons 1951:474). This quotation, and Parsons' approach more generally indicates that he held an apparently contradictory theoretical perspective towards medical knowledge. On the one hand, Parsons assumed that medical science is a universal value-free knowledge which is not suitable as a subject for sociological scrutiny. On the other hand, he believed that applied medical knowledge was not completely scientific (yet). As a consequence, in his view applied or clinical medical knowledge did warrant sociological investigation.

It is apparent, then, that Parsons did not accept uncritically the assumptions of medical positivism, as implied by some critics of traditional medical sociology (Wright & Treacher 1982, Bury 1986). Parsons did assume that the content of scientific medical knowledge was objective and universal, and beyond the influence of society. However, he recognized that the institutionalization of science within medical practice was far from complete, as medical practice was influenced by personal, social and other non-scientific considerations. Thus, while the Parsonian perspective excluded the content of medical science from sociological scrutiny, when this knowledge was applied to problems of health and illness, in medical practice, it became suitable as a topic for sociological enquiry.

Freidson's phenomenological perspective

I move now to analyse Freidson's perspective in some depth, as his work has been most influential in problematizing the social construction of applied medical knowledge. Freidson's (1970a, 1970b, 1983, 1989) work was strongly influenced by Berger and Luckmann's unique style of phenomenological sociology. Their study, *The Social Construction of Reality: A Treatise in the Sociology of Knowledge* (Berger & Luckmann 1967) remains the most influential phenomenological study in the sociology of knowledge. Phenomenological sociology, in its various forms, aims generally to provide greater understanding and description of everyday life, of the social life-world. The phenomenological trends in sociology, such as symbolic interactionism, labelling theory and ethnomethodology have derived, to differing degrees, from phenomenological philosophy as developed earlier in this century by Edmund Husserl (1970) and applied to sociology by Alfred Schutz (1967).

The significance of phenomenology for sociology has been attributed to two principal factors: firstly, to the way the phenomenological perspective 'illuminates the human world' and secondly, because phenomenological method enables detailed description of concrete human experiences (Luckmann 1978:7). In Freidson's (1970a) core treatise in the 'sociology of applied medical knowledge' the twin concerns were setting and perspective. Freidson emphasized that one could only understand the socially constructed universe of medical practitioners through understanding the social organization of their work.

Freidson's early work in medical sociology, as in *Patients' Views of Medical Practice* (1961), takes Parsons' work as its starting point. Its main theoretical argument is that a sociological perspective which recognizes conflict is more appropriate in analysing doctor/patient relations than Parsons' structural-functionalist perspective. Freidson contends that conflict is endemic in the doctor-patient relationship because of two important factors: necessary differences in perspectives between doctors and patients and secondly, uncertainties inherent in the routine application of medical knowledge to human problems. This endemic conflict becomes visible when patients, on the basis of their 'lay perspective', attempt to have some control over doctors' actions.

Freidson's main thesis is that the separate worlds of experience and reference of patients and doctors are always in 'potential conflict' with one another. Problems are seen to arise because these parties may not agree on definitions of patients' problems, or on the means by which goals should be achieved. Freidson asserts that medical practice is sociologically problematic because of the fact that medical scientific knowledge is never complete and because medical treatment may be worthless or inadequate. It is pointed out that there are likely to be diseases that are unrecognized by contemporary diagnostic knowledge. For example, the distinction between typhoid and typhus was not known until 1820, and medical science did not distinguish between gonorrhoea and syphilis until later in the 19th century. Thus, for Freidson the first problem stems from the incompleteness in contemporary medical science. This problem becomes evident in the act of medical diagnosis. Even the most knowledgeable and well-intentioned doctor can mis-diagnose or ignore complaints because medical science is never complete.

The second sociological concern stems from the nature of medical practice, the arena in which abstract scientific knowledge is applied to concrete patient problems. Freidson recognizes that medical treatments can be ineffective, worthless or dangerous. A major concern is the way medical work takes on a routine character. Individual patient problems are interpreted as signs and symptoms within medicine's classificatory system, and thus treated as ordinary cases of particular diseases, such as upper respiratory tract infection, or cancer. Freidson's analysis of medical practice is particularly perceptive here:

> In so far as knowledge consists in general and objective diagnostic categories by which the physician sorts the concrete signs and complaints confronting him, it follows that work assumes a routine character. This is the routine of classifying the flow of reality into a limited number of categories so that the individual items that flow become reduced to mere incidences of a class, each individual instance being considered the same as every other in its class. (Freidson 1975:287)

Medical practice was viewed as a social arena within which human problems were categorized and classified by medical practitioners into problems amenable to medical diagnosis and treatment. Thus, the knowledge of medical practitioners is shaped with medical intervention in mind.

Weber's (1977) view of how knowledge is constituted, that is in terms of 'value relevance' and 'cultural significance' is useful here. According to Weber, social knowledge is always a function of the knower or observer's cognitive and cultural interests. In the often quoted essay, 'Methodology of the Social Sciences' Weber (1978:76–83) did not advocate that the social scientist should abstain from all value-commitments. Rather, in one's role as a scientist a particular subvalue system must be paramount for the investigation. Parsons (1977:59) has suggested that this subvalue system emphasizes conceptual clarity, consistency and generality in theoretical approach. In the empirical sphere, empirical accuracy and verifiability are the valued outputs of social scientific investigation. Weber held that social scientists should differentiate between their roles as value-free scientists and as value-laden participants in a culture. This enables social scientists to attain the 'objectivity' necessary to select out those factors which are essential to the scientific purpose, using *value-relevance*, from those *value-judgements* which stem from their own value systems which are irrelevant to the investigation.

The basic epistemological assumption which underlies the thought of Weber and Freidson is the neo-Kantian assumption, derived from Rickert, that social reality cannot be grasped objectively by the human mind. Any view of the social world, Weber held, must be limited and partial. The social world differs from the natural world and cannot be explained with holistic laws of cause and effect. For Weber:

...there is no absolutely 'objective' scientific analysis of culture...or of social phenomena independent of special and one-sided viewpoints according to which expressly or tacitly, consciously or unconsciously, they are selected, analysed and organised for expository purposes. (Weber 1977:24)

Following Weber, Freidson drew a distinction between the natural world of diseases and bodies, which is most appropriately comprehended by medical experts, and the social world of medical practice which is appropriately analysed by sociologists.

In the preface to *Profession of Medicine*, Freidson asserts:

Knowledge and expertise, whether accepted or rejected, tend to be seen as things existing in and of themselves rather than as abstractions which are realised by the activities of men organised in occupational careers and groups. (Freidson 1970a:*xi)*

His aim, then, is to examine sociologically connections between the professional organization of medical practice and medical knowledge. These, for Freidson, are analytically and, indeed, practically distinct social phenomena. The contrast with Parsons' theoretical approach is clear. Freidson does not accept the medical profession's own definition of its work, its expertise and its 'science' as Parsons did. On the contrary, Freidson sees the medical profession as a special type of 'occupational organization' in which a certain perspective thrives and which, by virtue of its social power, comes to transform 'if not actually create the substance of its own work' (Freidson 1970a:xix). Thus, the organization of professional medical work and the perspective of medical practitioners both influence the nature of medical concepts and knowledge. Clinical medical knowledge reflects the interests of medical practitioners, in attempting to control this or that disease or aspect of biophysical reality. Applied medical knowledge and concepts are not universal, but reflective of particular organizational structures, practices and interests.

Applied medical knowledge is also historically relative for Freidson. In examining the history of the medical profession, he points out that medicine did not become a 'true consulting profession' until the late 19th century when, 'having developed a sufficiently scientific foundation', its work seemed superior to that of irregular healers (Freidson 1970a:12). He is critical of most histories of medicine which selectively focus on great discoveries and those pieces of information that are now considered to be 'scientifically true'. In acknowledging the importance of a systematic scientific foundation for medicine he emphasizes that the discovery, in 1860, of the bacterial aetiology of anthrax was of critical significance in the history of medicine because, as Ackernecht observed, 'for the first time in history, causes of numerous diseases became known' (cited in Freidson 1970a:16). The germ theory of disease opened the way for a replacement of symptomatic or empirical medical treatment because it had demonstrable therapeutic efficacy in key categories of sickness.

In this phenomenological perspective, knowledge about biophysical reality is bracketed out from sociological consideration, in keeping with the phenomenological method of *epoche*. The phenomenological perspective on medical knowledge, as developed by Freidson, rests on a heuristic distinction between the 'natural' world of biophysical reality, which is most appropriately comprehended by medical experts, and the 'social life-world' of medical practice which is appropriately analysed by sociologists. The basic epistemological assumption which underlies Freidson's perspective, and the thought of Weber, is the neo-Kantian contention that social reality is distinct from nature, and cannot be grasped objectively with the methods of the natural sciences. Any view of the social world, Weber (1978) held, must be limited and partial. Thus, the social life-world and the natural world require different methods of scientific analysis.

Three related sociological concerns or issues emerge from Freidson's work and they are, first, the differing perspectives of doctors and patients, second, the unequal power relation between doctor and patient, and third, the potential for the medical perspective to be imposed on the patient. From a phenomenological perspective the problem is that the medical construction of reality is privileged over the lay perspective. The principal practical implication that can be drawn from Freidson's work is that health care consumers should have a greater say in how their health problems are defined and managed. However, the methodological approach of *epoche* means that Freidson excluded medical knowledge about biophysical reality, that is current scientific knowledge about the body, from sociological scrutiny.

Foucault's postmodern perspective

As Michel Foucault was a historian and philosopher of ideas, rather than a sociologist, it is not easy to locate his work within the theoretical traditions of sociology. Foucault's oeuvre has been variously labelled as 'post-modernist' and as 'post-structuralist'. This former term aligns Foucault's work with post-modernism's rejection of the Enlightenment ideal of progress towards a truly rational society (Fraser 1989, Wickham 1990). The latter term is more specific. It associates Foucault's work with that of other contemporary French philosophers, linguists, psychoanalysts and feminists whose work destabilizes the structure of hierarchical binary oppositions such as brain/heart, man/woman, masculine/feminine (Delacour & Short 1992). In particular, Derrida's (1978) notion of *difference* and the process of 'deconstruction' incorporate a rejection of these binary structures of thought and truth. Derrida brings our attention to the repression of difference. The work of Cixous (1981) and other contemporary French feminists (Sawicki

1991) examines the repression of the feminine in western thought. Deconstruction examines ways in which discourses, that is ways of thinking, have been constructed. Deconstructive, or post-structuralist, analyses bring the naturalized, glossed-over and unarticulated presuppositions in language to our attention. The process of deconstruction destabilizes the constructed truth of powerful, monolithic and patriarchal discourses and acknowledges multiplicities of truths.

One such truth that deconstruction challenges is the notion of the 'subject' that emerged in the West following the Enlightenment. Foucault's work on knowledge/power configurations locates the production of the subject in particular 'regimes of truth'. A key work in this regard is 'The politics of health in the eighteenth century' (Foucault 1991). While previous historical accounts had traced the development of modern medicine from a personal relationship between doctor and patient to a collectively organized public health (Rosen 1958), Foucault contends that both private and socialized medicine derive from a common politics of health.

> In primitive communities, down to the Middle Ages, society's defence against sickness, physical or mental, was to *isolate* or *destroy* the patient; later came the endeavour to *heal* the sick so as to prevent them from infecting or harming their fellowmen or becoming a burden on society; and finally the establishment of the positive *protection of the healthy* from the dangers of disease.
>
> (Marti-Ibanez 1958:16)

Foucault's work can be understood as a challenge to structuralist accounts of history, and in this case public health accounts, which view medical history as progress towards the bacteriological revolution and the era of preventive medicine.

Foucault offers a de-centred or dispersed notion of knowledge/power relations, rather than one which gives primacy to any one structure or pattern of power relations. His work points to multiple sites for the operation of power and for resistance. This contrasts with the centred or structuralist notion of power in Marxism and much feminism, which sees power residing with the ruling class or with men in general. While Foucault's work points to a complex array of local resistances and to the need to identify specific sites of struggle, the latter tend to 'totalize' and to seek total transformations. Indeed, the central goal in Foucault's (1982) work over a twenty year period was to create a history of the different ways in which human beings are seen as subjects in our culture. His work deals with three particular ways in which human beings were transformed into subjects, through: the human sciences; the professions of psychiatry, medicine and the law; and through the domain of sexuality. In each mode power is exercised through knowledge and human beings are individualized as subjects. Foucault's (1982:216) central goal was '...to promote new forms of subjectivity through the refusal of this kind of individuality which has been imposed on us for centuries.' We turn now to examine the discourse of medicine which objectifies and transforms human beings into passive and compliant patients.

The conditions in which appeared the experiment and the whole clinical terminology—'the first scientifically structured terminology devoted to the individual'—have been brilliantly described by Foucault in *La naissance de la clinique*. (Jamous & Peloille 1970:127)

Foucault's central contribution to the sociology of medical knowledge is encapsulated in the above quotation. Foucault's (1975) history of medical ideas in *The Birth of the Clinic* delineated the discourse of clinical medicine, and associated its birth with the rise of the university-hospital system in France following the French Revolution. For the purposes of this Chapter the important breakthrough is that Foucault removed the brackets that had previously excluded medical scientific knowledge from sociological scrutiny.

Foucault linked the new clinical discourse with the creation of university-hospitals in which clinicians gained access to a new and diverse range of clinical material.

Modern medicine has fixed its own date of birth as being in the last years of the eighteenth century. Reflecting on its situation, it identifies the origin of its positivity with a return—over and above all theory—to the modest but effecting level of the perceived. (Foucault 1975:xii).

Three other organizational factors contributed to the rise of the French clinical school and the 'clinical gaze' at the beginning of the last century: the concentration of hospitals in Paris; the foundation of a system of selection and apprenticeship in the hospitals which was designed to create a kind of 'medical elite'; and the fact that the medical faculties chose their instructors from among the elite and highly qualified clinical experts from the hospitals (Jamous & Peloille 1970:128). 'Thus it was in the hospital wards, these 'natural laboratories', that medical science was born and fashioned' (Jamous & Peloille, 1970:130).

The post-modernist perspective towards medical knowledge that has been discerned here is evident in the work of Bloor (1976) and Nicolson and McLaughlin (1988). Their work is *Foucauldian* insofar as Foucault's (1974, 1975) work has been crucial in encouraging them to scrutinize the content of medical discourse. Bloor's (1976) case study on adenotonsillectomies is particularly significant because it questioned the *ontological* status of disease entities. It differed from the Parsonian and phenomenological work, because it scrutinized the *content* of medical scientific knowledge about a biophysical phenomenon, tonsillitis. Bloor stated that the content of medical scientific knowledge should become a subject for sociological inquiry, rather than simply a resource.

More recently, Nicolson and McLaughlin's (1988) study revealed that the skills, knowledge and backgrounds of protagonists in the debate about the causes of multiple sclerosis shaped the *content* of the knowledge produced about multiple sclerosis. Their study described how multiple medical scientific truths about multiple sclerosis were constructed. It is important to note, however, that in this constructivist or relativist approach to the sociology of knowledge, one does not make judgements about the truth status of the knowledge under sociological scrutiny. In this relativist stream of postmodernist theorizing the implication is that knowledge that has been socially constructed could have been constructed differently, under different circumstances. The main conclusion to be drawn from this perspective is that the content of medical scientific knowledge *could* be different.

Towards a critical sociology of medical knowledge

Habermas' theory of cognitive interests, or interests that guide knowledge, also explodes the myth of authorless, objective scientific knowledge. Habermas' (1971, 1978) framework of knowledge and human interests exposes the connection between scientific knowledge and human interest which positivism conceals. It reveals that the general orientation guiding the natural sciences is rooted in a deep-seated *cognitive interest* in predicting and controlling events in the natural environment. He calls this intellectual interest the 'technical interest'.

Habermas' notion of cognitive interests extends the sociological critique of positivism one step further than the perspectives examined above. Habermas' critical theory reveals that science is value-neutral in appearance only; because it actually takes a partisan position in favour of progressive scientific and technological control. Thus, medical scientific knowledge is not value-neutral. It not only reflects the cognitive interests of the scientific community. Its interest can be summarized as an interest in controlling and predicting the natural environment. For Habermas (1971:55)

...the professional practice in question [medicine] will always have to assume the form of technical control of objectified processes.

Understood in this way, it can be argued that the appropriate response to the problem of medical positivism is cultivation of the understanding that scientific knowledge is one type of knowledge which reflects the intellectual interests of the medical scientific community. Ironically, it is just this type of critical analysis which positivism blocks, and in so doing it conceals the social and intellectual interests that actually determine the content of medical scientific knowledge.

This critical perspective towards medical knowledge has developed principally in work located in the Marxist (Figlio 1982, 1985, Richards 1986, 1988) and socialist feminist traditions (Kaufert & McKinlay 1985). The critical perspective views medical scientific knowledge as a cultural product which reflects the particular values and material interests of researchers in the name of universal truth. In Figlio's (1982, 1985) work on miners' nystagmus, an occupational disease, medical science is seen to be problematic for two reasons. Firstly, because the values implicit in the medical scientific knowledge about miners' nystagmus encouraged miners to accept unhealthy working conditions and occupational diseases as if they were natural, necessary and inevitable. Medical science as ideology was problematic also because it legitimated the knowledge and power of the medical profession, and the mine owners for whom they worked, in the name of universal truth and knowledge.

Richards' (1986, 1988) study on vitamin C revealed that the medical researcher is a partisan participant in the research process, rather than an unbiased arbiter of scientific truth. Richards contends that medicine's monopoly over health research should be challenged, and that the process of therapeutic evaluation should be revised to reflect the values and interests of non-medical parties, through the participation of non-medical experts, patients and members of the public at large.

Kaufert and McKinlay's (1985) research on hormone replacement therapy (HRT) reveals that medical researchers used their knowledge about oestrogen replacement therapy as an ideology in order to protect clinicians against the threat of legal action from dissatisfied users of HRT.

These critical studies provide evidence of competing medical 'truths', and these medical truths, or ideologies, reflect the particular intellectual and material interests of researchers, in the name of universal truth. Whilst a Foucauldian perspective views these different truths or discourses in a non-judgemental or relativistic way, a critical sociological perspective views these medical truths, as examples of ideologies which mask and legitimate medical power. Medical science as ideology has the effect of masking the dominant position which medical researchers have over other groups in the social production of health knowledge.

The Foucauldian and critical perspectives examined here lead to different political conclusions. The Foucauldian perspective concludes that medical knowledge could be produced in a different way, within a different regime of truth. The critical perspective, in contrast, argues that health knowledge *should* be produced in a more emancipatory way. It challenges the freedom from outside scrutiny that medical researchers have traditionally enjoyed, and calls their monopoly over the production of health knowledge into question.

The contrast is clear, while relativism eschews evaluation, critical sociology demands political analysis and engagement (Fraser 1989). Critical sociologists make judgements about the knowledge under investigation, or more precisely about the social context within which the knowledge under investigation was constructed. The principal question guiding critical research is was the knowledge constructed under conditions free from unnecessary domination? If the answer is no, then the implication is that the knowledge *should* be constructed under more equal or democratic circumstances. Whilst the relativist concludes that the knowledge under investigation *could* be constructed differently, the critical sociologist posits that it *should* be constructed under more just conditions.

From the epistemological point of view, both the Foucauldian and the critical perspectives differ from Parsons' perspective because they reject the positivist epistemological assumption that scientific medical knowledge is universal and objective, and hence unsuitable for sociological scrutiny. Epistemologically, they differ also from the phenomenological perspective because they reveal that scientific medical knowledge is value-laden and partial. This revelation breaks down the utility of the distinction between uncertain, subjective clinical knowledge and reliable, objective scientific knowledge, which characterized the phenomenological perspective.

Neither the Foucauldian nor critical approach accepts that the content of medical scientific knowledge is universal and objective. Both approaches subject medical knowledge to sociological scrutiny. Both examine the social production of biophysical knowledge, through analysing the complex interactions between medical experts, biophysical reality and the social life-world. They reject the positivist assumptions implicit in Parsons' perspective and the distinction between objective scientific knowledge and subjective clinical knowledge which is implicit in Freidson's perspective. Foucauldian and critical examinations of the social production of biophysical knowledge reveal, instead, a two-way interaction between the knower and the known that is always mediated by culture.

Conclusion

This Chapter has revealed that post-positivist health sociology neither accepts that the content of medical scientific knowledge is true, nor excludes it from sociological inquiry. It has also indicated that sociologists' willingness to scrutinize the *content* of medical scientific knowledge rests on a critique of medical positivism, such as that developed in the work of Foucault (1974, 1975) or in Habermas' critical sociology (1971, 1978). In drawing on critical sociology, and Habermas' work in particular, sociologists can see that medical scientific knowledge is value-neutral in appearance only; because it actually takes a partisan position in favour of progressive scientific and technological control over biophysical phenomena, such as cells, diseases and bodies.

The sociological scrutiny of medical scientific research and the concomitant challenge to the monopoly position of medical researchers has two implications for the politics of medical research: it implies either that the process of medical research can be different or that it should be different. On the one hand, sociologists conclude that the social process of health research can produce different and equally valid and useful results (Bloor 1976, Nicolson & McLaughlin 1988). This conclusion is consistent with a Foucauldian or relativistic sociological perspective. In these studies, and in the relativist program in the sociology of science more generally, sociologists do not attempt to evaluate the truth, falsehood or rationality of statements; they search for the conditions of possibility which have enabled that knowledge to be constructed. This calls for an even-handed or symmetrical approach towards all knowledge. In this relativistic approach, all knowledge is socially constructed and treated with equal respect. These sociologists do not take sides. Relativists undertake non-evaluative investigations. The theoretical potential of their analyses is not linked with political analysis or engagement.

In contrast, critical sociologists contend that the social process of health research should be different (Kaufert & McKinlay 1985, Figlio 1982, 1985, Richards 1986, 1988). These critical sociologists have challenged medicine's monopolistic position in medical research and called for an opening up of the 'health' research process to non-medical experts, such as sociologists and health care consumers. These studies reveal that the interests of women, workers and consumers have been ignored or negated in the medical production of knowledge about oestrogen replacement therapy, miners' nystagmus and vitamin C. This critical or emancipatory perspective towards the sociology of medical research concludes that the social production of health knowledge should be opened up to greater lay scrutiny, evaluation and participation. This critical approach links theoretical conclusions with political analysis and engagement, and thus calls for a more open and participatory research process.

While Freidson's challenge to the autonomy of medical practitioners led sociologists over the last twenty years to suggest that patients should have a greater say in the way health problems are managed, the challenge to the autonomy of medical researchers implicit in the fourth theoretical perspective identified in this Chapter indicates that non-medical experts and health care consumers should have a greater say in the way health problems are researched in the future.

REFERENCES

Berger P, Luckmann T 1967 The social construction of reality: a treatise in the sociology of knowledge. Anchor, New York

Bloor M 1976 Bishop Berkeley and the adenotonsillectomy enigma: an exploration of variation in the social construction of medical disposals. Sociology 10(1):43–61

Bury M R 1986 Social constructionism and the development of medical sociology. Sociology of Health and Illness 8(2):137–169

Cixous H 1981 Where is she? In: Marks E, de Coutivron I (eds) New French feminisms. Harvester, Sussex

Delacour S, Short S D 1992 Nursing, medicine and women's health: a discourse analysis. In: Gray G, Pratt R (eds) Issues in Australian nursing 3. Churchill Livingstone, Melbourne

Derrida J 1978 Writing and difference. University of Chicago Press, Chicago

Figlio K 1982 How does illness mediate social relations? Workmen's compensation and medico-legal practices 1890–1940. In: Wright P, Treacher A (eds) The problem of medical knowledge: examining the social construction of medicine. Edinburgh University Press, Edinburgh

Figlio K 1985 Medical diagnosis, class dynamics, social stability. In: Levidow L, Young B (eds) Science, technology and the labour process, vol 2. Free Association Books, London

Foucault M 1974 The archaeology of knowledge. Tavistock, London

Foucault M 1975 The birth of the clinic. Vintage, New York

Foucault M 1982 Afterword: the subject and power. In: Dreyfus H L, Rabinow P (eds) Michel Foucault: beyond structuralism and hermeneutics. Harvester, Brighton

Foucault M 1991 The politics of health in the eighteenth century. In: Rabinow P (ed) The Foucault reader: an introduction to Foucault's thought. Penguin, London

Fraser N 1989 Unruly practices: power, discourse and gender in contemporary social theory. Polity, Cambridge

Freidson E 1961 Patients' views of medical practice. Russell Sage Foundation, New York

Freidson E 1968 Medical personnel: physicians. In: International encyclopedia of the social sciences, vol 10. Macmillan, New York

Freidson E 1970a Profession of medicine: a study of the sociology of applied knowledge. Dodd Mead, New York

Freidson E 1970b Professional dominance: the social structure of medical care. Aldine, Chicago

Freidson E 1975 Dilemmas in the doctor/patient relationship. In: Cox C, Mead A (eds) A sociology of medical practice. Collier-Macmillan, London

Freidson E 1983 Viewpoint: sociology and medicine: a polemic! Sociology of Health and Illness 5(2):208–19

Freidson E 1989 Medical work in America. Yale University Press, New Haven

Habermas J 1971 Technology and science as ideology. In: Toward a rational society. Heinemann, London

Habermas J 1978 Knowledge and human interests. Heinemann, London

Husserl E 1970 The crisis of European sciences and transcendental phenomenology: an introduction to phenomenological philosophy. Northwestern University Press, Evanston

Jamous J, Peloille B 1970 Professions or self perpetuating systems? Changes in the French university hospital system. In: Jackson J (ed) Professions and professionalisation. Cambridge University Press, Cambridge

Kaufert P, McKinlay S 1985 Estrogen-replacement therapy: the production of medical knowledge and the emergence of policy. In: Lewin E, Olesen V (eds) Women, health and healing: towards a new perspective. Tavistock, London

Luckmann T (ed) 1978 Phenomenology and sociology: selected readings. Penguin, Harmondsworth

Marti-Ibanez F 1958 Foreword. In: Rosen G A history of public health. M. D. Publications, New York

Nicolson M, McLaughlin C 1988 Social constructionism and medical sociology: a study of the vascular theory of multiple sclerosis. Sociology of Health and Illness 10(3):234–61

Parsons T 1951 The social system. Routledge & Kegan Paul, London

Parsons T 1977 Value-freedom and objectivity. In: Dallymar F R, McCarthy T A (eds) Understanding and social inquiry. University of Notre Dame Press, Notre Dame

Richards E 1986 Vitamin C suffers a dose of politics. New Scientist 109(26)46–9

Richards E 1988 The politics of therapeutic evaluation: the vitamin C and cancer controversy. Social Studies of Science 18:653–701

Rosen G 1958 A history of public health. M. D. Publications, New York

Sawicki J 1991 Disciplining Foucault: feminism, power and the body. Routledge, New York

Schutz A 1967 The phenomenology of the social world. Heinemann, London

Weber M 1977 Objectivity in social science and social policy. In: Dallymar F, McCarthy T 1977 Understanding and social inquiry. University of Notre Dame Press, Notre Dame

Weber M 1978 Methodology of the social sciences. In: Runciman W G (ed) Max Weber: selections in translation. Cambridge University Press, Cambridge

Wickham G 1990 The political possibilities of postmodernism. Economy and Society 19(1)121–51

Wright P, Treacher A 1982 The problem of medical knowledge: examining the social construction of medicine. Edinburgh University Press, Edinburgh

16. Health technology policy and sleep disorder centres

Evan Willis   Jeanne Daly

The search for technological means to diagnose and treat ill health is an old one. This Chapter deals with policy issues surrounding the diffusion of medical technologies. The specific instance of sleep disorder centres is used to illustrate the difficult policy decisions that have to be made about the application of technologies to the improvement of human health.

At first glance, it may seem unusual to talk of 'medical technology policy'; surely medical technologies are introduced if they work and aren't if they don't! The problem is more complex. If we accept that there are limited health resources and many competing demands, how are we to choose knowledgeably between spending these resources on medical technologies as against other health programs? How do we know that a medical technology works? How are we to choose rationally between one technology and another which has the same or similar purpose? What weight should be given to considerations of cost, safety and possible social and ethical implications? Whose views are to carry weight in setting policy? What are the implications of all these choices in promoting access for those who require it?

The purpose of this Chapter is to argue that there is much more to the process of generating policy regarding medical technologies than purely technical considerations of what works. Indeed our argument is that a sociological perspective on policy setting for medical technology facilitates a focus on social justice considerations in this field and provides an opportunity to reflect on the broad social context of health care in Australia.

The concept of social justice is a difficult one to define. As the introduction to this book makes clear, at its most basic, policy settings with the aim of creating a just society aim at maximizing the opportunities for all individuals to benefit from advances in health care including those involving medical technology. This is a laudable aim. The difficulty is that an avowed aim towards social justice may represent an ideology that is useful for legitimating political programs as well as a discourse in which to cloak vested interest.

The social context of medical technology policy

We take *medical technologies* to mean the application of machines, devices, procedures or techniques as a means of achieving control over problems of ill

233

health. Medical technologies can range from the extremely simple to the very complex. *Diagnostic* technologies aim to identify existing disease and may range from a thermometer for diagnosing fevers to Positron Emission Tomography (PET) scanners for diagnosing metabolic disorders. *Therapeutic* technologies are used to treat health problems and range from aspirin through to chemotherapy for cancer and procedures like heart-lung transplants. *Preventive* technologies aim to reduce the risk of ill health and may range from condoms for reducing the likelihood of contracting sexually transmitted diseases to mass vaccination or screening programs. Hospitals and health care systems are becoming increasingly dependent on *information* technologies for processing health data.

All health technologies have in common a *material* or *technical* component but, less obviously, this is located within a *social* context. At the micro-level the social context consists of the people by whom and on whom the technology is used. At the next level are the social groups to which these people belong—the medical profession or consumer groups. At the macro-level there are broad social issues which impinge on the use of technology, for example, economic interests and the role of the State in maintaining and funding an effective health system.

Within the health system there are a large number of technologies which have been well established in clinical practice for many years. Other technologies are still new or in the process of being introduced. It is useful to distinguish where along a continuum a technology is located; from the new and experimental through the routine and well established to the old and out-dated. The concept of a medical technology having a 'career' is useful one (see McKinlay 1982). New machines or techniques with the potential for improving health are constantly being developed (invention). Some of these technologies will be seen as promising improved control over ill health and innovation occurs when some practitioners take up and use the technology. Diffusion occurs when more practitioners take up and use the technology as well. The social process of the career of a technology may not end there however. Once technologies have diffused into clinical practice, they may be found to be unsatisfactory so that diffusion is slowed and, in some cases, even with an established technology, disillusionment sets in so that the technology may be discontinued. In theory, health technology policy can seek to intervene at any stage along this career path, but in practice it has been primarily focused on the control of new technologies by stopping or slowing the diffusion of the technology, usually by not providing reimbursement for the cost of the procedure.

The methodological technique developed for attempting to resolve these questions of health technology policy, is itself a technology. The field of technology assessment has become a large one. In the health arena, whole academic journals and many conferences are held on this issue. Many countries in the world have developed specialized governmental agencies to advise governments and make decisions on which medical technologies should be introduced and how this should be done.

The conventional health technology assessment criteria are effectiveness (does it work?), cost, and safety. Equity of access for all consumers in need of the technology is an overriding concern. Technology assessment techniques have been most successful in controlling the proliferation of drugs by instituting mandatory testing procedures at the stage of innovation. Outside of this field, success has been patchy. The first problem encountered has been that it is unexpectedly difficult to establish that a technology is effective in achieving its technical purpose. This may be for a variety of reasons. Many technologies are used in conjunction with other interventions so that it is not clear what one particular technology contributes. In many cases the contribution to improved health for the patient is not clear and may need to be assumed. Diagnostic technologies, for example, pose the problem that more than one test is commonly used; if these tests together lead to a more accurate diagnosis, this may lead to a change in treatment which, in turn, may lead to improved health for the patient. How is any improved outcome to be assigned to one test? If the tests only confirm the doctor's diagnosis or show that the patient is *not* suffering from a particular disease, how is this outcome to be assessed in term of benefit to patients? Importantly many technologies are evolving rapidly so that the assessment of a technology may be out of date before it is completed. Ideally, evaluation should be based on the long term effect but this may not become apparent for 20 years or more by which time the technology will have been superseded many times over. Technology assessment procedures therefore have to be flexible, aiming at producing the best possible answer within these constraints.

Technologies can proliferate and become well established in practice without there being any evidence of effectiveness. This is true of many technologies in use at the present. Indeed, there is evidence that some technologies have proliferated when there is evidence that they are *ineffective* (Lumley 1987). This points to the problem that the reasons for the proliferation of a technology may be based not only on technical factors but also on social factors which may contradict or even override the conclusions of an evaluation. This social context involves what we call the social relations of medical technology. So despite the new emphasis on evaluation based health technology policies, in practice the direct effect of this evaluation on the proliferation of health technologies is still to be evaluated.

The social relations of medical technologies, which may operate to promote either their proliferation or discontinuation, include the diverse interests of groups of social actors in the setting of health technology policy. Issues of social justice are prominent in the arguments advanced.

Patients are obvious stakeholders, rarely represented directly but influencing policy setting in two ways. The influence comes directly from individual patients who have serious health problems or from patient support groups promoting a technology (such as the group 'Friends of IVF') to ensure access for patients who see themselves as needing this help. In extreme cases, they may pressure governments to allow access to unevaluated technologies in order to treat patients suffering from serious or distressing conditions for which there is no alternative treatment. This creates ethical dilemmas for clinicians who have doubts about the long term benefit of the treatment. The problem is particularly difficult if procedures are already available in other countries and very ill patients are spending large sums of money to go there for treatment. The consumer perspective may also be presented through wider consumer groups specifically established to represent consumer interests in matters of health policy setting such as the Consumers' Health Forum. In this case, the input to policy may be less concerned with the interests of individual patients and more with the interests of consumers as a whole.

Professional groups are another major stakeholder, not only individually but also through their professional organizations. Individual clinicians may well wish to do whatever is possible in treating an ill patient. Indeed, it could be argued that it is their ethical responsibility to do so irrespective of the cost to the community or social justice issues concerning access for other patients. The profession as a whole may respond to increasing concern about malpractice suits brought by patients by endorsing defensive medicine including the use of an ever increasing array of diagnostic tests. More subtly, a professional reputation may depend upon having access to the latest in diagnostic and treatment technologies since these are seen as setting the 'gold standard' for good clinical practice. This gives rise to what has been called the phenomenon of 'me too-ism'. The argument is that if one health care facility has a particular technology then others, if they are not to fall behind in providing the best care for their patient, must have one as well. Convenient access to the best technology can be important to consumer groups and, in a number of metropolitan centres in recent years, consumers have joined clinicians in public campaigns to raise money to buy big-ticket items such as CT scanners.

In addition, in this context, the process of proliferation may be accelerated when consortia of private medical specialists as entrepreneurs privately purchase big-ticket items and provide private services utilizing the technology. Whether in private or public practice, once a technology is acquired, a 'financial imperative' operates to make full use of an expensive machine. Doctors may gradually relax the indications for which patients are referred in order to maintain the 'throughput' of patients. The problem which arises is that the benefit to these patients may become doubtful.

Industry is also a stakeholder in that treating illness is a source of profit. Manufacturers of a technology not surprisingly have a stake in selling their product and having it widely used. There must be profits if manufacturers of health technologies are to stay in business. Pharmaceutical companies are perhaps best known in this regard, but all manufacturers of health technology promote the proliferation of their products. While, clearly, promoting the sale of existing technologies is a necessary step in the development of new and better technologies, problems arise when a technology is promoted to consumers in a manner which exaggerates benefits and minimizes risk. The media may aid this process when a revolutionary 'breakthrough' in the fight against disease, still at the experimental stage, is reported as effective and imminent.

The final stakeholder is the State[1] itself. Pursuing explicit social justice aims has been a feature of State policies in the last decade with the legislative arm being occupied by Labor governments of a social democratic type. For the State, seeking to balance the various social justice objectives, the cost implications of continual health technology innovation have been seen as substantial in the context of a national health insurance service such as Medicare and its predecessor Medibank. As new health technologies have appeared (the invention and innovation phase), pressure has commonly been exerted on the State health bureaucracy (at the federal level) by various groups above, and sometimes all in concert, to include the use of the technology under the Medicare scheme. Indeed securing a Medicare schedule number has often been crucial to the process of diffusion of that health technology.

There exists also a particularly Australian version of 'me-too-ism' which is known as 'state's rights'. 'If it is good enough for the large states to have this technology, it is good enough for smaller ones as well' is how this is usually expressed, even if the international evidence suggests that two or maybe three facilities are sufficient for a country the size of Australia.

The quest for a just health technology policy involves considerations that are relevant to both sides of this question. More facilities will promote equity of geographical access as patients do not have to travel interstate for complicated medical procedures. On the other hand, concentrating the availability of the procedure in a few centres may maximize the cost effectiveness of the resources used, as well as the safety aspects associated with potentially higher skill levels of practitioners performing a larger rather than a smaller number of the procedures. Balancing these considerations in the setting of policy is a difficult task.

The State response has been to establish its own health technology advisory body. The National Health Technology Advisory Panel was formally established in 1982, serviced by the Commonwealth Department of Health. Responsibility for supporting the panel passed to the newly established Australian Institute of Health in 1987. In 1991 this was restructured under the auspices and control of the National Health and Medical Research Council and renamed the Australian Health Technology Advisory Committee (AHTAC).[2] Technical support is provided by the Health Technology Division of the renamed Australian Institute of Health and Welfare. The role of AHTAC is to formulate guidelines and other measures to further the appropriate use of health technologies. In effect however, our interpretation is that one of the most significant aspects of this role in practice, is to attempt to slow the proliferation of new health technologies while technology assessment considerations can be considered and thus restrain the cost implications of health technology innovation for the national health service.

This committee bases its considerations not only on technical and economic criteria, but also on social and ethical criteria of which social justice considerations loom large. 'If a technology works, should it be offered to everyone and anyone, and if so under what conditions and with what restrictions?' is the sort of question that is frequently asked. The role of the committee is thus to balance these sort of considerations against the specific interests of the groups of social actors involved with the technology.

Social justice considerations go further than considerations of who should get access to the health technology under what circumstances and at what cost however. A crucial issue is the one of *equity of resource allocation*. In a situation of finite health budget allocations, particularly in an era of reduced State involvement, social justice considerations loom large in making decisions in making the budgetary allocations. Some would argue for greater expenditure on prevention rather than treatment but this shift can only be justified if prevention programs have themselves been evaluated and shown to be more cost-effective than the treatment option. The issues involved can be difficult and contentious. An example is coping with HIV\AIDS. The decision involves the relative balance between treatment facilities for people with AIDS versus public education campaigns to minimize the spread of the virus, especially when, in the current state of knowledge, prevention is the only certain way of stopping the spread of the disease. Obviously both the prevention and treatment aspects have a justified claim on funding allocation; the difficult social justice question is the relative importance of one against the other.

The question of whether monies would be better spent on other health priorities is an important one. Spending large amounts of money on high profile, big ticket items of diagnostic and curative health technologies may not be the best use of scarce health care monetary allocations. Paradoxically, the very extensive use of small scale technologies like pathology tests may constitute an even greater cost than the big ticket items, but how is their relative worth to be assessed?

These questions of resource allocation are difficult ones. It is the representation in this particular instance of the central sociological question about the relationship between the individual and society. How can the needs of sick individuals whose lives depend on massive technological interventions such as a liver transplant at the cost of $40 000–100 000 each, or a heart transplant at $80 000 each, be balanced against the needs of whole populations, such as for instance the Aboriginal population of Australia where life expectancy is approximately 20 years less than white Australians (Social Justice Collective 1991:209–10)? Such conundrums and the attempts to resolve them in the social and political context of the various stakeholders is what health technology policy is all about.

The case of sleep disorder centres

In this second section of the paper, the general issues of the setting of health technology policy in the quest for a just society are examined in relation to the particular case of Sleep Disorder Centres. In this instance the technology is *diagnostic*; its purpose is to investigate, monitor and diagnose disorders in sleep that individuals may experience. Individuals for whom sleep disorder assessment is ordered by a general practitioner or medical specialist, sleep overnight in a type of hospital ward or laboratory. During this time, their sleeping patterns and a number of basic functions (such as pulse, breathing rate, etc) are continuously monitored and their sleep disorder assessed.

The material component of a Sleep Disorder Centre is a diagnostic clinic using an adaptation of computer technology called a *polysomnograph*. Costing approximately $A300 000, it is a machine to which individuals are connected by a series of electrodes to simultaneously record as many as fourteen physiological variables (see Johns 1991:304). The machine produces material data in the form of a tracing which is interpreted according to criteria of what is considered to be a normal sleep pattern. The task of interpreting the results, and interpreting their meaning for sleeping patterns, is a fairly complicated one requiring the skills of a medical specialist in thoracic medicine. The material and the social component together comprise the technology which is known as *polysomnography* which occurs in these sleep disorder centres. It is not a treatment technology; on the basis of the assessment, the treatment for the individual will be decided separately.

Sleep Disorder Centres, involving the use of the technology of polysomnography were begun in Australia probably about the late 1970s, having evolved out of academic research on sleep begun in the 1960s (see John 1991:303) Although the individual tests which are possible utilizing this technology were not new, bringing together the measurement of bodily signs which could be measured in a polysomnogram, was. It is now an established technology, well into the proliferation stage of its career, that is widely considered by the medical profession to have value in diagnosing more serious sleeping disorders as a preliminary step to treatment. The question of how those diagnosed as having the disorder are to be treated and how effective the treatments are, is still being evaluated. Nevertheless, by 1990, the number of SDC's had grown to 17 and by early 1992 to 21 with another five under construction. Sixteen of these or 76% are in the public health sector and the remaining five (24%) in the private sector. Sleep disorder centres are now available in all states and the ACT with an overall rate of 4.8 sleep evaluation studies per 100 000 of the population although not all these are full studies (National Health and Medical Research Council 1992).

The technology is costly too. An attempt has been made to estimate the annual cost of a centre. Taking a four bed centre in a hospital, with one staff specialist and making no allowance for profit on investment in the technology, unpublished estimates from the AIHW estimate the annual cost to be $584 000 for each centre or just over $15 million dollars in a year, total cost for the whole of Australia. This may seem a large figure to spend on one technology, but is it? The reference to evaluate the technology originally came to a different committee, which AHTAC subsequently subsumed. There was concern about the cost implications of the widespread proliferation of the technology as well as the requirement of equity of access; that the technology be made available to all who need it. If people have a debilitating or life-threatening disorder, should they not have ready access to appropriate medical treatment? In order to gain some insight into the social meaning of this disorder, we need to examine the prevalence and significance of sleeping disorders as a health problem. We then need to look at the evidence for arguing that Sleep Disorder Centres can and do make an effective contribution to treating this disorder and, ultimately to patient outcome.

Sleeping disorders

Sleep disorders are very common, as many as half the population may be affected at some time in their lives. In medical terms, sleep disorders fall into four major categories: disorders of falling and staying asleep (insomnias); disorders of the sleep-wake schedule (such as jet-lag); disorders causing excessive daytime sleepiness such as sleep apnea syndrome (discussed below), periodic leg movement in sleep, and narcolepsy (falling asleep during the day); and parasomnias such as sleepwalking, night terrors and nightmares (Thorpy 1990).

Disturbances in the normal pattern of sleeping may be thought of as occurring along a continuum from the minor at one end such as insomnia which is very common, along the continuum to the other end which is represented by less common serious disorders with the potential to be life threatening.

At the minor end, sleeping disorders such as insomnia are self treated by such means as giving up coffee intake in the evening, drinking valerian tea before retiring or buying a specially shaped pillow to reduce snoring. If that fails, moving along the continuum, general practitioners evaluate and treat less minor sleep disorders, usually with drugs. Some sleeping disorders towards the serious end however are argued to need more specialized investigation and these patients may be referred to sleep disorder centres for polysomnography.

At the serious end of the continuum is the condition of *sleep apnea syndrome* (SAS) which is the most common of the range of sleep disorders studied using this technology. This is a condition in which breathing stops momentarily many times during the night accompanied by gasps and snorts (raising social justice considerations for bed partners!). There are different types of SAS and the condition is commonly classified as mild, moderate or severe. The National Health and Medical Research Council (1992) has estimated the incidence of clinically significant SAS to be 1–2% of the population.

The main risk factors are gender and age. In a retrospective survey of 200 patients undergoing polysomnography in a Melbourne private Sleep Disorder Centre, men outnumbered women three to one, with nearly three quarters over the age of 40 years (Johns 1991:305). Other risk factors have been identified as obesity and alcohol and sedative abuse (Bonekat & Krumpe 1990, Stradling & Crosby 1991).

This raises a difficult problem. If sleep disorder assessment is shown to be effective, will there be a tendency to exclude overweight men with a history of heavy alcohol and sedative consumption on the grounds that there is no point in diagnosing what might be defined as self-inflicted harm? This might be justifiable in terms of the welfare of the community but it might be unfair to the individual by further marginalizing people who may experience extreme difficulty in overcoming these lifestyle problems.

The major consequence of having SAS for individuals is sleepiness during the day which reduces the person's effective functioning in society; their productivity, social interaction and general quality of life. There is also evidence that the sufferer may be a hazard to themselves and others with greater incidence of motor accidents amongst sufferers than others (Bearpark et al 1989, Finley et al 1989), as well as possibly more industrial accidents (Lavie 1983). There is also a suggested relationship, at least in severe cases between SAS and cardiovascular diseases and thus life expectancy however whether the relationship is causal, or both are the result of obesity, is unclear.

The use of the diagnostic technology of polysomnography conducted in sleep disorder centres for sleeping disorders at the serious end of the continuum is well established and seen as uncontroversial amongst doctors but this appears to be based more on professional consensus than on evidence that the diagnosis leads to improved patient outcome. The appropriateness of the use of the technology for sleeping disorders of a less serious nature is more controversial. Medical opinion differs as to whether insomnia should be evaluated by polysomnography. Some, including the two medical associations with a direct professional interest, agree that insomnia alone does not justify referral for sleep monitoring. On the other hand there are also medical views that sleep disorder centres might appropriately conduct insomnia management programs. The effectiveness of these programs has not yet been evaluated.

The stakeholders

How has health technology policy in this particular case study been set? What has been the role of the stakeholders? Patients do not appear to have been involved other than very indirectly through consumer representation on AHTAC.

The medical practitioners who specialize in the diagnosis and treatment of sleep disorders are specialist physicians in thoracic medicine. Collectively they are involved in two organizations: the broader Thoracic Society, though the Thoracic Society includes many other respiratory physicians who are not specialists in sleep disorders; and the more specialized Australasian Sleep Association which is an association solely of sleep disorder specialists. Along with the manufacturers of the technology they have been involved in lobbying Government for greater recognition and availability of the technology. The target of their lobbying is the State, first directed at the Health Insurance Commission which administers the Medicare scheme. Following submissions made by the Thoracic Society, a Medicare benefit of $455 was made available for polysomnography in late 1989, but only for the investigation of SAS under the supervision of a specialist in thoracic medicine. Private sleep disorder centres charge $740 per sleep disorder study leaving patients a gap of $285 to meet from their own resources. According to the Health Insurance Commission, the cost of claims for this schedule item has almost doubled each financial year to cumulatively total $5.6m since its introduction.

The second target of lobbying at the level of the State has been the AHTAC and its predecessors, to provide guidelines which would facilitate the orderly development in the proliferation of the technology. The Thoracic Society proposed that there be one, four bed sleep centre for each half million of the population, requiring a total of 34 for Australia. This figure was based on the American evidence on availability. The society sought a judgement that up to this number should be established. The AHTAC imprimatur was sought to facilitate the aim of securing a form of targeted funding within hospitals known as block funding.

The AHTAC response, endorsed by the full council of its parent body the NH&MRC(1992) was that

> While AHTAC recognises the significance of sleep disorders, and the importance of their diagnosis and treatment, it considers that preparation of guidelines for sleep disorders is not yet appropriate. AHTAC notes that multidisciplinary SDCs are high cost facilities, which are staff intensive and have limited patient capacity. It is unclear what proportion of the Australian population would be at significant risk as a result of sleep disorders, what proportion of cases would require such comprehensive facilities, and how many could be treated by respiratory physicians in other ways. The committee therefore feels unable at this stage to endorse the proposal by the Thoracic Society of Australia and New Zealand that there should be one multidisciplinary SDC per 0.5 million population.

The statement goes on to call for quantification of benefits and further details of costs and effectiveness. In other words, while the technology has already significantly been diffused, AHTAC has attempted to restrain any further proliferation at this stage, with indications that the matter will be reviewed in the future. Specifically it declined to accept the American availability ratio as the appropriate standard for the Australian context. It has taken the view that not enough evidence is available that the technology actually contributes to better patient outcomes by making patients' lives better. In other words the judgement is that in terms of the expenditure required, the proponents of the diagnostic technology of polysomnography have not demonstrated that it makes a sufficient impact on the management and treatment decisions involving sleep disorders so that better patient outcomes result.

Just health?

How does all this relate to the 'just health' considerations which are the focus of this book? There are several aspects to consider, the pursual of which would not always have the same outcome. On one hand, from a consumer viewpoint, in theory at least, if an individual's sleep disorder is serious, and if the technology can be demonstrated to make a beneficial contribution to that person's health, then it should be available regardless of the individual's ability to pay. (AHTAC's position has been that neither criteria for severity nor evidence of beneficial impact are sufficiently established as yet).

On the other hand, there exists a technological and financial imperative to use the technology and to expand its use to patients whose sleep disorders are less severe than agreed upon indications such as SAS. Confronted by patients whose quality of life is affected by more common sleeping disorders such as insomnia, it is not surprising and indeed to be expected that individual doctors attempt to help those people. Indeed it is a normative expectation of the doctor-patient relationship to do so. The financial consequences of proliferation however are considerable, in the context of a universal health scheme that is sensibly available to all regardless of availability to pay.

The consequence of this technological imperative to widen the uses of the technology up the continuum towards less serious forms of sleeping disorders has to be considered. Equity of resource allocation questions have to do with alternative uses to which this public money might usefully be put. These might include developing really effective programs for reducing the risk factors for sleep disorders or they might be health programs addressing more pressing health needs in the community.

As the situation stands at present, there are equity of geographical access considerations associated with the uneven distribution of sleep disorder centres currently existing. According to unpublished data from AIHW, the variation in the number of sleep disorder studies conducted is considerable ranging from 14.2 sleep disorder studies per week per million of the population in New South Wales, to only 5.3 in Victoria. For instance, of the $5.6m cumulatively claimed from the Health Insurance Commission under Medicare, 70% of claims were from the state of New South Wales (with about 34% of the Australian population) and only 4% from the state of Victoria (with 25% of the total population). Unless it can be shown that the prevalence of sleep disorders is greater in some states than in others, there is considerable imbalance, though of course opinions vary on whether New South Wales has too many or Victoria too few.

Conclusion

The field of health technology policy and assessment is a complicated one. There are a variety of stakeholders with various and sometimes contradictory and competing claims often in the name of what is in the best interests of the patient. In this chapter, the specific instance of sleep disorder centres and the diagnostic technology of polysomnography have been analysed in order to demonstrate the complexities of health technology policy. Balancing policy objectives such as social justice against the interests of the different groups of social actors involved in the process of technological innovation, is a complex task. As a decade of reasonably explicit concern with social justice at all policy levels gives way to a greater emphasis on market forces to allocate health and financial resources with a consequent reduction in the level of activity by the State, there is a danger that such concerns will be heard less in the clamour of stakeholders to pursue the enlightened self-interest which is claimed to be the strength of the new order.

NOTES

1.   We are following the convention of using the term 'state' to refer to individual Australian geopolitical entities such as Victoria and Queensland and 'State' to refer to the more general notion of the capitalist State.
2.   The first author (EW) is, in 1993, currently a member of this committee, the nominee of the Consumers' Health Forum. All views expressed in this paper are, of course, personal ones.

REFERENCES

Bearpark H, Fell D, Leeder S 1989 Road safety and sleep apnea. Australian and New
    Zealand Journal of Medicine 19:645a
Bonekat H, Krumpe P 1990 Diagnosis of obstructive sleep apnea. Clinical Review of Allergy
    8(2–3):197–213
Connor S, Kingman S 1989 Search for the virus, 2nd edn. Penguin, London
Findley L, Unversagt M, Suratt P 1989 Severity of sleep apnea and automobile crashes. New
    England Journal of Medicine 320:869–869
Johns M 1991 Polysomnography at a sleep disorders centre in Melbourne. The Medical
    Journal of Australia 155(Sept2):303–307
Lavie P 1983 Incidence of sleep apnea in a presumable healthy working population: a
    significant relationship with excessive daytime sleepiness. Sleep 6:312–318
Lumley J 1987 Assessing technology in a teaching hospital: three case studies. In: Daly J,
    Green K, and Willis E, (eds). Technologies in health care: policies and politics. Canberra,
    Australian Institute of Health
McKinlay J 1982 From promising report to standard procedure in technology and the future
    of health care. MIT Press, Cambridge Mass
National Health and Medical Research Council 1992 Statement on sleep disorders.
    Canberra
Social Justice Collective 1991 Inequality in Australia. Heinneman, Melbourne
Stradling J, Crosby J 1991 Predictors and prevalence of obstructive sleep apnoea and snoring
    in 1001 middle aged men. Thorax 46(2):85–90
Thorpy M 1990 Handbook of sleep disorders. Marcel Dekker, New York
Thorpy M, Lederich P 1990 Medical treatment of obstructive sleep apnea syndrome. In:
    Thorpy M (ed) Handbook of sleep disorders. Marcel Dekker, New York

17. Medicalization, marginalization and control?

Julie Mulvany

Deinstitutionalization has dominated mental health policy since the 1950s. The number of mentally ill being treated in large mental institutions has declined and the average length of stay of patients in mental institutions has decreased (see Office of Psychiatric Services 1987). Increasing numbers of the psychiatrically disabled are being 'cared' for in the community (Australian Health Ministers 1992).

A policy development closely associated with this process of deinstitutionalization is the compulsory treatment of some mentally ill people within the community. Victoria and New South Wales have provisions for compulsory community based treatment in their mental health legislation. Neither England nor Wales have such provisions although various forms of this treatment have been operating in states in America for several years.

As a result of the Mental Health Act 1986 (Victoria), Community Treatment Orders (CTOs) were introduced in Victoria. Under these orders patients live in the community and are supervised by medical practitioners. A person can be returned to hospital as an involuntary patient if he/she fails to comply with the order or is 'no longer suitable for a community treatment order and requires in-patient treatment or care'. Although the initial order must not exceed twelve months, it may be extended if the patient is still seen to meet the prescribed criteria.

A number of arguments in favour of the use of compulsory community based treatment are advanced by proponents of this policy. These orders are seen to facilitate the treatment of patients with severe psychiatric illness in the 'less restrictive' environment of the community. Compulsory community based treatment enables 'a compromise between the mentally ill's right to liberty and their need of care and supervision' (Scheid-Cook 1991:43). Proponents of this treatment point to the fact that some patients, who respond well to medication while in hospital, relapse when released from hospital because of a failure to continue taking their medication. Without a CTO, community treatment staff are powerless to change this situation (Applebaum 1986, Dedman 1990, Mulvey et al 1987, Scheid-Cook 1991). Community based treatment, it is argued, leads to a decrease in frequent short term hospital admissions (Appelbaum 1986, Scheid-Cook 1991). In addition their application is a means of avoiding the costs associated with long-term hospitalization.

Enforced medical treatment, whether in the community or in hospital must be regarded seriously. The use of these orders in Victoria seems to be increasing and more recipients are remaining on the orders for several years. Despite the claims regarding the advantages of this form of treatment few attempts have been made to evaluate the effectiveness of CTOs (Van Putten et al 1988, Zanni & de Veau 1986). Attempts to differentiate between categories of chronically ill patients and their respective suitability for involuntary outpatient treatment have not been made (Geller 1990). None of the research has focussed on the recipients' assessment of the positive and negative affects of these orders. As the category of patients placed on CTOs tend to be those who suffer from chronic and severe psychiatric disabilities, policies directed towards their treatment and care should be closely scrutinized.

SOCIOLOGY AND MENTAL HEALTH POLICY

The use of a sociological perspective directs us to analyse the use of CTOs in a number of ways. By drawing on sociological theory and research the operation of the policy of compulsory community based treatment and the assumptions underlying its development will be analysed. The chapter will conclude with a discussion of the practical implications of such an analysis for an assessment of this social policy response to the management of the chronically mentally ill.

Dominance of the medical model in treatment responses

Of particular interest to sociologists is the fact that treatment in the community, of people diagnosed as suffering from a mental illness, consists largely of the prescription of medication. For many CTO recipients attendance at a mental health clinic once a month to be given an injection of anti-psychotic medication by a psychiatric nurse is the only 'treatment' received.

Sociologists working from within a symbolic interactionist framework have shown that conceptualizations of a social problem will differ depending on the backgrounds of the 'definers' (see Parton 1985). These conceptualizations are based on differing assumptions regarding, for example, the cause of the 'problem' and the most appropriate ways of dealing with it. The views of medical personnel regarding conceptualizations of the nature of mental illness and its treatment dominate community treatment policy. The patient is seen as an organism or object suffering from a debilitating disease. The way the patient behaves, the way he/she perceives the world around him/her, is seen to be a direct consequence of the illness. In terms of the medical model, the patients' problems are seen to be a direct result of their mental illness and consequently emphasis is placed on the central role medication should play in the treatment process.

Writers have expressed concern regarding the dominance of the medical model in the treatment of the mentally ill in the community. The importance of addressing both the social and the clinical disability of those being treated and the danger of seeing treatment only in terms of drug therapy has been raised (Thornicroft & Bebbington 1989). Scull (1984) has expressed concern that overmedicated patients are becoming institutionalized in their own homes.

In contrast to the medical model a 'social' model makes a distinction between the 'disorder' and the person (Barham 1992:94). The patient is seen as firstly a self-reflecting individual who is continually reacting to, and making sense of, his/her social environment and only secondly as a person who also suffers from some form of mental illness. This model does not deny the possible existence of physical causes of the illness but also acknowledges that some of the patient's 'symptoms' result from his/her social circumstances, including the nature of the medical treatment received (see, for example, Barham 1992, Goffman 1961, Link et al 1987).

The concept of treatment under the social model is not limited to pharmacological means but extends to the provision of a range of social support networks within the community, the provision of educational and leisure opportunities, appropriate accommodation, occupational services, geographic accessibility of services, and the provision of support for primary care givers (Browning Hoffman & Foust 1977, Scheid-Cook 1987).

Korr (1988) points out that the reason patients might have had multiple admissions to mental institutions (often a criterion used to place someone on a community treatment order) is the lack of support systems within the community. A number of participants in a study of community mental health clinics (CMHC) in America, carried out by Scheid-Cook (1991:49), claimed that most patients who failed to attend clinics for treatment lacked social supports such as 'transportation to the CMHC, money for medication, or family support'.

Barham (1992:88) argues that a focus on drug therapy has retarded the development of social services and in one sense 'the very need for drugs has been fuelled by the failure to tackle the social problems of former mental patients'. Drug usage provides a means of surviving in a hostile social environment. He urges (1992:147) that rather than focussing on the in-adequacy of the person we should examine 'the structurally produced inadequacy, the social forces that conspire to render the person with a history of mental illness incompetent and demoralized'.

Medical dominance

How do we explain the dominance of the narrow medical focus in the treatment of the CTO recipients? Much has been written about medical power, control and dominance. A number of writers (see, for instance, Freidson 1970, Willis 1989) have shown how the medical profession has been highly successful in restricting the involvement of related occupations in the health area and in maintaining autonomy and freedom from accountability. Freidson (1971:22) relates the power of the medical profession to its position of autonomy which enables it to control such activities as entry to the profession, its exclusive right to work in particular areas, standards of training and professional self regulation. Foucault (1973) has argued that there is a relationship between the use of specialist language or discourse and the exercise of power. Members of professions by their use of highly specialized and technical language are able to control conceptualizations of particular forms of human activities and behaviour which in turn influences what is seen to be the 'appropriate' handling of that behaviour. The medical profession has been particularly successful in establishing a specialized discourse and body of knowledge which it used to justify its unique right to deal with illness, both physical and mental (Turner 1987, Daniel 1990).

The focus on therapeutic considerations in the decision making process regarding the imposition of CTOs results in 'a lessening of emphasis on legal procedures or on the control of medical discretion, since any action taken is justifiable on the basis that it is *in the patient's best interests* (Peay 1981:164). The failure of the legal criteria to 'specify objective measures of behaviour' (Peay 1981:164–65) results in a reliance on factors such as the patient's insightfulness which are seen as falling within the expertise of the medical personnel to assess.

Decker (1987:170), commenting on the relationship between the foundation of the mental hospital and the professionalization of psychiatry, concludes that 'the professional power of psychiatrists continues to reside in their position of control over patients and knowledge within these total institutions'. The superior position that hospital based psychiatrists assume within the medical hierarchy has implications for the way CTOs are used. Despite the fact that the case manager of the CTO recipient is usually based within the community, the decision to impose the order is made by the hospital doctor often without consultation with the community case manager. The power of hospital based doctors to influence the form community treatment takes is significant.

Coercive medical treatment: legal and medical models

Sociologists, in their attempt to differentiate the assumptions and practices of those working within the legal and medical arenas, have constructed ideal types or models to summarize the key features of legal and medical approaches. Under a legal model the individual is seen to be capable of making decisions regarding right and wrong. Legal control 'is a moralistic style that aims to punish offenders' (Horwitz 1990) who knowingly engage in behaviour deemed illegal. Nonetheless, 'such punishment should be proportional to the interests violated and should not unnecessarily interfere with the individuals' rights. The law should be minimal and limited by the notion of due process' (Parton 1985:15).

In contrast within the medical model individuals are not held responsible for their behaviour; they are seen rather as 'victims of an illness process beyond their control' (Horwitz 1990:78). A major aim is to restore the individual to a state of health rather than to reassert moral values. Despite the differences between the two models of human behaviour the response to the mentally ill frequently involves components of both these models.

The use of State coercive powers to control the mentally ill is justified on two grounds (Shah 1989:238–239). The safety of citizens is protected through the use of 'police power'. In addition the State adopts a paternalistic role by using legislation to protect those psychiatrically disabled who are believed to be unable to care for themselves or who are thought to be in danger of exploitation. CTOs represent a paradox in which the law intervenes purportedly to protect rather than punish. The combination of these powers, however, can result in the abuse of the rights of the mentally ill. As Shah points out:

> persons who are ostensibly the object of benevolent and therapeutic handling may well experience longer deprivations of liberty ('therapeutic sanction') than would have been possible under the punitive sanctions of the criminal law. Yet, some of the legal safeguards typically available in the criminal law are not deemed relevant since 'therapeutic' rather than 'punitive' objectives are involved. There is, therefore, not just a combining of the two rationales, but indeed what could be characterized as their confounding (Shah 1989:239).

Control systems as social constructs

How might we explain the compulsory treatment of the mentally ill within the community? Sociologists have demonstrated how social, economic and political factors influence legal and medical ideologies and practices (Busfield 1986, Edwards 1988). Conceptualizations and practices relating to the treatment of the mentally ill differ between different cultures and even within the same society over time (Edwards 1988, Horwitz 1990). It was not until the 1830s that the mentally ill were treated in large asylums; previously they had been cared for in the community (Felton & Shinn 1981). Although these institutions were initially seen as benevolent places in which the mentally ill could be 'cured' and returned to society as functioning individuals, they soon became large, overcrowded custodial institutions. From the mid 1950s a policy of deinstitutionalization developed in most western nations. (See Busfield 1986, Rothman 1971, Scull 1984 for a detailed historical analysis of the development of psychiatric policy.)

Writers have argued that policies of deinstitutionalization have been initiated by governments seeking to avoid the costs involved in maintaining large psychiatric institutions. An additional advantage to state governments is that the mentally ill in the community are forced to rely on federally funded welfare benefits such as sickness benefits, the invalid pension and Medicare (Scull 1981). Scull argues that the development of more comprehensive federally funded welfare benefits in the post war period has meant that the psychiatrically disabled can be treated more cheaply outside the institution (Scull 1981). Warner (1989:25) argues that such policies were also influenced by the 'demand for labour'. On the basis of an examination of the development of policies of deinstitutionalization in a number of countries he argues that labour shortages 'can be a stimulus to the rehabilitation of the marginally functional mentally ill' (1989:24). In the United States, for example, high unemployment exists, responsibility for health policy is divided between different levels of government, and there is little commitment to the provision of comprehensive health care. Policies of deinstitutionalization are, not surprisingly, popular.

It may be argued that economic and political circumstances, more than professional philosophy or technological innovation, have shaped our mental health care system (Warner 1989:27).

The use of CTOs, including their increased use, must also be seen as taking place within a particular socio-political environment. As a result of deinstitutionalization policy fewer hospital beds are available thus increasing pressure on hospitals to discharge patients. In Victoria in 1989/90, for example, the average length of stay of patients in metropolitan state psychiatric hospitals was 22.9 days (Buckingham 1992:79). Why, though, do we have compulsory treatment in the community for some psychiatrically disabled?

Criticism of the policy of deinstitutionalization has increased over the last decade. The policy, it is claimed, has resulted in major neglect of the needs of the mentally ill living within the community. This neglect is largely attributed to the lack of availability of community support services (Scull 1981). Increasingly critics argue that deinstitutionalization has resulted in the 'revolving door' process wherein, for a particular category of the mentally ill, frequent short term crisis admissions have replaced long-term admissions (Warner 1989). In Victoria approximately one third of admissions are 'by people having two (or more) admissions within that year' (Buckingham 1992:79). As a result of deinstitutionalization, some critics argue, the number of mentally ill amongst the homeless has increased. (See Bachrach 1984 for a summary of this literature.) It is also claimed that the number of mentally ill being admitted to prison has risen (Abramson 1972). In addition the media has portrayed the untreated ex-mental patient as potentially dangerous and violent (French 1987).

In this climate of criticism the use of a CTO to ensure compliance with medication may be seen by policy makers as a means of overcoming the 'revolving door' process, the criminalization of the mentally ill, and the threat posed by 'dangerous' untreated mentally ill. The discharge of a patient on a CTO, with its mandatory monitoring requirements, provides a safety net for staff who may feel compelled, because of diminishing hospital resources, to discharge patients after only a short admission. The use of CTOs places pressure on community members, rather than hospital staff, to care for the patients.

In theory the CTO enables the control and monitoring of the behaviour of those psychiatrically disabled who are seen to pose a risk to either themselves or others when released into the community. The instigation of legislation enabling compulsory community treatment can be seen as an attempt by policy makers to overcome some of the unintended negative consequences of deinstitutionalization.

COMPULSORY COMMUNITY TREATMENT AND SOCIAL JUSTICE

People with a history of mental illness face greater discrimination and stigmatization and are more likely to experience poverty and neglect than individuals suffering from most forms of physical illness (Campbell & Heginbotham 1991, Warner 1985). The above sociological analysis suggests that the policy of enforced treatment of the mentally ill within the community is being used principally to meet a combination of social control and economic objectives at the cost of the well-being of the psychiatrically disabled. Research suggests that ex-mental patients require access to many community supports if they are to live fulfilling and satisfying lives outside the mental institution (see, for example, Kennedy 1989, Lieberman & Test 1987). The argument of this chapter is, however, that the CTO is being used merely to enforce medication.

The dominance of the medical model in the treatment of the mentally ill results in what Conrad (1979) calls the medicalization of the problems of the psychiatrically disabled. Medicalization, by focusing on the characteristics of individuals, leads to a simplification of complex social problems, disguising the contribution of the 'system' to the 'problem' (Conrad 1979). By relying on medication in the treatment of CTO recipients, attention is diverted from an examination of the lack of availability of alternative community based resources. The contribution these resources can make to the quality of life of the psychiatrically disabled is ignored. Critics of deinstitutionalization (see, for example, Bachrach 1976, Scull 1984, Thornicroft & Bebbington 1989) drawing on American and English experiences have argued that, unless appropriate community resources are made available to cater for the specific needs of the psychiatrically disabled being treated outside hospital, their reintegration into the community will be unsuccessful.

Although CTO recipients may remain out of hospital and receive basic welfare benefits they have little control over their lives and are defined principally in terms of their psychiatric disability. 'Isolation and segregation from the non-patient community, custodial care, stagnation, and dependency continue' (Estroff 1981:121–122). The role of patient is perpetuated, stigmatization continues, and patients lacking dignity and self-esteem have little control over treatment decisions (Estroff 1981:126). The result is that 'an attempt is made to reproduce in the community the concepts and styles of patient domestication and management that derive from the hospital setting' (Barham 1992:123). This trend is exacerbated by the lack of cooperative and coordinated relationships existing between large psychiatric institutions and local community mental health clinics (Bleicher 1967) and maintains the dominance of hospital staff in the conferring of compulsory community treatment (Miller 1988).

The analysis in this chapter suggests that the almost exclusive focus on drug therapy is likely to continue given the power of the medical profession to determine the nature of community based treatment and the advantages drug treatment appears to offer governments concerned to cut health and community services budgets.

Community Treatment Orders provide a handy tool for those who may be tempted to reduce the complexities of community provision for people with mental illness to the mechanics of drug delivery. Once such legislation appeared, cost-conscious health managers and accountants may be drawn to the view that a Community Treatment Order 'provides much better value for money than the provision of staff and facilities to build up trust so that people can take medication voluntarily' (Barham 1992:125–126).

Compulsory community based treatment entails two conflicting goals: the attempt to provide the patient with a less restrictive treatment environment (and hence a concern with individual liberty) while at the same time ensuring control over the patients' compliance with treatment (Scheid-Cook 1991:44). In light of evidence of the side effects of anti-psychotic medication, particular concern is expressed at the removal of the right of patients' to refuse treatment (Bursten 1986, Mulvey et al 1987). Ironically, over the last decade there has been a movement to enshrine in legislation the right of patients to make decisions regarding the medical treatment they desire. The 1986 Mental Health Act (Victoria) explicitly identifies this protection as an important goal of government psychiatric services. Should a person who is no longer suffering from psychotic symptoms be compelled to take medication indefinitely when the negative symptoms of the illness such as lethargy, lack of motivation, blunting of emotional responses can be exacerbated by medication (Barham 1992)?

The danger here is that the pressure on psychiatrists to come up with cost-effective solutions may lead them to understate the adverse effects of continuous medication (Barham 1992:127).

The argument that refusals by patients to take medication result from lack of insight into their condition, reflects a disregard of the ability of individuals to identify the side effects of medication and to make choices regarding their life experiences.

A recent backlash against compulsory community based treatment has emerged. Legal scholars are concerned with the possible infringement of the liberty and privacy rights of the mentally ill (Miller 1992:79). Critics argue that such treatment will broaden the social control net by increasing the number of patients subject to compulsory treatment and thus lead to the depletion of limited community treatment resources. These orders are seen particularly by consumer groups to be social control rather than treatment (Wilk 1988a). It is contended that under certain circumstances the purpose of the CTO is to control the positive or overt symptoms of the illness and so ensure that the individual is not disruptive within the community. Vigilance is urged in ensuring that the use of legislation to force compliance with medical treatment (see Cohen 1985, Rose 1986) does not merely result in the curtailment of the liberty of increasing numbers of people with no concomitant gains to their health and well-being.

Also the 'burden of care' on relatives of those psychiatrically disabled living in the community must be considered. A number of writers (see Finch & Groves 1983) have pointed to the increasing responsibility the female relatives of patients have been forced to carry. For those whose relations have been placed on CTOs 'the burden of care' may well be extended to ensuring compliance with medication and assuming the responsibility to report non-compliance.

A practical consequence of the intrusion of the legal model into the treatment of the mentally ill is the dilemma mental health professionals face in engaging in case management and counselling with patients who do not want to be treated (Wilk 1988a:136). The 'benevolent coercion' (Mulvey et al 1987:575) associated with compulsory community treatment leads to the constant use of threats in the treatment process. This coercive treatment may produce resentment, anxiety and agitation that in turn may mitigate against improvement in the patient's condition. Many treatment staff see such an approach as counterproductive and contend that an effective staff patient relationship should be based on trust rather than coercion (Scheid-Cook 1991:47). An Australian psychiatrist has asserted that hospital staff are more enthusiastic about the use of CTOs than community health clinic staff (Dedman 1990:464).

The supervision of CTOs places major demands on community mental health agencies and their resources through excessive case management loads (Wilk 1988b). Unless the increased cost of monitoring and treating these patients is provided the work loads of staff will increase and even less support will be provided for the CTO recipient (Wilk 1988a:136).

Conclusion

Placement on a CTO should not be an end point in the treatment process. The use of CTOs to facilitate the movement of patients into the least restrictive treatment environment must be examined. Research is required which identifies the categories of people being placed on these orders, the reasons for their placement and the treatment they receive while on the order.

Dedman (1990:464) suggests that in Victoria CTOs are effective only in 'persuading the persuadable'. In a limited number of cases patients 'are impressed or intimidated by the CTO'. In many other cases the CTO is merely a means of facilitating hospital admission in cases of non-compliance. Potentially CTOs could be used to ensure that appropriate community resources are provided for the mentally ill. It is for sociologists, amongst others, to monitor and research the process of deinstitutionalization and the use of CTOs to ensure that the policy does not dilapidate into the continued medicalization, marginalization and control of those diagnosed as suffering from a chronic mental illness.

REFERENCES

Abramson M F 1972 The criminalization of mentally disordered behaviour: possible side-effect of a new mental health law. Hospital and Community Psychiatry 23:101–105

Applebaum P S 1986 Outpatient commitment: the problems and the promise. American Journal of Psychiatry 143(10):1270–1272

Australian Health Ministers 1992 National mental health policy. Australian Government Publishing Service, Canberra (April)

Bachrach L 1976 Deinstitutionalisation: an analytical review and sociological perspective. US Department of Health, Education and Welfare, NIMH, Rockville, Maryland

Bachrach L 1984 The homeless mentally ill and mental health services: an analytical review of the literature. Report prepared for the Alcohol, Drug Abuse and Mental Health Administration, Washington, DC: US Department of Health and Human Services (April)

Barham P 1992 Closing the asylum. Penguin, London

Bleicher B K 1967 Compulsory community care for the mentally ill. Clev-Mar. Law Review (January):93–115

Browning Hoffman P, Foust L L 1977 Least restrictive treatment of the mentally ill: a doctrine in search of its senses. San Diego Law Review 14:1100–1154

Buckingham B 1992 Access to acute inpatient care in metropolitan Melbourne. Public Psychiatry 1(3):76–84

Bursten B 1986 Posthospital mandatory outpatient treatment. American Journal of Psychiatry 143(10):1255–1258

Busfield J 1986 Managing madness. Hutchinson, London

Campbell T, Heginbotham C 1991 Mental illness prejudice, discrimination and the law. Dartmouth, Aldershot

Carney T 1986 The mental health, intellectual disability services and guardianship acts: how do they rate? Legal Service Bulletin 11:128–131

Cohen S 1985 Visions of social control. Polity Press, Cambridge

Conrad P 1979 Types of medical social control. Sociology of Health and Illness 1(1):1–7

Daniel A 1990 Medicine and the State. Allen & Unwin, North Sydney

Decker F H 1987 Psychiatric management of legal defense in periodic commitment hearings. Social Problems 34(2):156–171

Dedman P 1990 Community treatment orders in Victoria, Australia. Psychiatric Bulletin 14:462–464

Edwards A 1988 Regulation and repression. Allen & Unwin, Sydney

Estroff S 1981 Psychiatric deinstitutionalization: a sociocultural analysis. Journal of Social Issues 37(3):116–132

Felton B J & Shinn M 1981 Ideology and practice of deinstitutionalization. Journal of Social Issues 37(3):158–172

Finch J, Groves D eds 1983 A labour of love: women, work and caring. Routledge & Kegan Paul, London

Foucault M 1973 The birth of the clinic. Tavistock, London

Freidson E 1970 Profession of medicine: a study of the sociology of applied knowledge. Harper & Row, New York

Freidson E 1971 Professions and their prospects. Sage, Beverley Hills

French L 1987 Victimization of the mentally ill: an unintended consequence of deinstitutionalization. Social Work (November/December):502–505

Geller J L 1990 Clinical guidelines for the use of involuntary outpatient treatment. Hospital and Community Psychiatry 41(7):749–755

Goffman E 1961 Asylums: essays on the social situation of mental patients and other inmates. Doubleday, New York

Horwitz A V 1990 The logic of social control. Plenum Press, New York

Kennedy C 1989 Community integration and well-being: toward the goals of community care. Journal of Social Issues 45(3):65–77

Korr W S 1988 Outpatient commitment: additional concerns. American Psychologist (September):748–749

Lee J 1992 Community treatment orders: the Victorian experience. Unpublished paper, Mental Health Review Board, Victoria

Leonard D 1992 The bed state crisis and you. Public Psychiatry 1(2):42–47

Lieberman A, Test M 1987 Health care practices and health status of the mentally ill in the community. Health and Social Work (Winter):29–37

Link B C, Cullen F T, Frank J, Wozniak J F 1987 The social rejection of former mental patients: understanding why labels matter. American Journal of Sociology 92(6):1461–1500

Miller R D 1988 Outpatient civil commitment of the mentally ill: an overview and an update. Behavioral Sciences & the Law 6(1):99–118

Miller R D 1992 An update on involuntary civil commitment to outpatient treatment. Hospital and Community Psychiatry 43(1):79–81

Miller R D, Fiddleman P B 1984 Outpatient commitment: treatment in the least restrictive environment? Hospital and Community Psychiatry 35(2):147–151

Mulvey E P, Geller J L, Roth L H 1987 The promise and peril of involuntary outpatient commitment. American Psychologist 42:571–584

Office of Psychiatric Services 1987 Psychiatric services in Victoria: service dimensions and descriptive indicators. Health Department, Victoria

Parton N 1985 The politics of child abuse. Macmillan, Hampshire

Peay J 1981 Mental health review tribunals: just or efficacious safeguards? Law and Human Behaviour 5(2/3):161–186

Rose N 1986 Law, rights and psychiatry. In: Miller P, Rose N (eds) The power of psychiatry. Polity Press, Cambridge

Rothman D J 1971 The discovery of the asylum: social order and disorder in the new republic. Little & Brown, Boston

Scheid-Cook T L 1987 Commitment of the mentally ill to outpatient treatment. Community Mental Health Journal 23(3):173–182

Scheid-Cook T L 1991 Outpatient commitment as both social control and least restrictive alternative. The Sociological Quarterly 32(1):43–60

Scull A 1981 Deinstitutionalization and the rights of the deviant. Journal of Social Issues 37(3):6–19

Scull A 1984 Decarceration, 2nd edn. Polity, Cambridge

Shah S A 1989 Mental disorder and the criminal justice system: some overarching issues. International Journal of Law and Psychiatry 12:231–244

Thornicroft G P, Bebbington P 1989 Deinstitutionalisation: from hospital closure to service development. British Journal of Psychiatry 155:739–753

Turner B S 1987 Medical power and social knowledge. Sage, London

Unsworth C 1987 The politics of mental health legislation. Clarendon Press, Oxford

Van Putten R A, Santiago J M, Berren M R 1988 Involuntary outpatient commitment in Arizona: a retrospective study. Hospital and Community Psychiatry 39(9):953–958

Warner R 1985 Recovery from schizophrenia. Routledge & Kegan Paul, London

Warner R 1989 Deinstitutionalization: how did we get where we are? Journal of Social Issues 45(3):17–30

Wilk R J 1988a Involuntary outpatient commitment of the mentally ill. Social Work 33:133–137

Wilk R J 1988b Implications of involuntary outpatient commitment for community mental health agencies. American Journal of Orthopsychiatry 58(4):580–591

Willis E 1989 Medical dominance: the division of labour in Australian health care, 2nd edn. Allen & Unwin, Sydney

Zanni G, de Veau L 1986 Inpatient stays before and after outpatient commitment. Hospital and Community Psychiatry 37(9):941–942

18. Just care-giving: whose work, whose control?

Rosemary Cant

A growing number of women act as unpaid carers to those with disabilities. There are several reasons for this. The first is that government policies have changed with a newer emphasis on the private home as the appropriate context of care. The second is that medical science has been very successful in saving lives: those of premature babies, those damaged by accident, and those afflicted by mental or physical disease. However, it has not been as successful in preventing disability.

Social justice considerations have led to an emphasis on the necessity that care be given in a way that allows those with disabilities to live as autonomously and independently as possible. Social justice considerations have not until now extended these principles to caregivers. How can we ensure that carers also have their needs for autonomy met? How can we ensure that whatever their age, gender or social position, carers have the same access to leisure and paid work, that those who do not meet the dependency needs of others are able to enjoy? These are not easy questions, but the analysis that follows suggests that orthodox answers to the problems of care-giving will not suffice. It also suggests that when those who are carers are mothers, the problems with orthodox answers are more often overlooked because of cultural assumptions about appropriate ways of meeting dependency in children. 'A good mother will gladly sacrifice her interests for the interests of her children', the cultural prescription goes. The principles of collective responsibility for children are rarely invoked. When the children are disabled, the principles of collective responsibility are most often applied as professional control to ensure that mothers play their roles appropriately.

Philosophies of economic rationalism applied to health care systems have reallocated most of the care of the physically dependent from hospitals and other institutions to women at home. Attempts to ration services have lead to increased monitoring, while moves to professionalize the allied health groups have extended controls.

A major issue which has been explored by feminists is the role of ideology in defining care-giving as the work of women (Barrett & McIntosh 1982, Finch & Groves 1983, Graham 1984, Bryson 1985, Bryson & Mowbray 1986, Pascall 1986, Dalley 1988). The state has formulated policies of community and family care for children who are disabled based on this assumption. The constraints imposed by ideologies of caring and resulting policies are in themselves important forms of control of women (Wilson 1977, Land 1976, 1977, Tulloch 1984, Shaver 1983, Edwards 1988), but over and above this is an increasing measure of direct regulation of women's care-giving work. Provisions for parental choice in terms of the type of care that the child receives is related to this issue. In Australia and Britain, the state increasingly claims the right to 'assess' the need for both long term residential care and support services provided for children tended at home. Many of the professional services are not only providing support but also are 'tutelary' since they provide supervision of care-giving work, especially those parts designated as educational or therapeutic.

The regulation of mother's work

The way in which the institution of motherhood is structured, facilitates the regulation of women's activities. Rich (1976) points to the lack of 'symbolic architecture' or visible embodiment of authority or power associated with motherhood and the contrast with other structures of power (such as universities, hospitals and courts). She notes the hidden connections between other institutions, which are supposedly independent such as 'the institutions of medicine and professional expertise, law and the public bureaucracies' (Rich 1976: 274). Edwards (1988) concurs with this analysis which acknowledges the importance of institutions such as medicine in moulding the child rearing process.[1] In her book, *Regulation and Repression,* she sketches the various mechanisms, techniques and forms of control which are characteristic of each, though Rich's analysis is more pointed in locating control with gender divisions. The basis of control lies in the elements of the institution of motherhood which she argues includes lack of alternative child care, 'the chaining of women in links of love and guilt', the enforced dependence on a man, 'the psychoanalytic castigation of the mother' and 'the pedagogic assumption that the mother is inadequate and ignorant' (Rich 1976: 274). It can be seen that she is describing the social restriction and subordination enforced by the ideology of motherhood, but she goes further and hints at something more. Inadequacy and ignorance assumed by the ideology, must be alleviated by supervision and education. The activities of mothers must be regulated. In an historical account, Reiger (1985) has traced the rise of many Australian organizations before the Great War aimed at reforming women's activities as housewives. She observes:

Reformers as various as churchmen, urban planners and public health and welfare workers who disagreed on many other political aspects of urban reform showed considerable unity when it came to discussion of women and their family responsibilities. They were engaged in nothing less than a project of 'housewifery reform', seeing poor living conditions and poor housekeeping as twin evils.

...the 'experts' on home and family, whilst ostensibly promoting the separation of sexual spheres and the privacy of the home, were invading it at every point, demanding that women learn and apply the principles of the capitalist industrial world. (Reiger 1985:36, 55)

Medical authority, professionalization, bureaucratization and the regulation of care-giving work

Where a child is disabled, the regulatory mechanisms are strengthened and there is increased threat to the autonomy of women at home carrying out care-giving work. These threats come from three main sources. First, from traditional medical authority. Second, they emanate from the move to professionalization of the so-called caring professions. Nursing, the therapies and social work lay claim to the control of care-giving work in their attempts to professionalize. Finally they come from what can be loosely designated as growing rationalism or bureaucratization. These strands of control are woven into a braid in the helping agencies of the state that binds women into a position of subordination to their 'helpers'. Marshall (1970) suggested approvingly that 'the professions are being socialized and the social and public services are being professionalized'. But precisely these trends and the resulting nexus between professional power and bureaucratic control allow tight surveillance over those needing state provided professional services.

Medical authority and the medical gaze

Medical control is the focus of many analyses of patient-practitioner relationships (Parsons 1951, Friedson 1970, Illich 1977, Navarro 1980, Willis 1983 among others). For this analysis, the mother's position in the doctor/mother/child triad and her subjection to medical authority is the issue at point. Her position is somewhat ambiguous, since she is co-provider of medical services to her child, as well as a co-client of the doctor. In both roles, however, she is subject to the doctor's authority.

One of the main methods of medical science is careful and detailed observation. The observations of the child by the mother must be relayed on request to the doctor. Her observations and the doctor's examination of her account are parts of the medical gaze. Sociological theory has always included a thread which has interpreted the 'gaze' as being regulatory (disciplinary) in its effect. Cooley's 'looking glass self' incorporates the notion of the disciplinary effect of the self judging the ego's actions in the way it supposes others to do—and pre-judging mentally rehearsed or planned action. The symbolic interactionist school incorporated these notions within its theoretical framework. The writing of Michel Foucault has emphasized the gaze of science and the way that knowledge based on observation constitutes a powerful disciplinary force. Medical 'science' has emphasized observation both as a means of enlarging its knowledge base and as a method of routine clinical practice (as in 'he is in hospital for observation'). Medical professional power is based on these surveillance practices as well in the social structures of society.

Donzelot (1979) has offered an historical analysis of the transformation by which women were required to relinquish their own medical skills and become subject to the tutelage of medical practitioners. He quotes the hygienist Fonssagrives in 1876,

...my purpose here is to teach women the art of domestic nursing. Hired attendants are to true nurses what professional nursemaids are to mothers: a necessity and nothing more. It is my ambition to make women into accomplished nurses who are understanding of all things, but who understand most of all that their role is there with the sick, and that it is exalted as it is helpful. The role of the mother and that of the doctor are and must remain distinct. The one prepares and facilitates the other; they are, or rather they should be, complementary to each other in the interests of the patient. The doctor prescribes, the mother executes. (Fonssagrives 1876 in *Dictionnaire de la Sante*, quoted by Donzelot 1979:18)

Some one hundred years later, paid labour is considered less appropriate than maternal care for both sick and physically dependent children, but maternal work must be carefully regulated by doctors and other health professionals. In a study of care-giving (Cant 1991), medical appointments were regarded by many mothers as examinations of their care-giving work that were inflicted on them monthly. Being seen as a good mother was a test that mothers faced continually as they interacted with nurses, teachers, doctors, therapists and other health professionals.

Mrs L: It's just—you know, you're tested like that all the time—do this, this and this and this—with the implication that with everything, you haven't been doing it, and you've got to sit down and tell them 'Well—you're asking an awful lot of me and I don't know that everything is going to be well if I do.'
Mrs P: There's constant assessment—you as well as your child. Mothers of normal children are judged by their behaviour while mothers of disabled children are judged by their performance. It's your test too.

Some mothers believed doctors deny the parental expertise they believed they had developed, and to deny to mothers their rightful place in the determination of the treatment of their children. Four mothers commented on the hostility which greeted their attempts to discuss alternative programs for their children other than those the professional had specified, and the way they were made to feel silly for suggesting these. Some said they were unable to raise such issues.

Mrs P: I'm not brave enough to talk about it with him. I just go my own way.

In a Foucauldian analysis, Riessman (1989) has considered the 'fit' between the interests of women and the interests of doctors which has resulted in an extension of medical definitions and medical jurisdiction into the lives and experiences of women. She argues that the 'fit' has been tension-filled and fraught with contradictions for women, who have both gained and lost with each intrusion that medicine has made in their lives. Medical regulation of family life with a disabled child has resulted in parallel gains and losses for the women involved. Their problems are recognized at the same time that their lives are made public and their autonomy reduced.

The newer health professions and professionalization

Public regulation of women's work by professionals belonging to what Gouldner (1979) has called the new middle class has increased with the growth of the therapies, social work, domestic science and 'special' education. Medical authority reinforces the control exercised by this new class (Edwards 1988).

Discourses which construct mothers as 'natural' carers have allowed policies to be put into place which privatize care by re-locating it into the home. Activities, formerly performed as paid work by nurses and other health professionals in the public domain, have been moved into the household where they are carried out unpaid by mothers as 'shadow work',[2] work largely hidden from public view. Hence the state only needs to provide supervision.

Since physical disabilities create functional deficits, which require support in the activities of daily living and intensive therapy and education to achieve greater independence in the longer term, professional control of daily life is ubiquitous for these families. Daily life is exposed to the professional gaze. Thus, occupational therapy has as a major area of study, 'activities of daily living'. Occupational therapists visit the homes of children with disabilities to 'advise mothers' and 'assess the problems'. They suggest alterations to the fabric of the house and also to the patterns of household life. One parent in my study of care-giving, likened her home to an institution, capturing the pervasiveness of this scrutiny and its concomitant de-privatization.

There gets a point where you can't cope with any more services. You can't take any more of that intrusion. Effectively my home is an institution and not only John but my two daughters, my husband and myself are also institutionalized.

Physiotherapists and speech therapists required daily regimens of exercises and teachers put into place 'early intervention programs' to be carried out by the family. Day surgery and early discharge results in more nursing tasks to be carried out in the household, and in the case of chronic conditions, these continue unless the child is able to take over medical procedures for him/ herself. Professional discourses define this care as the 'duty' of mothers and fail to recognize their legitimate claims to self development and the preservation of self identity.

Nursing and the therapies have been struggling for recognition as professions. Friedson (1970) emphasizes that the distinctive feature of a profession is the right of control of its work. This autonomy is ultimately 'secured by the political and economic influence of the elite which sponsors it through the activity of the state' (Friedson 1970:73). Another important feature of the professionalization process with regard to care-giving work is the efforts of developing professions to 'traditional intellectuality' (Larson 1977:xv), the cognitive base which enables it to lay claim to expert knowledge. To do this they require the broad scientific moorings offered by the modern university (Larson 1977:34). Thus in Australia, in the past two decades, the therapies and special education moved first into Colleges of Advanced Education and later into the universities. The 'symbolic architecture' of university and hospital, some in the form of towering institutions, others as prestigious, traditional, Gothic architecture bolsters the professions' claims to authority.[3]

Authority implies a supervised category. Both clients and those tending them are supervised. It is a taken-for-granted aspect of authority, that the greater the number of those supervised, the more important the role. Larson (1977:38) has argued that it is difficult to find a profession other than medicine which controls a sufficiently large group of underlings to achieve significant authority. The argument I put here is that the household and its workers while a small group nevertheless are underlings, which the health professions can in turn supervise. This offers them the option of keeping only the higher status work, adding to it the managerial functions of regulation and supervision of their discarded work now performed by mothers in the home.

In Hughes (1971) original essay, he used the phrase 'dirty work' to describe the actions of those subordinate to gangsters and others who were required to brutally enforce the orders of their masters. This carries the same connotations of 'doing someone else's dirty work' a phrase in common parlance. Later, he extended the notion to cover the relationship between doctor and nurse. Painful medical therapy and physiotherapy is dirty work which is often delegated to the mother as medical co-worker, often causing continual everyday conflict between mother and child. It is interesting to contrast the warning in an article written by two medical practitioners in the *Medical Journal of Australia* of the danger of **fathers** being caught up in this scenario. It warns of children with diabetes who may become phobic about repeated injections and the possibility that girls may see them as 'symbolic sexual attacks' where given by the father with the undesirable result of 'overemphasis on the girl's submissive, normally masochistic role'(Maddison & Raphael 1971:1268–1269). Hence the article offers advice which permits fathers to avoid this dirty work and the conflict with the child caused by medical therapy.

Where the mother resists the care-giving role, she herself may be seen as needing treatment. The same article suggests,

> The increased dependent needs in the child may reactivate the mother's own unresolved dependency conflicts, and these may be a further source of resentment and guilt. Overt or covert rejection of the child may result, as evidenced by unnecessary hospitalisation, the delegation of his care to others, or subtle negligence in his management. (Maddison & Raphael 1971:1267)

The likelihood of being considered sick if the care-giving role is played unenthusiastically is a possible outcome for either parent. Maddison and Raphael (1971:1268) define stress in either parent as lack of 'mature adapting' requiring 'psychological management'.

In my Australian study, the parents of children with spina bifida usually referred to incontinence management as one of the greatest problems and one that the professions do not address adequately, if at all. The reasons for this neglect by professionals seems to lie in its definition as dirty work, or mother's work, with which they need not concern themselves. Techniques of catheterising were taught to parents by nurses, but help in techniques of management of bowel incontinence was most often obtained from other mothers. It seems that because bladder incontinence management methods involved equipment it was seen as a technical problem and thus was suitable nursing work. However because it was routinely required, it was not seen as exclusively nursing work, but a task which could become the responsibility of the family, under supervision. In an analysis of medical professionalism, it has been argued that the physician is able to retain his position because he has a 'right hand man' [sic], a nurse, who if necessary will perform the tasks of those below her in the medical hierarchy—or those outside it (Hughes 1971). In their search for professional status, nurses and others from the semi-professions in health related fields are in their turn 'dumping' such tasks. Routine work is also defined as not requiring the 'expert' knowledge which is seen as the mark of a profession (Borremans & Illich 1978, Larson 1977, Daly & Willis 1988).

A British example of care-giving work being defined as inappropriate for health professionals is the statement in a policy document that:

> These changes should take into account the present level of dependence on occupational therapists as the main service providers for people with a physical disability *and allow better use of their skills*. (Caring for People 1989:84 emphasis mine)

An important development is that the appearance of control is blunted by the style of the new experts. Professionals present themselves as friendly rather than authoritative (Sapsford 1990). Compliance needs to be ensured and since a friendly manner encourages this, it should be employed to this end. As Billig et al aptly put it:

> The modern experts have to be experts in human relations, and this means presenting themselves in a non-authoritarian manner, as if they were the friends of the non-experts. However, the friendliness is itself a part of their expertise, and, as such, a part of their egalitarianly presented authority. (Billig et al 1988: 147)

There are two common ways in which resistance to professional authority can be exercised. One is to avoid health professionals and medical encounters whenever possible. The second is to ignore or 'misunderstand' their advice. It was significant however that in my study of care-giving, it was the single mothers who seemed more likely to avail themselves of these forms of resistance. The patriarchal authority of male partners appeared to buttress medical authority so medical advice was more difficult to ignore.

The regulatory activity of the state

Apart from professional surveillance exercised by some of its employees, the state claims control of care-giving work on the bases of stewardship of money and of children. Requirements of responsible expenditure give public officials a gate-keeping role and a surveillance role. This is explicit, for example, in an Australian policy document, the Richmond Report (NSW), which recommends setting up multidisciplinary teams to consider care plans for those with disabilities. The surveillance of families is justified by appeals to the discourses of community care and de-institutionalization, whilst the gate-keeping role of the assessment teams is made explicit for those families who attempt to choose not to provide the necessary care to meet the increased dependency needs of their disabled children. The alternatives for these children, to live outside the household in an institution, in a group home or to be fostered, need support from state funds. The wording in this report, which speaks of 'determining priorities' for residential places, acknowledges that there will be an unfulfilled need for residential care.

> The Inquiry therefore considers that as soon as community teams are established in every Region, admission to all Health Department residential services and ultimately all government services be filtered through such an assessment service. Funding and where appropriate licensing of non-government residential care facilities and nursing homes specialising in the care of the developmentally disabled should be conditional on their acceptance of a preadmission assessment process.
> In order to ensure that most effective use is made of available residential care, each Region should establish a Residential Placement Committee, involving service providers, to determine priorities for community residential places. (Richmond 1983:2:35)

The British Report, *Caring for People* (HMSO), speaks of 'securing places' (p26) and in a similar way to the NSW Richmond Report sets out the gate-keeping roles of public officials.

> From April 1991 local authorities will be responsible, in collaboration with health care professionals, for assessing the needs of new applicants for public support for residential or nursing home care. (HMSO 1989:26)

The claim for the need to assess is linked in this case quite specifically to the provision of 'public support'.

For parents, particularly mothers, the price of relief by the state from care-giving, either regularly through services or by institutionalization of the child is often admission of failure. The following advice to doctors is offered in the *Medical Journal of Australia* in an article entitled 'Handicapped children: let's be more positive and practical'.

> The only time to institutionalize is when both parents have tried to cope by themselves, and are *forced to admit* they cannot do it. (Green 1981:403 emphasis mine)

The threat to parents' identities through such judgements of inadequacy is apparent, as is the assumption of a legitimate continual monitoring role of family life by doctors.

Where services for children cared for in the community are scarce, the same criteria apply to their provision. Services available for support are limited and rationed, and bureaucrats are charged with ensuring they are utilized 'equitably' and 'efficiently'. This leads to monitoring of families in need in order to assess the 'coping' capability of carers. Rationing requires continuous assessment of need, and help is often only offered when inadequacy is conceded (Nicholson 1983, Graham 1985). As governments press on with their 'reforms' based on the ideologies of economic rationalism, rationing becomes ubiquitous. Rationing requires assessment, and the more assessment, the greater the surveillance and the de-privatization of family life and the greater the stress felt by the carer.

Privacy is an important liberty which is denied to the parents by this surveillance. Those philosophers who support this proposition do not argue that this privacy covers all one's affairs but argue that it should be extended to those pieces of information which are apt to pose a threat to identity. Kleinig speaks of the need for 'moral space' in non-intimate relationships. Where details of the carer's affairs or interpretation of her acts affects her standing, then her autonomy is at risk.

> People in these situations are likely to feel that the circumstances are inimical to their own initiative. Consciousness of (the likelihood of) others' knowledge of one's person and affairs can so intrude upon one's understanding of the social meaning of one's acts, that they come to be carried out in response to a viewpoint which is alienated from one's own...if our awareness of what others know or are able to come to know concerning ourselves places us under considerable pressure to restructure our self-presentation, lest it acquire an unwanted significance, or causes us shame and embarrassment, then our ability to achieve and maintain a unified awareness of ourselves as autonomous agents will be endangered. For we will no longer be free to be ourselves, to be our own person in relation to others. (Kleinig 1980:151–52)

Carers lack this freedom to be themselves. Their identities are under continuous threat from medical and bureaucratic monitoring. Caregiving work tends to isolate mothers from friends and neighbours and professional contacts often form a large proportion of their social interaction with adults (Cant 1992).

While the first basis of state control rests on stewardship of money, the second basis of state control appeals to notions of the state as the protector of children—all children, the healthy as well as the sick, both normal and disabled (Platt 1977, Davin 1978, Donzelot 1979, Reiger 1985, David 1985, Deacon 1985, Carrington 1989, Knapman 1990, Sapsford 1990). While mothers are 'naturally' fitted for child care, they need to be taught what to do and supervised carefully. Schools and other child-care agencies monitor the performance of mothers. Thus teachers, as they monitor the capabilities and the well-being of children, also judge the competence of mothers (David

1985). Supervisory roles claimed by the state are often invested in health care personnel where medical claims to authority bolster the control (Deacon 1985, Reiger 1985, Edwards 1988). A prototype for such surveillance is the Australian infant health services in each state (variously named), later termed the Early Childhood Service in New South Wales as it broadened its range of attention from babies to all young children, and from their physical well-being, measured by weight gain in the early months to social and psychological development (Deacon 1985, Reiger 1985, Knapman 1990). For children with disabilities, the same claims to legitimacy of those exercising control are made on the basis of professional knowledge. The assessment teams put in place in the mid-eighties in New South Wales are largely drawn from the ranks of health care personnel. The establishment of these teams is justified on the basis of the protection of the true interests of children and families.

The Richmond Report stresses the importance of managing parents so they will accept their roles as the providers of the added care necessary to support children with disabilities.

> The evidence clearly indicates that with early support and counselling families can be supported to accept the handicap, to deal with their own guilt and grief, and to continue to care for their child with the availability of appropriate back-up support and respite care. The evidence available on the positive benefit for both child and family of this approach and the negative effects of early institutional care on the child's subsequent development clearly point to the need for formal and comprehensive assessment as early as possible and certainly prior to admission to residential care. (Richmond 1983:2:35)

De-institutionalization has meant that surveillance of children has been broadened to include their families, principally their mothers. As Edwards (1988: 95) puts it, this 'de-structuring' process is accompanied by 'dispersion' or 'diversion' of social control. The removal of the child from the family of origin is not based on choices made by that family nor is it based on the needs of the principal carer as the quotation above makes clear. Instead it depends on judgements about lack of competence of the family and carer. On this basis, assessment of competence is the primary function of the 'child saving' experts (Carrington 1989). One mother I interviewed, spoke of her irritation at the constant reiteration of the question, 'Are you coping?'. The significance of it was lost to her, but it is of the essence of the function of the experts, their attempts to assess competence. The autonomy of the family comes to depend not on legal or civil rights, but on competence and successful child raising. Through the 'failures' of families, the welfare state finds the means to legitimize intervention. It does so selectively, and families with children who are disabled are onerously policed.

Critiques of control of household activities and empowerment

There are a number of critiques which decry the authority claimed by the state in the private sphere of the home. They originate from two different theoretical stances. The first is that of Lasch (1977) and Donzelot (1979) who either implicitly or explicitly confront the state's assumption of patriarchal authority. Donzelot's thesis is that patriarchal authority has weakened and the power of women increased, in the private sphere, through their alliance with medical authority.

The second theoretical stance is that of feminist writers such as Ehrenreich and English (1978), Pascall (1986), Fraser (1987) and Edwards (1988) whose stance is that women should seize control of their own labour. Their work addresses the way in which the movement of the boundary between state activity and family responsibility has strengthened regulation of women's family work. There is however, some ambivalence in women's writing as it acknowledges the extension of this state activity. Those such as Pateman (1988) and Dalley (1988) accept this extension and remind us that feminist social reformers early in the century fought for it, while others such as Fraser (1987) deprecate the control of bureaucrats and professionals which follow in its wake. Pateman argues that the *public* nature of the client role in which women are placed, defends them against the heavy hand of state functionaries. In this way it is preferable to the alternative of the out-of-sight capriciousness of private dependence. Fraser does not concur with this analysis of the benign nature of state activity, characterizing the welfare system as a juridical-administrative-therapeutic state apparatus (JAT) aimed very much at women. Certainly, it can be argued that for the families in this present study, the expert child development discourses referred to earlier, empower the professionals employed by the JAT to closely supervise the mothers. At the same time, they set them an impossible task in terms of child rearing. It is impossible because normality is an unattainable goal and in any event, no matter how much effort is invested, it can always be increased. Illich uses similar imagery to describe the growth of control by the new experts arguing: '(Most professionals) not only increase tutelage over the citizen-become-client, but also determine the shape of his world-become-ward' (Illich 1977:17).

A different but parallel argument is put by Yeatman (1990:42) who distinguishes between market citizenship and social citizenship. Social citizenship entitles carers to resources through the activity of the welfare state. Market citizenship is available to those with adequate economic resources who can buy the services they need in the open market. It is usually denied to carers and it entails a degree of freedom and power not granted to those positioned outside the market. Male carers that I interviewed sometimes referred to this distinction. One patted his pocket significantly when asked about the most important forms of support for him and his wife and said: 'My best friend is my pocket'. Empowerment of mothers perhaps can best be achieved by giving them better access to the market.

Policies are shaped by current rehabilitation discourses which are anchored around notions of 'normalization', 'community care' and 'rights of the disabled'. Political philosophers (McClosky 1980, Kleinig 1980) have argued closely the right to life, liberty and the development of self for those with handicaps. What is needed is the development of a similar exposition of the rights of those who tend them—an issue which is usually touched on in discussions, but not explored in depth.

The distinctions between 'negative' and 'positive' liberties has formed part of such philosophical debates on the right to liberty. The first consists of the absence of interference. The interference to women carers as they carry out care-giving, both from bureaucracy and from the professions, has been highlighted here. Liberty in a second, stronger sense consists in being in control of one's destiny, rather than 'being a plaything of forces outside of one's self' (McClosky 1980:99). This right to liberty involves the right to self-development. Those discussing the nature of the rights of those with disabilities have placed emphasis on the potential and capabilities of the individual, which must not be prevented from developing into actual talent and skill. The same right to self-development must be accorded to their carers.

While the focus of this chapter is the control of care-giving work carried out by women mothering their children, similar controls exist for other care-giving work—care given in private homes to those with schizophrenia or dementia, those recovering from surgery or acute illness, and the frail elderly. The extent of this work is increasing as governments try to contain costs by deinstitutionalizing the elderly and those with physical or psychiatric disabilities, limiting access to hospitals for 'low tech' cases, and reducing the length of hospital stays. 'Just care-giving' is therefore an increasingly important issue.

NOTES

1. Psychology and education have claimed child-rearing knowledge as part of their professional ambit.
2. A term used by Illich to describe work carried out in the private sphere where its shape and extent is only partially visible.
3. Rich (1976) notes the way in which the architecture of the academy reinforces authority.

REFERENCES

Barrett M, McIntosh M 1982 The anti-social family. Verso, London
Billig M, Condor S, Edwards D, Gane M, Middleton D, Radley A 1988 Ideological dilemmas: a social psychology of everyday thinking. Sage, London
Bryson L 1985 Sharing the caring: overcoming barriers to gender equality. Australian Quarterly 57(4):300–309
Bryson L, Mowbray M 1986 Who cares? Social security, family policy and women. International Social Security Review 2:183–200
Cant R 1991 Tending work: caring for children who are disabled. Unpublished doctoral thesis, University of Newcastle, Newcastle
Cant R 1992 Friendship, neighbouring and the isolated family: the case of families with disabled children. International Journal of Sociology of the Family 22 (Autumn): 31–50
Carrington K 1989 Manufacturing female delinquency: a study of juvenile justice. Unpublished doctoral thesis, Macquarie University, Sydney

Dalley G 1988 Ideologies of caring. Macmillan Education, London

Daly J, Willis E 1988 Technological innovation in health care. In: Willis E (ed) Technology and the labour process. Allen & Unwin, Sydney

David M 1985 Motherhood and social policy—a matter of education. Critical Social Policy 12:28–43

Davin A 1978 Imperialism and motherhood. History Workshop 5:9–65

Deacon D 1985 Taylorism in the home: the medical profession, the infant welfare movement and the deskilling of women. Australian and New Zealand Journal of Sociology 25(2):161–173

Donzelot J 1979 The policing of families. Hutchinson, London

Edwards A 1988 Regulation and repression: a study of social control. Allen & Unwin, Sydney

Ehrenreich B, English D 1978 For her own good: 150 years of the experts' advice to women. Anchor Books, New York

Finch J, Groves D (eds) 1983 A labour of love: women, work and caring. Routledge and Kegan Paul, London

Foucault M 1973 The birth of the clinic: an archaeology of medical perception. Tavistock, London

Fraser N 1987 Women, welfare and the politics of need interpretation. Thesis Eleven 17:88–107

Friedson E 1970 Profession of medicine, a study of the sociology of applied knowledge. Harper and Row, New York

Gouldner A W 1979 The future of intellectuals and the rise of the new class: a frame of reference, theses, conjectures, arguments, and an historical perspective on the role of intellectuals and intelligentsia in the international/class contest of the modern era. Macmillan, London

Graham H 1984 Women, health and the family. Wheatsheaf Books, Brighton

Green C 1981 Handicapped children: let's be more positive and practical. The Medical Journal of Australia 1(8):402–404

HMSO 1989 Caring for people: community care in the next decade and beyond. London

Hughes E C 1971 Studying the nurse's work. In: The sociological eye: selected papers. Aldine Atherton, Chicago

Illich I 1977 Disabling professions. In: Illich I, Zola I K, McKnight J, Caplan J, Shaiken H (eds) Disabling professions. Marion Boyars, London

Kleinig J 1980 Privacy, personal identity and handicap. In: Laura R S (ed) Problems of handicap. Macmillan, South Melbourne

Knapman C 1990 Reconstructing mothering: policy and practice in infant welfare. Cumberland College seminar, University of Sydney, Sydney

Land H 1976 Women: supporters or supported? In: Barker L D, Allen S (eds) Sexual divisions and society: progress and change. Tavistock, London

Land H 1977 Inequalities in large families. In: Chester R, Peel J (eds) Equalities and inequalities in family life. Academic Press, London

Larson M S 1977 The rise of professionalism: a sociological analysis. University of California, Berkeley

Lasch C 1977 Haven in a heartless world: the family beseiged. Basic Books, New York

McClosky H J 1980 Handicapped persons and the rights they possess. In: Laura R S (ed) Problems of handicap. Macmillan, South Melbourne

Maddison D, Raphael B 1971 Social and psychological consequences of chronic disease in childhood. Medical Journal of Australia 2(25):1265–1270

Marshall T H 1970 Social policy. Hutchison University Library, London

Navarro V 1980 Work, ideology and science: the case of medicine. International Journal of Health Services 10(4):523–550

Nicholson N 1983 Home comforts. Health and Social Service Journal (March):356–7

Parsons T 1951 The social system: outlines of a conceptual scheme for the analysis of structure and process in social systems. Tavistock, London

Pascall G 1986 Social policy: a feminist analysis. Tavistock, London

Pateman C 1988 The patriarchal welfare state: women and democracy. In: Gutman A (ed) Democracy and the welfare state. Princeton University Press, Princeton

Platt A 1977 The child savers. University of Chicago Press, Chicago

Reiger K M 1985 The disenchantment of the home. Oxford University Press, London

Rich A 1976 Of woman born: motherhood as experience and institution. W W Norton, New York

Richmond D T (Pres) 1983 Inquiry into mental health services for the psychiatrically ill and developmentally disabled. Government Printer, Sydney

Riessman C K 1989 Women and medicalization: a new perspective. In: Brown P (ed) Perspectives in medical sociology. Wadsworth, Belmont

Sapsford R 1990 Family ideology and family discourse: paper presented to British Sociological Association Conference. University of Surrey, Guildford

Shaver S 1983 Sex and money in the welfare state. In: Baldock C, Cass B (eds) Women, social welfare and the state. George Allen & Unwin, North Sydney

Tulloch P 1984 Gender and dependency. In: Broom D H (ed) Unfinished business: social justice for women in Australia. George Allen & Unwin, Sydney

Wilson E 1987 Thatcherism and women: after seven years. In: Miliband R, Panitch J, Saville J (eds) Social register. Merlin, London

Yeatman A 1990 Bureaucrats, technocrats, femocrats. Allen & Unwin, North Sydney

19.   What is a health consumer?

Victoria M. Grace

There is no doubt that something called 'the health consumer' has emerged as a key player in debates about the provision of health care services in the last couple of decades. The language of consumerism in connection with health is used by groups of people who appear to have very different agendas, or interests, with respect to the provision of health care services. On the one hand there are numerous, often voluntary community based, health consumer groups dedicated to the cause of ensuring that our health care services are equitable, easily accessible to all members of the community, and that they place the needs of the consumer first. Health consumer groups in New Zealand and Australia typically oppose elitism and other forms of discriminatory practice in the delivery of health services and in the formulation of health-related policy. On the other hand there are the new marketers of health services for whom the emergence of the health consumer goes hand in hand with the new need to 'market health'.

A plan for the so-called 'reform' of the New Zealand system of health service delivery was introduced in July 1991 by the National Government. During 1992 and 1993 a special Directorate, located in the Department of the Prime Minister and Cabinet did the groundwork for the implementation date for the new system of July 1993. The discourse of the need for 'reform' and the process of changing to a new system appears to be driven by a market model of health services: there is a need to restructure the system in the interests of greater efficiency, greater effectiveness and increased consumer responsiveness. 'Better value for the dollar' is the favourite slogan.

In this discourse, being a consumer is associated with having more choice, being asked what you want, having the service catering entirely to your needs. This is supposedly in contrast to an era when the health system has been criticized by 'consumer groups' as catering to the needs of doctors, biomedical researchers, and drug companies, frequently at the patient's expense.

Is this new era of the health consumer genuinely empowering, and indicative of a better deal for people in need of health care and preventive health services? To answer this question it is necessary to examine critically the very notion of a health consumer and to develop an understanding of the concept in its institutional, social, economic and political context.

In what way is health a consumer product?

The limitations of the notion of 'consuming' health care services as if health care was a commodity like any other, have been central to the resistance to the 'reform' of the health system in New Zealand by health professionals and consumer groups alike. It has been pointed out in many fora that the consumer of health services does not have the information and expertise necessary to make informed decisions, and certainly the health care provider has superior knowledge. The health consumer is usually not in a position to repeat the purchase of whatever product or intervention she or he has received and thus make a better consumer choice on the basis of experience. The successful outcome of a health care service 'purchase' is usually, at least to some degree, dependent on the quality of the relationship between the doctor, or other health professional, and the patient; such a relationship lies outside of the economic equation calculating the value of an exchanged good or service. There are numerous other arguments refuting the appropriateness of the consumer model to the provision of health care services.

The argument is being made around the western world as health systems are being restructured in accordance with a market model, that health is not a commodity (Kuuskoski-Vikatmaa 1988). Baudrillard has argued in a number of books and articles that the object of consumption in our contemporary consumer society is not in fact a commodity, but a sign (Baudrillard 1968, 1970, 1972, 1973, 1981).

Prior to, and in the early stages of, industrialization in Europe, 'use' was understood as a key factor in determining the value of an item: how useful the item was to the person or group wanting to obtain that item determined its 'use value'. As industrialization progressed, the way value was determined also changed. By the middle of last century this was understood by various theorists (including Marx, the neo-classical economists and utilitarian philosophers) to be best defined as 'exchange value': a value derived from the strength of supply (embodying labour and capital), and demand (resting again on the notion of usefulness, or 'utility').

With the advent of mass consumption and the information age, Baudrillard has argued that objects are valued, not in terms of their use value, nor even in terms of their exchange value (as commodities) but rather in terms of their signifying value (as signs). Objects of consumption obtain value by virtue of their signifying a desirable or necessary item, event, experience. For example, clothes of a certain style and fabric obtain their value not because of the exchange value of the raw materials and subsequent production and marketing costs, but because of the fact that they signify, let's say, a sophisticated and yet casual image of the individual as someone who is in control of their lives, clearly makes a good living, is young, successful, popular. And of course these images, and their desirability, are constructed through the media. The entire business of marketing and competing for markets becomes one of image making, whether it is toothpaste (fresh, clean, healthy, sparkling), interiors (significations of a nostalgia for the security of the simple and beautiful life of another era and another place, through simulations of crockery and furniture from Provence, for example) to health care (signifying quality of service, and playing on people's insecurities and vulnerabilities when sick, offering 'hotel-like' surroundings for their hospital stay).

If the object of consumption is fully mediated in this way, indeed its very reality is mediated, the value of that object is not tied in any intrinsic way to the item itself. Baudrillard and others have referred to this phenomenon as the loss of the referent. The referent, or object referred to, no longer provides an anchor point for determining its own value nor provides the basis for its own definition. Rather, the object's reality and value are determined within a play of signs. The era of contemporary consumer society characterized by this logic of production whereby the play of signs precedes the value and indeed the reality of the object, Baudrillard has called 'hyperreality'.

A discourse analysis[1] of the concept of health articulated by health promotion professionals in New Zealand shows how health, as an object of consumption, can be understood as a floating signifier, consistent with Baudrillard's notion of the sign which, he argued, is at the heart of the political economy of consumer society. Insight into the nature of health, as consumer object, as sign, throws light on the contradictory positioning of the individual on the one hand 'liberated' to be a 'consumer' of health/health care services, but on the other hand entirely subject to the economic code of sign value constructing that consumer. In accordance with Bauman's argument (1988), the freedom of the consumer is not exactly the freedom the health consumer groups had in mind when campaigning in opposition to the medical dominance of health care provision and health care policy.

The positivity of health

We must have more health, longer life, healthier lifestyles, better quality health, healthier more-quality years of life.

In fact, for those who successfully manipulate the signs of employment, business, the stock exchange, and hence are the consumers in the supermarkets, in the world of fashion, computerized choices, consumer gadgets and simulated experiences of every conceivable shape, size and colour, *death* (and illness) feature as a kind of deviant blip on the otherwise smooth and fairly regular surface of accumulated existence. The value of health seems to be gradually replacing the values of right and wrong—to be healthy is a moral duty, to evaluate the 'rightness' of a policy, action, or discourse is to assess the way it impacts on health. To be healthy is a signifier of social status, of pure functionality, and also plays a role in locating 'good' (and safe) sexuality, against deviant and contaminated sex.

The momentum toward more health, more life, more...everything, (everything that is healthful, enjoyable, exciting, satisfying, rewarding, *positive*), leaves death in a kind of limbo place. Death, illness, deterioration, are the negative terms that somehow do not quite fit. As Woody Allen once said as a character in one of his own films: 'Die! What Do You Mean Die!' In other words, surrounded by the positivity of the consumer society in the heart of a bustling New York evening, the idea of death is virtually inconceivable—there is no cultural space for a concept of something so astonishingly *present* as a person to simply die, end, vanish, evaporate, disappear.

The denial of death and disease

The entire development of materialism, industry, exact science...has made us forget we are mortal. (Virilio 1983:124)

Imhof (1985) has considered the changing attitudes towards death implicit in medical approaches to the eradication of disease during the last four centuries.[2] He asked his reader to consider whether the eradication of one sort of disease, or cause of death, and its replacement with another is in fact a desirable exchange, and questioned the current lack of attention being paid to this issue. Imhof outlined some of the sociological features which have accompanied these changes in mortality patterns. These include large numbers of deaths now happening in the 'hidden' environment of the hospital, the secularization of 'life' and thus the 'shortening' of life (previously corporeal life on earth was just a brief phase in an eternal existence), and how the physical body has taken a corresponding appreciation in value. According to Imhof, the relationships between the changes in disease pattern, the attitudes towards and experiencing of death, the secularization of social life, and the attitudes towards the body and health are closely interlinked. He placed the final emphasis on the separation of life and death:

Life and death have become completely separated; at the moment they are two totally different things for us, hard to combine. As long as we are willing to accept only the first and to reject the other, we will remain in an unsolvable dilemma and continue to find ourselves—every time we are forced to attend a burial—in a situation like a blown-up soap bubble. (Imhof 1985:29)

McKnight (1986) commented on the denial of death in the health promotion context stating the importance of resisting this denial and analysing the political context in which it occurs:

We have not only the vitality of our healing but the capacity to suffer our mortality. This capacity to cope with suffering and finally celebrate our mortality is the foundation of culture. However, health without pain or death is the vision of a system whose tools are chemicals and plastic parts. In exchange for the power to cope and celebrate, we are offered chemically managed versions of therapeutic oblivion. (McKnight 1986:79)

Sontag (1978) discussed the denial of death in the course of her work on the metaphors associated with disease. The denial of death is closely linked with the denial of disease, both of which are understood as opposing life. Sontag also alluded to the importance of the loss of the 'religious consolations' about death in the process of changing attitudes towards death:

> For those who live neither with religious consolations about death nor with a sense of death (or of anything else) as natural, death is the obscene mystery, the ultimate affront, the thing that cannot be controlled. It can only be denied. (Sontag 1978:55)

Hence, the denial of death and disease is the corollary of the positivity of health.

The discourse of health promotion in New Zealand

> 'We want to move into prevention and promoting health, and promoting healthy lifestyles and enjoyment of life.' (Interview)

In 1988 I conducted a series of open-ended interviews with 23 individuals working in health promotion in New Zealand. This fieldwork, along with archival documents and conference papers, formed the empirical data for a critical analysis of the health promotion discourse in New Zealand.[3]

The discourse of health promotion professionals in New Zealand revealed health as a concept cast fully in the positive. The way in which this positivity appears, within a dualism of health and illness, casts illness into the negative. To focus on health in the positive does not serve to redefine or reposition 'health' with respect to the dualism, but shifts the focus from curing or treating the negative to producing or maintaining the positive. The positivity of health is evident in the following quotations taken from the interviews:

> It's wellness we're promoting; health

> Good health to all people. (Mission statement)

> Well-being is health, and enabling and empowering people to become healthy or maintain healthy states, and that's the definition of health promotion

> Try and promote quality of life, and I see that as a health promotion thing, you know, it's not just a matter of how physically well you are, it's how psychologically and mentally well you are that is just as important.

> There is another level on which health promotion is being talked about, which is very, very sort of new, and I think not very clearly conceptualized or clearly based in research, but it's that idea of trying to identify positive health, and indicators and trying really to promote positive health, and to get away from being defined in terms of disease classifications.

> Nurses from the first year right through, and right from the word go, I tell them that they're health promoters, that they're being trained not to tend the sick, but people in hospital need health promotion, sick people right from birth and right through to old age, they need health promotion, they need to have a sense of well-being and they need to know that life is for living and not for sort of wandering around.

> People think you get old, you get diseases, and you can't get across the idea that in fact you don't have to—I mean, sure you have to die from something in the

end, but you can actually get to old age without going through your life from one disease to another. (Interviews)

Health promotion experts have defined 'health' according to a number of different models. For example, Foss and Rothenberg (1987) used an adaptive, ecological model based on systems theory, viewing health as a state of equilibrium or balance of a dynamic system comprising interacting parts; Green, Kreuter, Deeds and Partridge (1980) used an instrumental model in which health is viewed as a resource that has utility and value as an instrument to achieve certain ends. However, the overwhelming conceptualization of health used by those interviewed was as a *state to be achieved*. Examples include:

...trying to impact health in a nation...

...there are so many contributing factors in health...

...total well-being; a total person concept...

...national health goals...

...to achieve health...

...important element for health...

...health impacts of various policies...

...measuring positive health...

...improve their health status...

...marketing of health...

...marketing of health behaviour...(Interviews)

The last two have a sense of health as a state to be 'acquired' rather than 'achieved'. Further analysis of the content of statements on health, and of the discursive positioning of health within the discourse as a whole, led to an expansion of the predominant concept of health to that of a *thing measured*. Health appeared as a kind of floating signification of measurement which actually does not make any other appearance in the discourse. Reading through the lists of statements in which the word 'health' appears, it is a thing which is 'impacted' and its 'status' is read off from a number of different indicators. Health is 'low', 'good', 'maintained', 'promoted', 'enhanced', 'conserved', 'better', 'improved', 'affected', 'changed'. Its status can be 'enhanced' by it being 'looked after'. It is 'a sense of well-being', which typically includes 'physical', 'social', 'mental' and 'spiritual' well-being, and also includes an absence of disease. This construction has a characteristic which typifies its discursive positioning and that is its positivity, as was mentioned above. This positivity is posed in relation to 'something'; health thus is positioned as *degrees* of well-being. These degrees of health do not exist in a vacuum, but rather on a scale which provides degrees of health in contrast to that which it is not—illness, or 'ill-being'. It is through this kind of reasoning that the problems associated with the positivity of health become evident and the political effects of the discursive negation of disease and death become available for analysis.

The assumption by health promoters that health exists as a referent of measurement (that object/event/process being measured), helps to explain how it is that health promotion is conceived of as an activity involving interventions to increase that measurement on the plus side of the scale, which will also mean a decrease of illness and death (see Lalonde 1974). Assessment of 'health' has been made primarily by examining morbidity and mortality statistics, but also more recently, by using self-report questionnaires and through collecting data on the amount of 'healthy' or 'unhealthy' products 'consumed' (Milio 1986). In the recent past, indicators of 'health status' which are not based on disease-related parameters have been, and are being, sought (early attempts include Andrews & Withey 1976, Campbell et al 1986, Krupinski 1980). This corroborates the loss of a referent and the generalization of health as a sign that floats among other signs discussed earlier. Health promotion is a business involving the 'increase of health', the 'improvement of health', the more 'equal distribution of health'. To enact this business, a model of 'health' *precedes* the action. There must be a prior construct of 'health' and this is then aimed at, produced, created. 'Health' is modelled and health promotion is an activity involving the attempt to make the 'reality' (that is, the objects(s) of the measurements) fit the model. A discourse of health which 'promotes healthy lifestyles' has a prior model of a 'healthy lifestyle'. An 'intervention' or 'program' is designed to increase 'health behaviour', to increase the 'healthy lifestyle', and the behaviour is not 'right', is not 'real health' until it conforms with the model. The 'real' is created or produced, and is only 'real' when it replicates the model. This phenomenon of the model preceding the reality to the extent that the model becomes the reality, is a central feature of Baudrillard's thesis of hyperreality and the political economy of the sign.

The precession[4] of the model

It is not right that people should get help after they need it; they've got to get it before they need it. (Interview)

Health promotion effectively models the consumer of health (Grace 1991). This process of 'modelling', or constructing a 'reality' in accordance with a model, is not simply referring to a process whereby a person intends to effect a certain change in a specific instance, acts and thus contributes to a transformation. It is referring to a particular process occurring in a particular historical epoch whereby the model of the change that is to occur is actually a reality that is structured in accordance with an economic code. This code involves a structural logic which opposes reversibility in a way which is all-pervasive and hegemonic. The sign is only positive; it excludes all negativity. The precession of the model is not simply a phenomenon of intentionality, but is related to the collapse of the polarity of signifier and signified.[5] The model, as a sign, becomes more real than that 'real' which it assumedly replaced, hence *hyperreality*.

Baudrillard used the word 'simulation' to refer to the process whereby the 'real' is simulated via the model. He introduced a discussion of the precession of simulacra by using an analogy of the relationship between the territory and the map. Instead of the territory preceding the map and the map being a replication or model of the territory which may or may not be accurate, the map now precedes the territory and the territory takes its 'reality' with reference to the map, or model. It is only 'real' if it reproduces the model. Thus the precession of simulacra threatens the distinction between 'true' and 'false', or between 'real' and 'imaginary'[6] (Baudrillard 1981:5). It is possible to see how the precession of the model is related to the 'loss of the object', as the dominance of the logic of sign value escalates. The 'collapse' of the poles of signifier and signified is related to the discursive disappearance of a referent.

The precession of the model is integral to the logic of sign value. As Baudrillard wrote:

Facts no longer have any trajectory of their own, they arise at the intersection of the models...This anticipation, this precession, this short-circuit, this confusion of the fact with its model (no more divergence of meaning, no more dialectical polarity, no more negative electricity or implosion of poles) is what each time allows for all the possible interpretations, even the most contradictory—all are true, in the sense that their truth is exchangable, in the image of the models from which they proceed, in a generalized cycle. (Baudrillard 1981:32)

The discourse analysis of the interview material provides ample evidence of the operation of the hyperreal mode in the discourse of health promotion. 'Health' does not appear as a product or commodity, but as a sign. The product is a hyperreal product. The signs of health are circulated—designed, produced, marketed and consumed, and the hyperreal health (of healthy lifestyles, healthy behaviours) is to be achieved, that is, it takes on value in its positivity as a sign. The entire discourse of health promotion pivots around the production of health in accordance with a model, through the implementation of programs, interventions or campaigns. This process is 'managed' in accordance with the marketing discourse. The linkage between the precession of the model with the management and marketing of health promotion appears in the interviews:

We know, or the commercial people know, that it is extremely difficult and long term to change people's behaviour, and I'm always reminded of a sentence which appeared in the *New York Times* on January 16th, 1983, where a tobacco company spokesperson...said that in this business people kill for the point differential. What he meant by this is that it is so difficult to capture even one tenth of 1% of the market share for any particular brand that you crack open the champagne when it happens. So they know that to achieve such a tiny behaviour change as 0.1% for a particular brand costs an enormous amount of money and you go to the ends of the earth in order to do it. Then I think health education should begin to appreciate the difficulty it [sic] is in changing people's behavioural patterns. (Interview)

The simulated nature of the market model is masked in this discourse of competition and strategy. The speaker fails to notice that the 'behaviour' that is so 'difficult' to change is modelled in the first instance in accordance with the marketing premise.

The health care consumer appears at centre stage of the discourse of health marketing, whether we are talking about medical care, preventive services or health promotion. For example, Moore (1992) described a model for maximizing health consumer, or client, satisfaction. The client becomes a 'target system' and the model delineates a process to administer the '7-Ms': matrix, measure, market, massage, manifest, monitor, manage. The target system is the dependent variable and satisfaction maximization measures are derived as a result of implementation of the model (in other words, degrees of satisfaction register on the consumer who is the passive component in the system). Consumer satisfaction is the product of health care delivery and the model creates it.

In another example, Nestor (1992) described both the important role of 'psychographics' in understanding the consumer market, and the need for health markets to concentrate on 'micro-marketing'. Nestor claimed that 'marketing in health care organizations in the 1990s will (be) transform(ed)' (Nestor 1992:28). Ironically, her article carries the title 'Marketing to consumers: unleashing technologies to help the public choose health service options'. The sacred icon of consumerism, choice, is modelled through an elaborate marketing system. Even the do-it-yourself health care consumer has been identified as a market niche. Profiled, surveyed, analysed, segmented, targeted, the do-it-yourself health care consumer has the freedom to choose exactly what he or she might want, and can be assured of 'satisfaction' (see Pinto & Gehrt 1991).

Conclusion

This analysis of the notion of a 'health consumer' has not resolved the contradiction between the health consumer as a manipulated component of a marketing enterprise and the health consumer as a radical opponent to a medically dominated health care system. Rather, we have seen how, as a 'consumer', the individual is 'programmed' in accordance with a model, the provider of the service no less than the consumer. If we pursue Baudrillard's analysis, the model is, at root, a logic of signification, that of sign value, which ensures its own hegemony by its non-reversibility. The sign, as Baudrillard depicted it, is fully positive, with no ambivalence. We saw how the positivity of health in the discourse of health promotion experts reflected this positivity characteristic of the logic of the sign. Health was located within the discourse as a floating signifier, consistent with the hyperreal mode of production and marketing of health.

Of course ambivalence cannot be eradicated. But this relentless progression of the hyperreal logic of signification into all areas of social life means that resistance and opposition is not recognizable by those functioning within the system. This resistance simply becomes characterized as yet another market niche, another psychodemographic market segment.

The conclusion that can be drawn from this analysis is that the health consumer striving for a more equitable, fair and empowering health care service is not commensurate with the health consumer who is an artifact of the health marketing system.

NOTES

1. The word 'discourse' is used instead of 'language' because discourse connotes the actively political and strategic role of words and the way they are connected to form sentences and construct meaning. This differs from understandings of 'language' which imply universal and fixed linguistic structures and meanings for words. An analysis of discourse is concerned with discovering how and under what conditions words and phrases have specific meanings and what can be learnt about the politics underpinning the structuring of a particular discourse at a given historical moment.
2. It is important to recognize that there is a substantial literature analysing the phenomenon of the denial of death in the discourses typifying western industrialized countries, especially those of medical institutions. (This literature expanded considerably from the 1970s onwards, e.g. Aries 1977, Morin 1977, Ziegler 1975.)
3. The method of discourse analysis used was lexicology. For a full description of the research methodology used in this project see unpublished PhD thesis *The Marketing of Empowerment and the Construction of the Health Consumer: a Critique of Health Promotion in New Zealand*, 1989, University of Canterbury.
4. 'Precession' is an astronomical term referring to the way in which the equinoctical point defining the beginning of spring moves in a slow retrograde way along the ecliptic with the result that each year the timing of the beginning of spring slightly precedes the previous year's timing. It seems that Baudrillard used this term to stress his point with regard to the way simulacra, or models, come to take place before the real, so to speak, and flip reality into a hyperreal mode in which reality is that which is felt and experienced according to a model.
5. To try and explain this concept in simple terms one might say that the polarity of the signifier and signified refer to the separation of the mark, or word, or representation code, and the thing it is referring to (strictly speaking, the concept it is referring to).
6. This observation was made by Lasch (1979).

REFERENCES

Andrews F M, Withey S B 1976 Social indicators of well-being: American perceptions of life quality. Plenum Press, New York
Aries P 1977 L'homme devant la mort. Le Seuil, Paris
Baudrillard J 1968 Le systéme des objets. Gallimard, Paris
Baudrillard J 1970 La société de consommation. Galliamard, Paris
Baudrillard J 1972 (trans 1981) For a critique of the political economy of the sign. Telos Press, St Louis MO
Baudrillard J 1973 (trans 1975) The mirror of production. Telos Press, St Louis Mo
Baudrillard J 1981 (trans 1983) Simulations. Semiotext(e), New York
Bauman Z 1988 Freedom. Open University Press, Milton Keynes
Campbell A, Converse P E, Rodgers W L 1986 Quality of American life: perceptions, evaluations and satisfaction. Russell Sage Foundation, New York
Foss L, Rothenberg K 1987 The second medical revolution: from biomedicine to infomedicine. New Science Library, Boston

Grace V M 1991 The marketing of empowerment and the construction of the health consumer: a critique of health promotion. International Journal of Health Services 21(2):329–343

Green L W, Kreuter M W, Deeds S G, Partridge K B 1980 Health education planning: a diagnostic approach. Mayfield Publishing, California

Imhof A E 1985 From the old morality pattern to the new: implications of a radical change from the sixteenth to the twentieth century. Bulletin of the History of Medicine 59:1–29

Krupinski J 1980 Health and quality of life. Social Science and Medicine 14A:203–211

Kuuskoski-Vikatmaa E 1988 Interactions of health policy, ethics and human values: a European perspective. In: Bankowski Z, Bryant J H Health policy, ethics and human values: European and North American perspectives. CIMS, Geneva

Lalonde M 1974 A new perspective on the health of Canadians. Information Canada, Ottawa

Lasch C 1979 The culture of narcissism. W H Norton, New York

McKnight J L 1986 Well-being: the new threshold of the old medicine. Health Promotion 1(1):77–80

Milio N 1986 Promoting health through public policy. Canadian Public Health Association, Ottawa

Moore S T 1992 Maximizing satisfaction and managing dissatisfaction in mental health and human services: a model for administrative practice. Health Marketing Quarterly 9(3/4):29–37

Morin E 1977 L'homme et la mort. Le Seuil, Paris

Nestor S E 1992 Marketing to consumers: unleashing technologies to help the public choose health service options. Topics in Health Care Financing 18(3):28–37

Pinto M B, Gehrt K C 1991 The do-it-yourself health care consumer: preliminary identification and marketing implications. Health Marketing Quarterly 8(3/4):97–106

Sontag S 1978 Illness as metaphor. Farrar, Strauss and Giroux, New York

Virilio P 1983 Pure war. Semiotext(e), New York

Ziegler J 1975 Les vivants et la mort. Le Seuil, Paris

20. Negotiations around health: do women as consumers have any choice?

Liz Eckermann

Serious debates about the future of health care are occurring all over the world. In the United Kingdom, the National Health Service is under review. In the United States, the Clinton administration has opened up the debate between privatized and nationalized health care and the medical-industrial complex is being subjected to growing criticism (Relman 1993). Australia is no exception to this international trend. Health was one of the key contentious issues in the 1993 federal election.

Context

These debates can be placed within the context of broader arguments about citizenship and social justice. The world-wide economic recession of the late 1980s and early 1990s has put health care on the agenda as a 'negotiable' resource. No longer can unlimited health care be regarded as an inalienable right. Choices are being made on a public policy level about distribution of scarce resources, and sectional interest groups lobby harder than ever to get their share of the health dollar (Sax 1990). Alongside these developments, and in opposition to them, is the rise of the health consumer movement (Palmer & Short 1989) and some serious challenges to medical dominance in the health field (Willis 1988). Although it is argued that these challenges have merely made medical dominance more covert (Willis 1993), health and the human body have become the canvas for political contestation in the closing years of the twentieth century (Turner 1992). This is especially evident in political debates about the demographic revolution towards an ageing population, ethical debates about reproductive technology and clinical debates about the re-emergence of infectious diseases (for example tuberculosis and AIDS) and environmentally induced illness (Turner 1992). The concept of risk (Beck 1992) provides a framework for understanding such changes, for understanding consumer decision-making and for examining the meaning of informed consent.

A plethora of public documents at an international, national, state and local government level has emerged in response to needs to restructure various sectors of health care. The national report on *The Future of General Practice* (National Health Strategy 1992) and the final national report on

Improving Australia's Health: The Role of Primary Health Care (National Centre for Epidemiology and Population Health 1992), both of which recommend radical changes to existing structures and practices in primary health in line with the recommendations of WHO's Alma Ata of 1978 and the Ottawa Charter of 1981, are germane to the current debate about social justice in the delivery of health care. The consumer perspective on the proposed changes to general practice appeared in three national documents (Broom 1991, Consumers' Health Forum 1992a, 1992b). At the local government level, local councils in Victoria have been charged with the task of preparing Strategic Health Plans for their areas. Geelong's municipality of the City of South Barwon's 1993 Municipal Public Health Plan recommends promotion of the community's self-sufficiency at both a personal and a collective level. One of the main recommendations of that report, is that 'a feeling of a degree of control over your own destiny' and 'a feeling that our community has some power' (City of South Barwon 1993:14) contribute greatly to a sense of community and individual well-being. To investigate the potential for such empowerment from a sociological perspective, I argue that we need to consider the health consumer as an embodied agent. We should not fall into the trap of the classical tradition in sociology of privileging the mind and rational reflection as the only site for the exercise of agency. Social actors are embodied actors and their bodies are in turn gendered.

In Australia the recent Human Rights and Equal Opportunity Commission case on the legitimacy and lawfulness of 'women-only' health services (Broom 1992) (Ch. 28) has raised important questions relating to the provision of services to women. The challenge to women's health services raised some interesting debates about citizenship and sectional calls upon the public purse as well as more general debates about what constitutes health and the sexed body. Thus the politico-socioeconomic context needs to complemented with an analysis of consumers as embodied and gendered subjects negotiating the health system. That agenda forms the focus of the research detailed below.

The research agenda

This chapter represents a work-in-progress report on research which I am undertaking in the field of consumer entry to the health system. Part of that research involves an evaluation project (under the auspices of the General Practice Evaluation Program) which examines consumer knowledge, opinions, satisfactions and perceived choices in primary health care provision. I am not yet in a position to report comprehensive results of the research as it is still in process. Those results will be published in due course (in conjunction with my colleagues in the research, Shane Thomas, Ian Steven, Colette Browning and Liz Dickens). However, I am able to provide the background to the research, a review of the existing literature and some preliminary results from one of the focus groups, attenders at a women's health centre.

In response to the above mentioned debates and calls for change, I address the following broad question: *Within the structural constraints of factors such as social class, gender, ethnicity, age, professional dominance, health insurance arrangements and geographical location, what are the opportunities for the exercise of individual and collective agency on the part of health care consumers?*

This question raises further questions of an ontological nature (what is health? what is the body?) as well as epistemological issues about the status of various claims to knowledge (including that of consumers) about health and primary health care. I seek to elaborate on a broad sociology of consumption model in the health field and apply the structure/agency debate, which is at the forefront of sociological theoretical debates, to health issues (Giddens 1984, 1991, 1992, Pescosolido 1992). I want to ascertain how people exercise personal power and mobilize institutional power in making decisions about care and maintenance of their bodies. This inquiry leads me into arguments about the extent to which bodies are regulated and controlled by external forces and by individuals themselves (Foucault 1980, Turner 1992) or subjected to the vagaries and chaos of 'risk society' (Beck 1992). I also seek to test, in an Australian context, the claims by Pescosolido, in her work in the United States, that social interaction has 'primacy in (the process of) decision-making' and that 'systematic patterning of interaction networks form the proper analytic focus for study' of decision-making about health care use (Pescosolido 1992:1098).

Literature review

Most of the early literature on consumer experience of the health care system from a sociological perspective concentrated on structural factors which influence the encounter between the consumer, the health system and the providers of health care (Koos 1954) and this tradition has continued in more recent work (Eisenberg 1979, Calnan 1988, Briscoe 1987, Greene et al 1980, Preston-Whyte et al 1983, Weisman & Teitelbaum 1985, Weiss 1988). Class, gender, ethnicity, age and geographical location are the dimensions which are often used to differentiate groups with distinct experiences of clinical encounters. Most of these studies concentrate on clinical encounters between general practitioners or specialists and their clients suggesting differential diagnostic rates and differential treatment regimes according to social class, sex of the client and practitioner, ethnicity, age and geographical location. Many use Parsons' 'sick role' (Parsons 1951) as the organizing principle of such encounters. Some provide critiques of the Parsonian framework arguing that negotiation between doctor and client more closely characterizes that relationship (especially in the case of chronic illness) than the exercise of expert power/knowledge (Arney & Bergen 1983, Stewart & Sullivan 1982). Very few studies question the epistemological framework of the medical model (Wright & Treacher 1983). There is a tendency to accept a foundationalist conception of health, illness and the human body and often the recommendations from the research are for redistribution of existing services. While most of these studies have been able to establish the conditions which circumscribe consumers' experiences of the health system, very few have addressed the role of consumers as agents, either collectively or individually, making decisions about their health care.

At the other extreme are those sociologists who emphasize the role of the sovereign individual acting within a rational action framework in making choices about health care (Lindenberg 1985, Friedman & Hechter 1988). Pescosolido suggests that this polarity between economic rationalism and structural explanations reflects the wider debate in sociological theory between agency and structure as deciding factors in social action. Research on help-seeking behaviour on health issues in the 1960s tended to utilize one of two models.

The Health Belief Model (HBM) (developed by Rosenstock 1966) focused on the social psychology of decision making, primarily the role of motivations, beliefs, and perceptions on individuals' decisions to seek formal medical care (Pescosolido 1992:1110).

Or alternatively:

The Socio-Behavioural Model (SBM) (Andersen 1968) (which) was more structurally oriented—focusing primarily on access to and 'need' for care (Pescosolido 1992:1110).

Pescosolido argues that these two orientations have drawn 'insights from each other and moved toward synthesis' (Pescosolido 1992:1110) however my search of the literature in the area suggests that this 'synthesis' has not been universal with many researchers still adhering single-mindedly to one or the other orientation.

A recent Australian attempt to overcome this conceptual hiatus between structure and agency, as the key factors in making health care decisions, is the research conducted by Peter Lloyd and colleagues (Lloyd et al 1991). The researchers addressed the issue of consumerism in the health care setting arguing that in many respects consumers of health care act as a unique market. Lloyd et al suggest that the concept of consumerism as applied to health is somewhat premature since their surveyed population (a cross-section of GP attenders in the outer western and northern suburbs of Sydney in March 1990) did not fit the neoclassical economic prerequisite of discerning, rational and sovereign consumers. By contrast, those surveyed were 'strongly attracted to the traditional model of medical care, which is characterized by the trusting and dependent relationship of patients with their doctors' (Lloyd et al 1991:194).

These findings reinforce the arguments put forward by Evans (1984) in his work on Canadian GP attenders, McGuire et al (1988) in Britain and Relman (1993) in the United States that a variety of factors militate against the existence of a 'pure' market in health care. Health is excluded from discretionary decision-making on the basis of the 'professional and commercial monopoly enjoyed by doctors' over service provision and medical knowledge along with the 'unpredictable nature of illness' making individuals 'particularly vulnerable at the very time when critical decisions are required' (Lloyd et al 1991:194-5).

Given the trend by both major political parties in Australia to view the health care system increasingly as yet another market and to apply economic rationalism to policy on health (see Hewson 'fight-back package' on health Nov 1991 and federal ALP policy on Medicare surcharge July 1991 (Commonwealth of Australia 1991)) there appears to be some substance to the researchers warning that:

the limitation to the neoclassical understanding of the concept of consumers should be borne in mind when assessing the ability of...(users of the system)...to behave consumeristically. (Lloyd et al 1991:195)

Lloyd et al also found that most people in their sample had not adopted the role of 'active' consumer in health care despite the fact that on the collective level consumer groups in Australia such as the Consumers' Health Forum had been quite active in the policy-making arena (Broom 1991, Consumers' Health Forum 1992a, 1992b). (See also Palmer & Short 1989:135 on consumer groups and health practitioner education.) Cost was not a primary concern, and consumers failed to evaluate independently the services of the doctor, perhaps because they were also found to have a limited concept of what, in medical terms, constitutes good or bad service. They were more likely to display blind trust and faith in their GP's competence than to display critical and discriminating attitudes (Lloyd et al 1991).

The researchers suggest that 'a smaller study focusing on qualitative data and using focus groups or interviews, could provide valuable insights into (clients')...tendencies towards consumerist behaviour in the health care setting' (Lloyd et al 1991:200). This is one of the challenges taken up by a consumer knowledge study which I am undertaking with several colleagues. However, I feel that we need to move beyond the agenda addressed by Lloyd et al to question the ontological and epistemological assumptions of the conventional medical model of health care and explore a variety of health care options including self-care.

Pescosolido suggests that researchers need to re-cast the 'agent' in health care choices as 'the agent in interaction' if they wish to move beyond a rational choice framework. I address this issue by examining the context and complexities of decision-making and by emphasizing the need to consider collective as well as individual agency. The 'connection between action, interaction and structure' (Pescosolido 1992:1107) is implied in the question posed above. With Pescosolido I agree that 'individuals are neither puppets of some abstract structure nor calculating individualists' since 'people both shape and are shaped by social networks' (Pescosolido 1992:1109). However, given contrasting health care arrangements between the United States and

Australia (especially with regard to universal health insurance) the applicability to this country of the 'social organization strategy' framework, proposed by Pescosolido to explain lay decision making about health care, is yet to be tested. Similarly, Pescosolido works with a disembodied notion of the social actor. However, I endorse Pescosolido's claim that to understand fully the 'social dynamics of how people seek help' we need to move away from discipline based 'arid debates and toward transdisciplinary, multilevel frameworks for understanding social action' (Pescosolido 1992:1126). This involves using both a diversity of theoretical positions and a multiplicity of methodological perspectives. Thus a thoroughgoing analysis of consumer choice would need to examine the phenomenology of the lived experience that consumers have of the health system and of their own bodies, an examination of the social roles consumers and providers play in interaction in the social system as well as a politico-economic analysis of the context of health care (Turner 1987).

Current research

Research on the extent to which consumers of health care services feel that they have genuine choice and control over decision-making in their use of primary health care is the focus of a project I am currently undertaking with several colleagues. The project (funded by the Commonwealth Department of Health, Housing, Community Services and Local Government and administered under the General Practice Evaluation Program) is entitled 'Consumer knowledge, opinions, satisfactions and perceived choices in primary health care provision' (S. Thomas, I. Steven, C. Browning, E. Eckermann and E. Dickens). This chapter focuses on the background literature which informed the research process and some preliminary findings on one of the groups informing the research project. The detailed findings of the project will be published elsewhere in 1994.

Methodology

There were several component studies in the project, each with its own distinct methodology.

1. A focus group study
2. Development of a consumer knowledge and opinion instrument
3. A validation study of the instrument

The last two studies are being conducted currently and involve large representative samples of the Australian population using ABS random sampling frames and employing ABS stratification variables (sex, age, residence, income, previous level of health care usage). We unashamedly incorporated both quantitative and qualitative methodologies in our research believing that they complement each other in providing an understanding of consumer decision-making in health care. We have all had research experiences in using the technique of triangulation of sources and methodologies (Denzin 1978, Thomas et al 1992). We were prepared to 'traverse the epistemological hiatus which opens up between the (qualitative and quantitative) research traditions' (Bryman 1984) and argue that both quantitative and qualitative data are needed to understand health issues fully and to develop appropriate services and policy. Rather than regard qualitative research as merely exploratory preparation or 'fodder' for the quantitative phase of research, we see the results of the qualitative stages of the research as having integrity in their own right (Silverman 1987, Oakley 1988, Baum 1992, Eckermann 1993).

The focus group study taps into the lived experience of consumers of health services and involves groups drawn from a wide representation of Australians. The study explored the dimensions of consumer knowledge, experience and opinions of primary health care. In this particular part of the project no attempt was made to achieve randomness in the samples. The focus groups were seen as constituting a sample of key informants who provided a 'comprehensive range of perspectives and ideas rather than as a means of estimating the relative frequencies of the numbers of people in a population who hold these perspectives and ideas' (Thomas et al 1992:10). Thus we were interested in 'analysing the constructs, ideas, feelings and motives' of our informants. There were 26 focus groups with 8–10 people in each. The groups were drawn from the following populations:

(a) Attenders at city general practices. Six groups formed from this category including frequent attenders and infrequent attenders from each of upper, middle and lower socioeconomic strata
(b) Attenders at 24 hour clinics
(c) Attenders at hospital accident and emergency departments
(d) Attenders at a general practice in a large country town
(e) Attenders at a general practice in a medium country town
(f) Attenders at a general practice in a small country town
(g) People 60 years and older
(h) Australian Aboriginal people
(i) Attenders at chiropractors
(j) Attenders at naturopaths
(k) People with Greek as their primary language
(l) People with Italian as their primary language
(m) People with Vietnamese as their primary language
(n) Attenders at community health centres
(o) Attenders at women's health centres
(p) Attenders at pharmacies.

The meetings were led by trained facilitators and videotaped.

The videotapes were transcribed and the transcripts subjected to various qualitative and quantitative analyses including protocol analysis and thematic analysis using computer packages such as NUDIST. These analyses yielded the required dimensions of consumer knowledge and opinion which form the basis for the second phase of the research program.

Key questions addressed in the focus groups covered the informants knowledge of the health system and the options available, their attitudes to, and evaluation of, the available options and their decision-making strategies (including the role of the lay referral and treatment system). A detailed coverage of the focus group methodology used is published elsewhere (Thomas et al 1992).

Preliminary results

I examine the lived and embodied experience of a group of women who attend a women's health centre and their assessment of the role they enter as 'patients' or clients of various health systems.

In contrast to the women informants in mixed focus groups who discussed their partner's or children's health status rather than their own, the informants from the women's health centre were far from reticent about discussing their own health issues.

I examined the decision-making processes that these women went through and looked at the kind of agency that they felt they exercised over entering the patient role whether it be to chiropractors, general practitioners, crystal therapists or counsellors.

There were eight women aged between 24 and 55 years. Three had Greek ancestry, four were physically disabled and all had experienced extensive contact with a variety of health providers and health systems.

The women had an enormous amount of knowledge of health systems. They knew the ins and outs of the allopathic medical system and most had a detailed knowledge and at least some first hand experience of a wide range of alternative or complementary healers including traditional healers from non-western countries. They prepared a social definition of health which went well beyond a medical model. They referred to community support, prevention and health as being more than just illness and sickness. One informant argued that literature and philosophy should be taught to health professionals to engender a more humane approach in the health professions. Several informants rejected the mind/body dualism in conceptions of health arguing that mind and body are inextricably entwined in all health issues. All informants emphasized the important role of self diagnosis and self treatment. Some used cross cultural examples to promote the idea of holistic healing. One informant argued that her experience of witchdoctors in New Guinea was that, for many illnesses, they were more effective than western style healers.

The individualistic notion of health as being about lifestyle, self management and coping was prevalent in the discussion. The word 'coping' cropped up regularly. However some informants were critical of such a stance arguing for a more structural model of health which took account of poverty, class, gender issues, education and nutrition policy. All members of the group agreed on the need to incorporate alternative practitioners into an expanded definition of health care.

Informants were clear about the point at which self care was no longer adequate and outside help was needed.

> Mary: I lost all colour vision in my left eye...
> Clara: It all depends on the level of pain...
> Pam: and the type of condition...

Most tried self care first.

> Sally: I try to ease the pain myself...I try massage and maybe pain killers...I personally would not go to the doctors unless I had some regular test for example diabetes...but for a cold...I would never go...I dread the idea of seeing a doctor unless...I have a broken bone...mostly I try to prevent illness.

Others were more pragmatic ('Depends on how close you are living to a public hospital') or went to doctors as a last resort: 'desperation sends you to the doctor' given that waiting times and lack of transport were prohibitive in attending outpatients departments at public hospitals. Most saw doctors and hospitals as 'insurance' or a 'safety net'. Kath: 'It is comforting to know in the back of your head that you are close to the children's hospital even though I never used it'. However a couple of informants were critical of the process of communicating diagnosis and prognosis that they had experienced. It had taken over seven years from the onset of symptoms for a positive diagnosis of MS for Mary.

> Mary: I just got so frustrated with the medical profession that I thought I might as well have a bash at alternative medicine...The doctor said I should go to a psychiatrist and I said 'all right'. I had not lost total faith in myself and I called him a few F and C's but the next three months I kept on having symptoms...that 99.9% doctor (he had said he was 99.9% sure that she did not have MS) started ringing me and told me to see another specialist...
> Chilla: I am really terrified of the medical profession...there is no trust there...how men got to be nurturers in such a profession I don't know, it is only the science part that men come in on...

Analysis of the informants discussions indicate that economic factors are central to decision-making about use of health care services and which services to use. Kath: 'I would like to use more alternative medicine but that doesn't cater for people on low incomes'. Mary:' It is hard when you go to the doctor and you are chronic with arthritis and the doctor says...I think you need physiotherapy and you don't go along because you can't afford it'. However individuals exercise a great deal of ingenuity in overcoming economic restraints on their choices. As noted above, all of health consumers interviewed in this focus group had knowledge about alternative health providers, for example acupuncturists and naturopaths, and many assessed these services favourably, but did not use such services because of the non-refundability of fees under current health insurance arrangements. However, some of the informants found their way around this problem by seeking out medical practitioners who use unorthodox methods of healing under the medical insurance arrangements.

Sally: I have a doctor who has gone above the ordinary doctor's degree to learn acupuncture and homeopathy...I go in as an ordinary doctor's patient and he will charge me as an ordinary doctor but he will do all the unusual things.

The concept of the relationship between their bodies and their selves was an overriding, and unsolicited, theme in the focus group discussion. The concept of knowledge about their own bodies and the ability to deal with their own bodies when they 'turned nasty' was central. Given hypothetical injury scenarios, all informants suggested that they would do everything in their power to deal with the situation themselves. In answer to the scenario of a hot fat burn on the leg producing a blister the size of a cup, none of the informants mentioned attending a GP clinic.(Lyn: 'I wouldn't dream of ringing the doctor up'.) The most outside help that was proposed was a visit to the local pharmacy for burn ointment or antiseptic cream. The scenario of paralysis after falling out of a tree was met with suggestions of first aid administered by lay persons followed by medical intervention.

The importance of self-knowledge and self-care was expressed in the following way.

Lyn: Doctors quite often don't really give you credit for actually knowing things about your own health, which is absolutely ridiculous because you live with yourself all your life, you live within your body.

The fragility of the relationship of the body to self-image was expressed by Sally who told of how her positive self image was destroyed by illness.

Sally: Prior to getting sick I thought of myself as reasonably healthy, and no one could tell me what was wrong with me. I just kept going to all these doctors and after a while my whole perception of my own health changed and I have never been able to regain that sort of confidence about being healthy or being able to be healthy...that sort of way of treating people can be really damaging.

Most members of the focus group claimed that they used friends as referral sources for health practitioners. Few acted consumeristically by shopping around for services. In many cases the reluctance to shop around reflected a resistance to having to repeat life and medical histories to a chain of different practitioners. However the informants claimed that they did not accept the practitioner's word as gospel.

Clara: Any diagnosis, I always question it...I certainly wouldn't take his word as law. I have learnt not to do that. I will go somewhere else if I feel a little bit dissatisfied.

The focus group decided that women make the best doctors because they listen and seem to understand. They wanted to be listened to, not prescribed to. Sue argued that what differentiated a good from a bad consultation was:

Sue: Information that I can understand. I don't want some bullshit fed to me that I know is wrong, and when I try to question it, I get talked down to...I need to have other areas of my life explored...get feedback information...be allowed to ask questions and get answers back that I understand.

There was strong criticism of doctors as 'representatives of pharmaceutical companies'.

The focus group reached consensus on the ideal type of health service as a multidisciplinary centre with a mix of mainstream and alternative services. They suggested that the cost of services be uniform and alternative therapy charges be eligible for Medicare refundability.

Conclusion

What emerges from the focus group analysis is that these women had an enormous amount of knowledge about the mainstream health system, the alternative services that are available and about caring for their own bodies. They only used outside professional services when absolutely necessary and when their self-healing repertoire did not extend to a particular condition. They did act 'consumeristically' in questioning their health practitioners' advice but argued that the prohibitive effects of cost and non-refundability limited their use of alternative health paradigms. They tended to use lay referral systems in choosing practitioners. Their assessment of practitioners included criticisms of lack of communication skills on the part of practitioners, the prohibitive effects of cost and their gate keeping role. These findings are in line with those of other research conducted on consumer satisfaction (for example Consumers' Health Forum 1992a, 1992b, van der Heide 1992). We need to look at these responses within the context of changes in health provisions for women.

The politico-socioeconomic context for women's health is never static. The Proudfoot saga in the Australian Capital Territory (Ch. 28) (Broom 1992), the actual and potential closure of women's health care centres around Australia and the general backlash which exists against affirmative action, equal opportunity policy and special services for women makes it crucial to conduct research on women's specific health needs. Research continues to show that although women live on average five to eight years longer than men, they have more reported illness (Australian Institute of Health and Welfare 1992). While women win on mortality, they lose on morbidity. Women use health services of all kinds more than men and therefore are in a position to judge the comparative effectiveness and user-friendliness of various services. Women are thus a key source of knowledge concerning consumer evaluation of health services.

Women as gendered subjects undoubtedly bring different experiences to the health arena from men as gendered subjects. Women are articulated by class, ethnicity, race, age, geographical location and disability/ability status. They therefore come to the health system with a complex arrangement of subject positions. The literature suggests that women are conceived of as inherently and potentially 'sick' (perhaps even neurotic) in comparison to men. Thus women are seen as consumers of health services, men as providers (Broom 1989). Their bodies are seen as having the potential to 'turn nasty' on them. This is seen as one of the disadvantages of inhering in nature rather than in culture (Martin 1987). However, as the above analysis suggests, women are not necessarily passive consumers. They do not only inhabit the natural world, the environment, along with 'disease'. They act as powerful embodied agents whose bodies have potential as well as limitations (Foucault 1980). The historical process of delegitimizing women's healing powers (Weedon 1987) has not been complete. Women still retain a reservoir of knowledge about self-healing which is often overlooked in research on utilization of health resources. Australian research on the amount of lay healing and treatment which occurs in the home and in informal healing networks is underdeveloped. Compendia of home remedies are often tacked on to recipe books or treated as quaint historical curios rather than as part of the data base of health practices in Australia.

To provide legitimation to the knowledge that women have of their own bodies and of their healing potential would be to undermine the current epistemological basis of what passes for health knowledge. The consumer revolt against allopathic health services is being led by women. In many ways women are acting as discerning consumers of health services. Rather than handing their bodies over to health professionals, they are deciding which ailments are appropriately addressed by self care and home remedies, which by alternative therapists and which by mainstream scientific medicine. To this extent women health consumers are abiding by the complementary framework of health services outlined by Willis (1989). In this process it could be argued that women health consumers are taking enormous risks by engaging in pre-diagnosis. However my research suggests that the risks taken are very much informed risks.

A problem arises in translating women's unique approaches to the consumption of health care into policy. It is hard enough to translate consumer perspectives generally into concrete policy proposals, although such a task has been done admirably in recent years in Australia (Broom 1991, Consumers Health Forum 1992a, 1992b).

Assumptions about health as yet another market may mask the extent to which demand from health professionals themselves and senior bureaucrats, rather than demand from consumers, influence the supply of health services (both quantity and type of services). This may be true not only of traditional forms of clinical medicine but also of 'new' public health (see Baum 1990).

It has been argued that in the next ten years in Australia we may witness a serious 'over-supply of health-care providers leading to a lot of provider-generated demand' (Considine et al 1991). The supply of medical practitioners may be only minimally affected by consumer demand.

In contrast to the arguments put forward by Lloyd et al (1991), Smith (1991) argues that there are advantages in viewing health as a commodity market:

Health care is a product offered like any other commodity or service and the wise consumer will shop around, demand comprehensive information, check the credentials of the provider, discuss the service with other women and expect to be treated with dignity and privacy. (Smith 1991:16)

The question arises as to whether this potential for consumeristic behaviour is being realized among all groups of health service users. If not, why not?

REFERENCES

Arney W R, Bergen B J 1983 The anomaly, the chronic patient and the play of medical power. Sociology of Health and Illness 5(1)1–24

Arrow K J 1963 Uncertainty and the welfare economics of medical care. American Economic Review 53(5):941–73

Australian Institute of Health & Welfare 1992 Australia's health 1992. AGPS, Canberra

Baum F 1990 The new public health: force for change or reaction. Health Promotion International 5(2):145–50

Baum F 1992 Deconstructing the qualitative-quantitative divide in health research. Methodological Issues in Qualitative Health Research Conference, 27th November, 1992, Deakin University, Geelong

Beck U 1992 Risk society. Sage, London

Briscoe M E 1987 Why do people go to the doctor? sex differences in the correlates of GP consultation. Social Science and Medicine 25(5):507–513

Broom D 1989 Masculine medicine, feminine illness: gender and health. In: Lupton G, Najman J (eds) Sociology of health and illness: Australian readings. Macmillan, Melbourne

Broom D 1991 Speaking for themselves: consumer issues in the restructuring of general practice. National Centre for Epidemiology and Population Health, Canberra

Broom D 1992 Adding insult to injury: the discrimination case against women's health centres. Refractory Girl April: 62–65

Bryman A 1984 The debate about quantitative and qualitative research: a question of method or epistemology? British Journal of Sociology XXXV(1) March: 75–92

Calnan M 1988 Towards a conceptual framework of lay evaluation of health care. Social Science and Medicine 27(9):927–33

City of South Barwon 1993 A profile of wellbeing 1993–1995: municipal public health plan. City of South Barwon, Geelong

Clark J A, Potter D A, McKinlay J B 1991 Bringing social structure back into clinical decision-making. Social Science and Medicine 32(8):853–866

Commonwealth of Australia 1991 Health care in Australia: directions for reform in the 1991–92 budget, budget related paper no. 9. AGPS, Canberra

Considine M 1991 Health care under siege. The Age (28 Nov 1991):11

Consumers' Health Forum of Australia 1992a Consumer perspectives on general practice restructuring. CHF, Canberra

Consumers' Health Forum of Australia 1992b Consumer views on reforming general practice. CHF, Canberra

Denzin N K 1978 The research act: a theoretical introduction to sociological methods. McGraw Hill, New York

Eckermann E 1993 Researching women's health. In: Colquhoun D, Kellehear A (eds.) Health research: political, ethical & methodological issues. Chapman & Hall, London

Eisenberg J M 1979 Sociologic influences on decision-making by clinicians. Annals of Internal Medicine 90:957–64

Evans R 1984 Strained mercy: the economics of Canadian health care. Butterworth, Toronto

Foucault M 1980 (ed. C. Gordon) Power/knowledge. Harvester, London

Friedman D, Hechter M 1988 The contribution of rational choice theory to macrosociological research. Sociological Theory 6:201–18

Giddens A 1984 The constitution of society: outline of the theory of structuration. Polity Press, Cambridge

Giddens A 1991 Modernity and self-identity: self and society in the late modern age. Stanford University Press, California

Giddens A 1992 Transformation of intimacy. Polity Press, Cambridge

Greene J Y, Weinberger M, Mamlin J J 1980 Patient attitudes towards health care: expectations of primary care in a clinic setting. Social Science and Medicine 14A:133–38

Koos E 1954 The health of Regionville. Columbia University Press, New York

Lindenberg S 1985 An assessment of the new political economy: its potential for the social sciences and sociology in particular. Sociological Theory 3:99–114

Lloyd P, Lupton D, Donaldson C 1991 Consumerism in the health care setting: an exploratory study of factors underlying the selection and evaluation of primary medical services. Australian Journal of Public Health 15(3):194–201

McGuire A, Henderson J, Mooney G 1988 The economics of health care: an introductory text. Croom Helm, London

Martin E 1987 The woman in the body: a cultural analysis of reproduction. Open University Press, Milton Keynes

National Centre for Epidemiology and Population Health 1992 Improving Australia's health: the role of primary health care, final report. National Centre for Epidemiology and Population Health, The Australian National University, Canberra

National Health Strategy 1992 The future of general practice, issues paper no.2. Treble Press, Australia

Oakley A 1988 Interviewing women: a contradiction in terms. In: Roberts H (ed) Doing feminist research. Routledge, London

Palmer G, Short S 1989 Health care and public policy. Macmillan, Melbourne

Parsons T 1951 The social system. Free Press, Glencoe

Pescosolido B A 1992 Beyond rational choice: the social dynamics of how people seek help. American Journal of Sociology 97(4) January: 1096–1138

Relman A 1993 The health report (interview). Australian Broadcasting Corporation Radio National 1 February

Sax S 1990 Health care choices and the public purse. Allen & Unwin, Sydney

Silverman D 1987 Communication and medical practice: social relations in the clinic. Sage, London

Smith A 1991 Women, consumer power and the health care system: rocking the cradle is fine, just don't rock the boat. In: Smith A (ed) Women's health in Australia. University of New England Press, Armidale NSW

Stewart D, Sullivan T 1982 Illness behaviour and the sick role in chronic illness. Social Science and Medicine 16

Thomas S, Steven I D, Browning C, Dickens E, Eckermann E, Carey L, Pollard S 1992 Focus groups in health research: a methodological review. Annual Review of Health Social Sciences 2:7–20

Turner B S 1987 Medical power & social knowledge. Sage, London

Turner B S 1992 Regulating bodies: essays in medical sociology. Routledge, London

Van der Heide G 1992 What consumers want from general practitioners: a consumers' voice in health policy development. Paper to The Australian Sociological Association Conference, University of South Australia, Adelaide, Dec 1992

Weedon C 1987 Feminist practice and poststructuralist theory. Basil Blackwell, Oxford

Weisman C S, Teitelbaum M A 1985 Physician gender and the physician-patient relationship: recent evidence and relevant questions. Social Science and Medicine 20(11):1119–1127

Willis D P (ed) 1988 The changing character of the medical profession. The Milbank Quarterly 66(2)

Willis E 1989 Complementary healers. In: Lupton G, Najman J (eds) Sociology of health and illness: Australian readings. Macmillan, Melbourne

Willis E 1993 The medical profession in Australia. In: Hafferty F, McKinlay J (eds) The changing character of the medical profession : an international perspective. Oxford University Press, New York

World Health Organization 1978 Alma Ata 1978: primary health care: report of the international conference on primary health care. WHO, Geneva

Wright P, Treacher A (eds) 1983 The problem of medical knowledge. Raven Press, New York

21. Caveat emptor and pain: acupuncturists and chiropractors

Arthur O'Neill

> The Artist too express'd the solemn State
> Of grave *Physicians* at a Consult met;
> About each Symptom how they disagree,
> But how unanimous in case of Fee.
> Whilst each *Assassion* his learn'd Colleague tires
> With learn'd Impertinence, the Sick expires.
>
> *The Dispensary,* Sir Samuel Garth (1699)

The medical establishment is unforgiving of those who presume to heal without its blessing. Alternative practitioners are denounced, even as they obtain popular endorsement. They must be put beyond the pale, so the argument goes, because they rely on exclusive dogmas, are unscientific and pose a danger to their clients. This is the line taken by the National Health and Medical Research Council (NH&MRC) in its reports on acupuncture (1988b, 1989) and by the Australian Medical Association (AMA) in its 1992 position paper on chiropractic.

On the other hand, alternative healers express indignation at being unfairly criticized; denied the recognition that is their due; opposed on specious grounds; and blocked by restrictive practices such as closed referral systems, disbarment from hospitals, and limitations on patient access to public health insurance reimbursement benefits for alternative medical services. They often look to establishment motives and purposes in order to explain their stigmatization: the likes of registered medical practitioners and physiotherapists are said to mount exclusionary campaigns because the alternatives threaten their interests. Or repudiation is interpreted as a failure to appreciate the significance of therapies that are not so much alternatives to the usual prescriptions as marked improvements on them. In which case, alternative practitioners associate themselves with a medical change project and accept their isolation as the usual lot of reformers. A chiropractor tells his colleagues:

> The pattern of [registered medical practitioner] criticism is invariably the same: condemnation of the procedures for their potential risk; challenging our clinical competence to detect (diagnose) underlying pathology which may require more aggressive intervention; attempting to refute any relationship between the reduction of symptoms and the therapy, often dismissing the therapeutic effect as being only 'placebo effect'. (Wood 1988:6)

Alternative practitioners are made into antagonists because the peculiar character of orthodoxy is that it admits of no exceptions. Acupuncture and spinal manipulation have been taken up by many conventional practitioners, but far from leading to convivial relations with traditional Chinese acupuncturists and chiropractors, the new users claim exclusive procedural rights. They say the public need not patronize unsafe and unscientific alternative practitioners because the services in question are available in the ordinary course—a proposition that is also found in the NH&MRC reports on acupuncture (1988b, 1989) and the AMA diatribe on chiropractic (1992). Hence, the exponents of alternative medicines are further distanced by their very success. Segregation is a policy that grows out of the incapacity of the privileged to extirpate their opponents.

Fuel is added to the fire of occupational dispute when alternative practitioners claim good results in dealing with conditions that are ordinarily defined as chronic and intractable (typifications which convert an inability to deal comprehensively with them into characteristics of the ailments themselves). All healers are challenged by pain; it is an amorphous misery, an untenanted category, that nevertheless offers expropriative prospects for all those who settle their causes on it. If orthodox practitioners fail in their curative attempts then they frequently assume that anything else on offer must be fraudulent. In addition, the legitimacy of the pain, or its intensity, is questioned.

The quotations used in this chapter do not relay the entirety of alternative and conventional practitioner opinions about pain (there are profound member differences within as well as between occupations) but they are indicative of shared assumptions and tendencies on either side of the alternative-conventional medical divide. Overall, my aim is to demonstrate that occupational insufficiencies are exposed by the treatment of pain; that the 'problem' frequently gets transferred off practitioners and onto patients (who are held to be at least partly accountable for their chronicity because of inherent failings); and that pain gives rise to treatment inequities and antagonistic occupational relations precisely because its sources and meanings are so often obscure.

The inequality of persistent pain

What is to be made of pain? Any description is insignificant beside the experience itself. Physical pain is an assault on consciousness, an overshadowing of existence. It demands to be understood and alleviated.

Medicine works a transformation in dealing with the subject. Pain ceases to be an existential state and becomes an appearance to be construed. It is 'by any definition a symptom of disease' says Patrick Wall (1986:1). Therefore to kill the pain is to do away with the clue. The job of medicine is to treat causes rather than symptoms of disease:

Indeed, medical students are taught that treatment of symptoms such as pain might make it difficult, if not impossible to arrive at accurate diagnosis. As a result, doctors have become reluctant to treat pain for fear that they might be regarded as practising inadequate or unscientific medicine (NH&MRC 1988a:33).

Pain does not easily reveal its diagnostic meaning. To translate feelings into data, this indicator of pathology is classified by duration, fluctuation, frequency, intensity and site; and it is verbalized, visualized and rated. Nevertheless, pain is as elusive for investigators as it is immediate for sufferers. The use of scales and instruments in order to quantify pain—so characteristic of scientific endeavour—leads to a fundamental misconception. Researchers like Tursky (1976) paint themselves into a corner by distinguishing pain from the response to it; by further dividing the experience into sensory or perceptual and psychological or reactive components; and by supposing that these can be specified accurately and consistently. He sets up a measurement scheme:

> The intensity scale is defined as a measure of *how much the pain hurts* in units of intensity, the reactive scale is defined as a measure of *how the pain feels* in units of reaction, and the sensory scale is defined as a measure of *what the pain feels like* in units of sensation (Tursky 1976: 215).

Relative scale values are then taken to be the thing itself. Subject responses to verbal descriptors of intensity, reaction and sensation become dimensions of pain. As it were, questionnaires are used to centrifuge the essence of pain out of sufferers. Pain is then robbed of its intimacy by the presumption that there is an object corresponding to the sensation. We are in pain but the presence of something with quantifiable features—of an independent entity—seems to be certified by our way of talking about pain.

However, there is a world of a difference between references to something like a tree and references to a sensation like pain. In the former case, an object is held to exist outside ourselves; in the latter, feeling is all. As Wittgenstein remarks, 'if we construe the grammar of the expression of sensation on the model of 'object and designation' the object drops out of consideration as irrelevant'; for 'You learned the *concept* 'pain' when you learned the language' (1958: §§ 293, 384). Uncovering mechanisms of neurological action is one thing but a semiology of pain is far from being attained.

So is effective treatment. Even though their complaints of pain are vivid, many patients are run through all the tests without any organic pathology being discovered. The very success of medicine in other spheres then creates its own strain:

> The doctor sees his role as the curer of disease and 'forgets' his role as a healer of the sick, and patients wander disabled but without a culturally acceptable mantle of disease with which to clothe the nakedness of their pain (Cassell 1978: 44).

One might block the sensation with pain killers but that is to give up on the assumption that pain is a diagnostic sign and on the brief to uncover its meaning as a preliminary to treatment. But what else to do 'if pain persists'?

The significance of pain sensations may be questioned, on the ground that they cannot be taken to represent interior conditions accurately. According to Bakan (1975: 197), 'the attempt to come to an understanding of pain is characteristically met at the doorway by the materialist objection that subjective states can, at best, be allowed only a secondary status in the realm of scientific reality'. In this case the status of chronic pain—its evidentiary rank—is diminished because it has to do with the self rather than with the medical object. Pain is not explained but spirited away—made into an epiphenomenon—on this reckoning.

Another course is to send patients on to someone more expert at discovery. Which can lead to a downward spiral of referrals. Wall notes that:

> The patient whose problems extend beyond the expertise of one specialty or even worse whose problems fail to respond to the therapy of the first specialist *has* a severe problem and *is* a severe problem. The historical development of the specialties established a hierarchy of power and preference for which specialist had first access. The hierarchy ran from the 'action men' on top down through medicine to symptomatic physiotherapy and the nearly taboo fields of psychiatry and psychology with the nurses and social workers out of sight. The sad sight of the all too common failed patients slipping down the hierarchy with thickening file and growing distress led to a reaction. The grand old tradition of the self-sufficient individual doctor trained and supported by his specialist colleagues has been a powerful factor in medical advance but has its limits and nowhere so obviously as with intractable pain patients (Wall 1986:1-2).

His answer is to reorganize medicine, for the treatment of pain is a co-operative undertaking 'with respect for the contribution of many experts and with the possibility of combined therapies and the need for a new forum to discuss the new approach' (1986:2).

Bakan (1975) provides another answer by concentrating on features of the doctor-patient exchange. He distinguishes pain sensations from sufferer interpretations of them and suggests that there is a voluntary pain response system (i.e. a means of choosing actions to handle the experience of pain). Anxiety is defined as a species of psychic pain that results from confronting the problem of dealing with the sensation (as it were, anxiety adds to the pain). Then Bakan suggests that alleviation of the original pain can result when the patient reduces anxiety by permitting a shift in control of it to a healer. This occurs because 'transfer of the volitionary function to others also allows the person in pain to suspend his own volitionary processes'. In reverse, a failure to yield control turns into a major factor associated with persistent pathological pain (because of 'the inability of the individual to allow sufficiently the transfer to others of the management of his condition'). Pain is a reminder to keep up the search for assistance:

> I would suggest, for example, that, in cases of intractable pain, where the physician cannot find any 'cause' for the pain, that the very information that the physician cannot find the cause of the pain may itself be part of the dynamic. The existence of the pain operates as a continuing prod to the volitional processes of

the patient to continue, at the very least, in his hunt for someone who is wise enough to help him, someone who yet might provide the adequate safety and therapeutic measures (Bakan 1975:205).

The trouble with this and many other theories is that the 'problem' of pain is shifted off those who presume to treat it and onto those who have the misfortune to experience it. Sufferers are caught coming and going by circular explanations that relate their pain to an excess or a deficiency. In providing a typification of the behaviourist school of thought on pain, Vrancken says:

> A *pain patient* is characterized as one who has some interest in complaining about pain and/or whose coping strategies have failed. The pain may give him an identity, or he may avoid situations which are cognitively linked to pain. A patient who has a weak back might have spared his back too much, instead of doing exercises to strengthen it. Conversely, a patient may be too active, thereby overloading a painful part of the body. The 'typical' pain patient shows advanced somatic fixation, has a longstanding medical history (doctor shopping) and uses a lot of analgesics. He is 'caught in the web of chronic pain', as one physician formulated it (Vrancken 1989:437).

So pain patients are their own worst enemies:

> As pain persists, pain behaviours and emotions associated with the experience of pain are likely to reinforce the notion of illness and the sick role, thus inhibiting coping and reducing the probability of effective treatment (Edwards et al 1992:268).

These representations frequently give the impression that therapists rate their patients against a presumptive stoicism and blame them for complaining about their pain. One of the authors of the NH&MRC reports on acupuncture relays such a heroic comprehension of pain:

> Acupuncture is said to be useful in anaesthesia. People having operations under acupuncture—why have expensive anaesthetists, why have big operating theatres with gas machines? If you were brave enough, and if I coached you for a short while, most of the operations that you need to have done can be done without any anaesthetic. I have myself operated on patients, deep into their bodies, where the anaesthetic was only in the skin. It's the skin that hurts—the muscles don't hurt. You can probe around the muscles and the patient won't know what's going on.
>
> You can move the viscera of the abdomen around; they don't hurt. It just looks ugly and dramatic when there's guts spewing out all over the Technicolour screen. There's drama but it doesn't hurt.
>
> You can do operations with minimal analgesic, and indeed it's not as if it's mystical and only the acupuncturist can do it...
>
> If you are gutsy and can grit your teeth, then you can go through most of these procedures without suffering pain, it's just that we're not accustomed to doing so. You're all a bunch of sooks! But if we had to—if we ran out of halothane, if we ran out of drugs—we could go back to it, for it was done that way in the past (Bogduk 1988:26).

And pain sufferers may exaggerate their pain for ulterior purposes:

> Chronic pain patients, almost by definition, usually show more disability than would seem reasonable for the amount of physical damage that can be detected. However, this seems especially true in the case of patients with head and neck pain, particularly when this pain is produced by 'whiplash' (hyperflexion-

hyperextension) injuries. Historically, this seemingly excessive disability has been ascribed to secondary gain, litigation-seeking, or frank malingering (Schwartz 1988:24).

Motives of the sort continue to be imputed to whiplash victims, by Awerbuch (1992), for example, and by some of the other contributors to a subsequent 'Letters to the Editor' debate in *The Medical Journal of Australia*. They put chronicity down to 'abnormal illness behaviour', relating it to psychological tension, medical prophecies of long-term disability—the placebo effect in reverse!—and prospective compensatory gain:

> My own conclusion following these events [a reduction of Victorian whiplash injury claims from 8000 in 1985 to 800 in 1992 allegedly brought about by legislative change] is that the majority of chronic whiplash sufferers are created by the system of compensation and that health care providers both contribute to and perpetuate their disabilities by providing constant treatment, admonitions to rest, and certification of continued inability to resume work (Kinloch 1993:71).

The error here is to suppose that a satisfactory psychological explanation of pain chronicity is enabled by a failure to discover organic pain foundations. In fact, the question of pain origin is left quite open by the absence of physical signs because 'the test of requiring actual positive evidence of such causative psychological factors is not met' (Degood 1988:2).

Other sources of care

So much for interpreters of chronic pain who point a finger at the secret knavery of the psyche. But there are people wanting relief. With great frequency they do not wait on medical reform or mental reckonings but go elsewhere for assistance—particularly to chiropractors, osteopaths, naturopaths and traditional acupuncturists—and (to the chagrin of those who have failed them) cures are announced.

Many alternative practitioners not only believe what their patients say but also endorse patient beliefs about pain having a meaning. Rather than attempting to uncover lateral significance and patient shortcomings, pain is taken seriously. Pain is telling you something about bodily malfunction; it has a real source; you are right to complain of it; something can be done about it:

> Pain is your body's *fire alarm*; turning the alarm off with a pain-killer will not put out the fire. Feeling unwell, pain and other symptoms will usually alert the women to a problem long before blood and urine tests or x-rays show that anything is wrong. The pain is *not* in your imagination!
>
> Chiropractors, Osteopaths and Naturopaths excel in the management of women's health problems. Firstly because their procedures enable them to detect problems at a very early stage; and second because the therapy silences the alarm (pain) by extinguishing the fire—without unpleasant side-effects (Wood 1990:21).

In addition, pain is not taken in isolation. Alternative practitioners represent themselves as offering an holistic approach to treatment and as using only natural methods. The patient has a full identity:

In traditional Chinese medicine finding out how the human organism functions means taking into account the physiological, emotional and mental activities of the entire person, all of which are constantly changing in response to internal and external influences.

While specifically treating both the cause and symptoms of illness, the emphasis is on the treatment of the whole person. This ensures that the patient does not become of secondary importance to the condition with which they present (Godel not dated).

Treatment is encompassing; at the same time, normal functioning is promoted: 'Physiological, emotional and mental activities are regulated [by acupuncture], and the body's own defensive system is strengthened' (Godel not dated).

Pain, then, is a point of divergence. Members of healing groups can be distinguished (and distinguish themselves) by the understandings they relay about it and the treatments they offer for its relief. Organizational and therapeutic features of the occupations concerned are indicated by failures and successes in dealing with pain. What counts in establishing alternative medical reputability, so many practitioners believe, is their ability to benefit the 'rejects' who end up with them—the cases whose former intractability is a proof of orthodox insufficiency.

The situation is quite opposite in the established medical estimation. What counts against the alternatives is their leaping in where conventional doctors fear to tread:

Practitioners on the fringe, such as herbalists and the like, love such disorders [chronic fatigue syndrome or 'yuppie flu']; badly treated by doctors, no single cause identifiable, no data on treatment and exacerbations and remissions provide the perfect scenario for alternative medicine ('Retractor' 1992:82).

The conventional wisdom is that patients are not 'rescued' by alternative practitioners after unsuccessfully searching for orthodox cures but are further let down. Besides, the victim-blaming presumption is that they must have something wrong with them to start with (labelled as 'pre-morbid personality, anxiety hypochondriasis') in order to become paid up participants in the chronic pain cycle (see Fig. 21.1).

Nevertheless, the failure cannot be manifest to patients since interest in medical alternatives and patronage of alternative practitioners has considerably increased. (See Leibrich et al (1987) for a New Zealand review; and Social Development Committee (1986) for surveys of Victorian usage. Hill (1987:125) comments that in the search for alternative meaning systems, New Zealanders have not rejected their simple materialism and pursuit of health and possessions in favour of thoughts of salvation, 'but have merely sought health and well-being of a more esoteric and individualistically attuned kind'.)

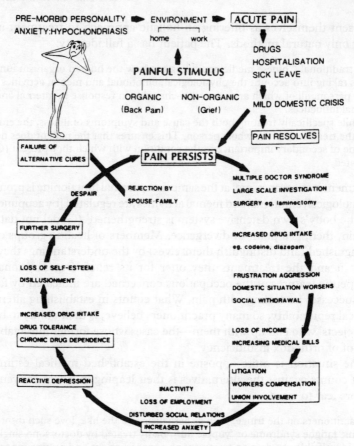

Fig. 21.1 The chronic pain cycle.
Reproduced from *Analgesic Guidelines* (Victorian Drug Usage Committee 1992) with
permission from the Department of Health and Community Services, Victoria.

Stemming the tide: chiropractic

The flight of patients to alternative healers is a standing challenge to
conventional practitioners. It is met by denigrating alternative medical
theories and practices; by casting doubt on reports of successes; and by
concurrently adopting popular alternative therapies like spinal manipulation
which now is in near universal use by physiotherapists and also has a large
regular medical following.

Therapeutic success does not lead to recognition for alternative
practitioners. The policy has been to deny medical interactions:

> The Australian Medical Association is of the opinion that medical practitioners
> may not act in consultation with, associate professionally with, conduct investiga-
> tions for, or refer patients to chiropractors or osteopaths (Australian Medical
> Association 1965:127).

There have been similar prohibitions in the United States — now legally overturned as a result of a successful antitrust suit mounted by five chiropractors (see Gevitz 1989, Wardwell 1992:168-178); and in New Zealand, where a government investigation reported that 'the opposition of the New Zealand medical establishment to chiropractic is, for all practical purposes, intense and absolute' (Commission of Inquiry into Chiropractic 1979:119).

Tolerant regular practitioners are perhaps now more easily found but the official position is little changed:

The AMA maintains that a medical practitioner should at all times practise methods of treatment based on sound scientific principles, and accordingly does not recognise any exclusive dogma such as homoeopathy, osteopathy, chiropractic or naturopathy (Australian Medical Association 1992:3).

Though they must complete five year qualifying courses of university education and have to be registered to practise, according to the AMA:

Australian chiropractors seek publicity for the benefits they claim to provide by their treatment of patients suffering low back pain, but avoid public acknowledgment of certain of their other claims (to treat organic illness by spinal manipulation). The AMA considers that this apparent coyness arises from chiropractors' recognition that such claims detract from their otherwise carefully nurtured political credibility. Practitioners of and apologists for chiropractic are equally reluctant to discuss the dangers and inappropriate uses of their techniques. The Australian Medical Association rejects chiropractic's self-seeking publicity and demands that its claims should be subjected to independent scrutiny (Australian Medical Association 1992:2).

Additionally, chiropractors are accused of engaging in misleading practices in the course of their public relations activities:

The first misrepresentation employed by chiropractors involves comparison of the treatment of back pain by spinal manipulation with its treatment by other means. Doctors and physiotherapists who use spinal manipulation similarly report that the results of their manual treatment of back pain can be superior to those obtained from other medical methods of management. Such trials demonstrate only the usefulness of spinal manipulation in treatment of back pain, *not* any special efficacy of chiropractic.

In the AMA's view, physiotherapists or physical medicine practitioners might easily provide equally effective treatment of back pain and would be likely to do so more safely than chiropractors. In this context, chiropractic represents only an unnecessary duplication of existing, competent services (Australian Medical Association 1992: 5).

A rather different comparison had been made twenty-five years earlier, when some Victorian physiotherapists met to discuss chiropractic dangers. Only men attended but it was 'DEFINATELY NOT [sic] an attempt to form an all male section of the APA [Australian Physiotherapy Association]. Any constructive thoughts coming from this evening's meeting would certainly be put to the 'girls' for their comments and recommendations' (Australian Physiotherapy Association 1967). An orthopaedic surgeon advised the chaps that physiotherapy incomes would drop by half 'if we do not take steps to advance our cause before unlicensed practitioners become registered'. He said physiotherapists had to give more attention to manipulation in order to meet this threat. One of the audience commented that 'Physiotherapists in general did not do much manipulation in their treatments despite the fact that all over the world this technique was reaching an important level'. American physiotherapists had realized this and were making efforts 'to stem the advancing tide of Chiropractors and Osteopaths'. Another attendee noted that Victorian physiotherapists were not doing their best because of a lack of knowledge and training in manipulation, 'whereas the opposition are more skilled operators'. 'However', he said, 'let us remember that the enemy can teach us a lot and we should not be slow to take advantage of this'. Some years later, an English pioneer of medical manipulation warned Australian doctors that it was idle to legislate against the 'lay' operators: 'the remedy is to render them superfluous' by replacing them with physiotherapists 'trained in hospitals [in manipulative techniques] by eminent medical men, and preserving an ethical code' (Cyriax 1973:1165).

What has happened, then, is that regular medical practitioners and physiotherapists have followed common business practice by borrowing the successful methods of their competitors in the pain market.

Stemming the tide: acupuncture

Needle acupuncture also has been taken up by physiotherapists and orthodox practitioners (together with a few chiropractors). Estimating use is difficult and is complicated by the wholesale adoption of procedural variants such as acupressure and electrical and laser stimulation of acupuncture points. An indication of popularity is given by records of reimbursed acupuncture services under the national health insurance scheme, Medicare. Some 3000 registered medical practitioners delivered 830 000 separate acupuncture services in the 1991-1992 financial year (Health Insurance Commission 1992). The vast majority of providers are in general practice, which means that 17% of GPs use acupuncture. (Based on the supposition that there are around 18 000 of them in active practice—see Committee of Inquiry into Medical Education and Medical Workforce (1988: 365-512) and National Health Strategy (1992 : 55-69) about complications in estimating numbers of doctors.) A small survey of Australian general practitioner opinions about alternative therapies found that 21% of the responding doctors had used acupuncture and another 38% said they would consider using it; the procedure was thought to be highly effective by 13% and moderately effective by 62% (Social Development Committee 1986: 214, 218). Similarly, 24% of respondents to a medical newspaper survey of reader opinions about alternative therapies believed the status of supporting scientific evidence for acupuncture was strong and another 45% believed it was moderate (Anon 1992:30–31).

The idea that acupuncture entered the general medical consciousness after it had been scientifically validated does not stand up to scrutiny. The National Health and Medical Research Council reports start with long chapters (drafted by Bogduk) on the neurophysiology of pain, which comprehend it in mechano-chemical terms and suggest that 'the abundant research that has been conducted into acupuncture analgesia strongly implicates mechanisms similar to those involved in morphine analgesia; involving the same pathways and transmitter substances as those involved in the descending nociceptive modulatory system' (NH&MRC 1988b, 1989:11). In other words, the existence of acupuncture analgesia can be allowed now because scientifically acceptable explanations have been found for its occurrence. However, those entertained by traditional acupuncturists are ruled out of court:

In the face of research developments there is no need for romantic or fanciful explanations of the basis of acupuncture analgesia. It is not necessary to invoke models involving meridians or other mystical explanations (NH&MRC 1988b, 1989:14).

Practitioners of acupuncture are similarly discriminated against. A society of registered physicians using acupuncture submitted to the NH&MRC review that 'the place of acupuncture in the management of pain is well accepted by the public and the medical profession' and that it also had a place in the treatment of disease and disability. A wide range of problems were said to respond favourably to acupuncture in the empirical experience of members of the society (Australian Medical Acupuncture Society 1987). These were listed under sub-headings, including: skin conditions, cardiovascular conditions, gastro-intestinal diseases, obstetric and gynaecological conditions, addictions, endocrine disorders, autonomic nervous system dysfunctions and genitourinary disorders. But the NH&MRC denied any acupuncture influence on organic pathology, asserting that 'Whereas neural and physiological mechanisms of acupuncture analgesia have been postulated...no such scientific rationale is available to explain a possible basis for the use of acupuncture as a primary clinical treatment for disease' (NH&MRC 1988b:51, 1989:57). In all that follows, the 'lay' and 'non-medical' practitioners of acupuncture (that is, everyone other than the conventionally qualified) are singled out for condemnation. As with the chiropractors, the effect is to represent traditional acupuncturists as ignorant, unscientific and unsafe whereas orthodox medical practitioners have all the virtues that can be endowed by clinical expertise and a proper education.

The effect of reviews

The targets of condemnation suppose a malevolent intent but the authors and authorizers of the AMA and NH&MRC papers are turned into the chicken-sexers of medicine by their occupational certitudes: they cannot help but damn the alternatives outright and unreservedly praise registered medical practitioners. They are preaching to the wrong audiences—to the medically converted and to cultists who are, axiomatically, irredeemable. The NH&MRC reports would have had a negligible public influence. A consumer information brochure was drafted but never issued. The AMA's chiropractic statement went out with its political newsletter, Australian Medicine, which is not usually stacked beside *New Idea* and *The Women's Weekly* in doctors' waiting rooms.

What, then, is the purpose of the AMA and NH&MRC documents? Perhaps to quell tendencies to 'go soft' on the alternatives by stiffening medical backbones but I doubt they are intended to keep competitors at bay and incomes up. Instead, notions of medical rectitude and quality are expressed by invoking the contrasting deficiencies of alternative theories and the dangers of alternative practitioners. Chiropractors and traditional Chinese acupuncturists are foils: the imperative is to maintain established authority, stability and unity by setting a *cordon sanitaire* about orthodox practice.

Those foolish enough to step outside it do so at their own peril. The NH&MRC's draft brochure says (capitals in the original):

> Acupuncture is a technique which CAN be helpful in relieving some forms of PAIN...If you use acupuncture, or any other form of treatment to relieve pain you should be aware that pain is a WARNING of some underlying condition. While the pain may be relieved the underlying CAUSE should not be ignored...
>
> Consumers who wish to use acupuncture for PAIN relief or management should be aware that there are NO AGREED STANDARDS of training or practice for its use and therefore NO SPECIFIC REGISTRATION of the practice of acupuncture. The RESPONSIBILITY for the use of acupuncture remains totally with the CONSUMER (NH&MRC 1988b, 1989:vii-viii).

This severe warning is followed by the customary elaboration of risks, a plug on behalf of 'reputable health professions' and another warning: 'you should be aware that it is unlikely a court of law would expect the same standard of care from an occasional acupuncturist or one with a limited training as it would from a frequent acupuncturist and/or one with medical training' (p.(viii)).

Why the onus has shifted from doctors to the recipients of medical services is explained in one of the five parts of the reports on acupuncture, entitled 'Acupuncture, politics and the health market place'. In the past:

> Health consumerism was only just evolving and health policy to a large degree was still dictated by a benign medical paternalism. Not only did the medical profession dominate health policy development, it accepted a responsibility to protect the public from alternative therapies that were unsafe or of unproven efficacy. This was expressed by prohibition (eg. banning the import of [a supposedly anti-cancer preparation called] Laetrile), by denial of financial support (denial of Medibank/Medicare rebates) and by denial of official recognition (registration) (NH&MRC 1988b:65, 1989:75).

Then medical consumer organizations entered the health policy forum and 'increasingly, they have demanded the right to have information on which individuals will make their own health choices'. Their intervention has consequences for medicine and for consumers:

Thus, in 1974 [when the NH&MRC issued its first report on acupuncture] it may have been acceptable to recommend a ban on lay acupuncture in the interests of public safety. In 1988, this is not acceptable as it is regarded as a relic of medical paternalism. In 1988, medical consumers demand information about the various alternative therapies available. Health servicing is no longer seen to be a monopoly belonging to conventional medicine. The very phrase 'health market place' was almost unthinkable two decades ago but it is now an accurate description of how people make health choices.

Having discarded medical paternalism the community is now faced with the principle of Caveat Emptor (let the buyer beware) in making health decisions and treatment choices (NH&MRC 1988b:66, 1989:76).

The possibility that consumer representation movements are founded on the existence of an unbalanced relation between doctors and patients is not allowed for on this interpretation. Rather, those who 'own' pain are free to hawk it around the market-place—a freedom that brings on attendant liabilities for consumers. What makes the explanation satisfying is the exteriorization of responsibility for any diminishment in the social place of conventional medicine *and* for the dilemmas facing patients in pain: problems of choice and any resultant burdens (of injury, even death) fall on them. It is as if the Church, having made its salvationary message plain and no longer possessing coercive powers, wipes its hands of those who pass up the offer. Why they might do so, and how it comes to be that the alternatives prosper, are questions that can safely be put aside.

Conclusion

'In what sense does my present painless state contain the possibility of pain?', asks Wittgenstein. He continues:

If anyone says: 'For the word 'pain' to have a meaning it is necessary that pain should be recognized as such when it occurs'—one can reply: 'It is no more necessary than that the absence of pain should be recognized.'
'But mustn't I know what it would be like if I were in pain?'—We fail to get away from the idea that using a sentence involves imagining something for every word (Wittgenstein 1958: §§ 448, 449).

My aim here has to been to consider several versions of the medical imagination of pain. One—often associated with conventional practice— involves finding something for the word 'pain' by attempted objectifications of it and by explaining non-organic chronicity as, essentially, a function of patient shortcomings. Another—commonly met amongst alternative practitioners—amounts to joining patients in affirmations of the reality of pain, rendering plausible explanations of it and offering confident treatment.

Since the institution of medicine is held to stand for patient interests, a common supposition is that treatment failures are a reflection on the sufferers, or on the state of knowledge, rather than on conventional practice.

It is true that 'the problems of cutaneous mechanisms in general, and pain in particular, have given rise to vituperation that is unparalleled in the biological sciences' (Melzack 1977:79). In addition to internal dispute over pain, the solidity of the established medical position is also eroded by social currents running counter to its system of authority. Against the advice of representative medical and physiotherapy associations, governments have recognized chiropractors and osteopaths by registering them and providing them with qualifying higher education. Now the same might be done for traditional acupuncturists (the offer of pre-service university courses in Melbourne and Sydney for primary contact practice having been already allowed). This most recent event reveals a critical flaw in the established medical stance. The medical argument implies that governments cause injustice not only by permitting but also by seeming to endorse practitioners whose activities are inherently dangerous. The public interest demands that they should be banned instead. Then again, public interest can be invoked to justify the opposite position: if the danger contentions are valid then why not give alternative practitioners proper training and practice regulation in order to make them safe? Chiropractic largely owes its recognition to the success of this argument and even the NH&MRC has been forced in the same direction by accepting an 'in the interests of public safety' case for approved training after yet another review which recommended higher education and registration for traditional acupuncturists (NH&MRC 1990).

Alleviating pain is a proper task for medicine. When medical groups convert a pain into a means of diminishing patients and other practitioners they do not contribute to the business of healing.

REFERENCES

Anon 1992 Alternative therapies fail to impress. Australian Dr Weekly 19 June, pp 30–31
Australian Medical Acupuncture Society 1987 Submission to the NH&MRC working party on acupuncture
Australian Medical Association 1965 Relations between the AMA and chiropractors. Australian Medical Association—The Fourth Federal Assembly. Medical Journal of Australia, Supplement 1(17):126–127
Australian Medical Association 1992 Chiropractic in Australia. AMA
Australian Physiotherapy Association 1967 Minutes: social evening held at the Royal Automobile Club of Victoria, 9 June
Awerbuch M 1992 Whiplash in Australia: illness or injury? Medical Journal of Australia 157:193–196
Bakan D 1975 Pain: the existential symptom. In: Engelhardt H T, Spicker S F (eds) Evaluation and explanation in the biomedical sciences. Reidel, Dordrecht, pp 197–207
Bogduk N 1988 Romance, magic, the dollar and truth. The Skeptic 8(2):23–26, 28
Cassell E 1978 The healer's art: a new approach to the doctor-patient relationship. Penguin, Harmondsworth
Commission of Inquiry into Chiropractic (Inglis B Chairman) 1979 Chiropractic in New Zealand. Government Printer, Wellington
Committee of Inquiry into Medical Education and Medical Workforce (Doherty R Chairman) 1988 Australian medical education and workforce in the 21st century. Australian Government Publishing Service, Canberra
Cyriax J 1973 Letter to the editor: registration of chiropractors. Medical Journal of Australia 1(23):1165

Degood D 1988 A rationale and format for psychological evaluation. In: Lynch N T, Vasudevan S (eds) Persistent pain: psychosocial assessment and intervention. Kluwer, Boston, pp 1–22

Edwards L, Pearce S, Turner-Stokes L, Jones A 1992 The pain beliefs questionnaire: an investigation of beliefs in the causes and consequences of pain. Pain 51:267–272

Garth S 1649 The dispensary, 9th edn (1725), Scholars' Facsimiles & Reprints (1975). Delmar, New York

Gevitz N 1989 The chiropractors and the AMA [American Medical Association]: reflections on the history of the consultation clause. Perspectives in Biology and Medicine 32(2):281–299

Godel D (not dated) Patient brochure: the information guide to your local natural medicine practice of acupuncture and herbal medicine. North Carlton

Health Insurance Commission 1992 Summary tables: Numbers of acupuncture providers by financial year and by State for 1990/1991 and 1991/1992; Numbers of acupuncture services by financial year and by State for 1990/1991 and 1991/1992

Hill M 1987 The cult of humanity and the secret religion of the educated classes. New Zealand Sociology 2(2):112–127

Kinloch B 1993 Letter to the editor. Medical Journal of Australia 158:70–71

Leibrich J, Hickling, Pitt G 1987 In search of well-being: exploratory research into complementary therapies, special report 76. Health Services Research and Development Unit, Department of Health, Wellington

Melzack R 1977 The gate theory revisited. In: Le Roy P, Boulos, M, Goloskov J (eds) Current concepts in the management of chronic pain. Symposia Specialists, Miami/ Stratton Intercontinental Book Corporation, New York, pp 79–92

National Health and Medical Research Council 1974 Acupuncture: a report to the National Health and Medical Research Council. Australian Government Publishing Service, Canberra

National Health and Medical Research Council 1988a Management of severe pain: report of the working party on management of severe pain. Australian Government Publishing Service, Canberra

National Health and Medical Research Council 1988b Acupuncture: report of the NH&MRC working party on acupuncture. Department of Community Services and Health, Canberra

National Health and Medical Research Council 1989 Acupuncture. Department of Community Services and Health, Canberra

National Health and Medical Research Council 1990 Report of the working party on the role and requirements for acupuncture education. Department of Community Services and Health, Canberra

National Health Strategy 1992 The future of general practice. Issues paper no 3 National Health Strategy, Canberra

Retractor 1992 An unforgettable patient with 'yuppie flu'. Australian Dr Weekly 25 September, pp 82–83

Social Development Committee, Parliament of Victoria (Dixon J Chairperson) 1986 report: inquiry into alternative medicine and the health food industry. Government Printer, Melbourne

Schwartz D 1988 Cognitive deficits. In: Lynch N T, Vasudevan S V (eds). Persistent pain: psychosocial assessment and intervention. Kluwer, Boston, pp 23–41

Tursky B 1976 The evaluation of pain responses: a need for improved measures. In: Spicker S F, Engelhardt H T (eds) Philosophical dimensions of the neuro-medical sciences. Reidel, Dordrecht, pp 209–219

Victorian Drug Usage Committee, Analgesic Guidelines Sub-Committee 1992 Analgesic guidelines, 2nd edn. Victorian Medical Postgraduate Foundation, North Melbourne

Vrancken M 1989 Schools of thought on pain. Social Science and Medicine 29:435–444

Wall P D 1986 Editorial: 25 volumes of Pain. Pain 25:1–4

Wardwell W 1992 Chiropractic. history and evolution of a new profession. Year Book. Mosby, St Louis

Wittgenstein L 1958 Philosophical investigations. Blackwell, Oxford

Wood M 1988 Letter to the editor. A.C.A [Australian Chiropractors' Association] News 15(10):6

Wood M 1990 Chiro care: every women [sic]. The Plenty Valley Town Crier, 36 (February)

PART 3

Inequalities in prevention

Introduction

Illness prevention. The term has such a strong positive connotation that it is difficult to see how it could be other than part of just health. 'Prevention' is often defined in terms of what is seen to be its opposite—cure. Hence the adage, 'prevention is better than cure'. This implies the treatment of disease which is the domain of biomedicine. However, prevention is taking on a broader meaning and is frequently used interchangeably with 'health promotion'. The chapters in this part are all centrally engaged with debates about the meaning, content and justice implications of illness prevention and of the closely related concept of health promotion.

Heightened concern with illness prevention and health promotion, both in Australia and overseas, arose in the 1980s and early 1990s and can be linked with the development of the so-called 'new public health movement'. This movement has sought changes not just in the physical environment (clean air and water, food, infection control and occupational health and safety legislation)—concerns of the 'old public health movement'—but also in those economic, political, social, and environmental conditions that are believed to augment health. During the 1980s, many government reports and World Health Organization documents argued that health advancement presupposes social justice and equity; that optimum health depends upon 'the creation of an economy, a society, and an environment conducive to good health, as distinct from disease' (Palmer & Short 1989:191). While there has been a continuing focus on the medical approach to disease prevention—preventing the occurrence of disease, or minimizing its effects—increasingly reference has been made to the potential of influencing health in the broadest sense by attention to individual lifestyles and to such larger factors as environmental pollution, the marketing and promotion of 'unhealthy' products and unsafe working conditions.

On the face of it, such a broad agenda would seem to challenge the individualistic, curative approach of medicine. It shifts the attention away from therapeutic interventions to encompass areas beyond those traditionally defined as health related, for example, housing, transport, industry, and arts. And, in rhetoric at least, it entails a greater sharing of power between different levels of government (Federal, State and local), and between government departments and private and community organisations. The catch-phrases of the new public health movement, 'community empowerment', 'healthy public policy', and 'the creation of supportive environments' certainly would seem to be pre-requisites of a more just, healthier society. But has the rhetoric been matched by reality, and is it likely to be?

The answer to these questions depends very much on one's theoretical framework, and in particular on one's assumptions about change (the desirability of change, the required areas of change, whether change should be individual or structural, and the extent and speed of change) and about how and when change should be measured. Some writers view prevention and promotion philosophies as progressive; as necessarily advancing health overall and reducing inequalities. Some see them as having contradictory effects in that they benefit some groups and not others. And others adopt a more sceptical viewpoint on the entire prevention/promotion enterprise seeing it simply as an extension of bureaucratic and expert intrusion into our everyday lives and/or as diverting attention from other, more fundamental, problems.

Many arguments centre on the question of what counts as a successful initiative when one moves away from biomedical and quantitative measures of normal health. If one accepts the prevention/promotion credos, then it makes no sense to apply conventional medical measures of success in terms of restoration to some norm of physical health. But exactly what measures should be applied? What should count as 'success'? And at what point in time can an intervention be said to be successful?

Some programs may be 'successful' by some criteria and not others. For example, health promotion programs which focus mainly on individual lifestyles may be 'successful' in changing individual behaviours but fail to change the social context within which 'unhealthy' lifestyle choices are made. They may also extract a price which outweighs their supposed benefits. It has been argued, for instance, that legislation making mandatory the wearing of bicycle helmets and random breath tests for drink drivers should not be supported because they represent severe infringements on individual rights. 'Success' is frequently little more than what politicians, bureaucrats and health promotion 'experts' define it to be, generally in terms of some quantifiable and short term outcome. The health promotion effort has been criticized on all these counts.

Like any issue, illness prevention and health promotion is subject to on-going contestation over the nature of 'truth'. And there is no single and objective standpoint from which to evaluate competing claims to truth. Different ideas are supported by different groups according to their own values, perceived interests and investments, all of which may change through time. And so it is that the following chapters reflect the debates and the diversity of viewpoints that exist within the broader prevention/promotion literature.

The authors of the first four chapters make a generally positive evaluation of the new public health.

In his overview of the contribution of the new public health to assisting those communities most affected by HIV and AIDS, Ross believes that strategies for reducing HIV transmission have by and large been 'extremely successful' (Ch. 22). A large part of this success, he believes, is attributable to the emphasis on change in the new public health: at the social, organizational, and individual levels. It has been a broad approach to health, and not one focussing on just a single factor. It is an approach which also has sought to empower the effected groups, and in this case particularly homosexually active men who are discriminated against both socially and, in some jurisdictions, legally. The problem of stigmatization of affected groups, Ross argues, should provide a major focus for change; for example, the decriminalization of homosexual behaviour between consenting adults. Where such decriminalization has occurred, this has strengthened the development of a community and community norms which is likely to support behaviours which reduce HIV transmission. Ross believes that, 'in the absence of a cure for HIV infection or AIDS, and the possibility that there will not be any cure in the foreseeable future, prevention of HIV infection is the only way of halting its spread'. But his broader message is that the new public health has placed issues of social equity and justice firmly on the health agenda.

Leonie Short and Alan Patterson's involvement in a project to reduce inequalities of oral health status leads them to believe that it is possible to create conditions for empowerment and community building in line with the new public health movement (Ch. 23). Their project was based in the Moree district of New South Wales where children, especially Aboriginal children, were known to require a particularly high level of dental treatment. It focussed, in particular, on oral health promotion strategies in infants and primary school students within the target communities. A significant outcome of this project, which the authors believe is a central tenet of the new public health, is the participation of the local community. It involved representatives of the health services, private and public dental practitioners, the local Aboriginal health services, school principals, Parents and Citizens Associations and the local Shire Council. And on this count, they believe, they have ensured 'a more widespread involvement in, and acceptance of, the programs which were implemented'. Although the project is (at the time of writing) continuing, early analysis has shown it to have been successful so far in terms of a reduction in the percentage of children urgently requiring treatment, and on a range of other criteria such as cost effectiveness and intersectoral collaboration.

Colette Browning, Hal Kendig and Karen Teshuva indicate a more qualified faith in the existing public health movement in their discussion of the health promotion of older people (Ch. 24). The scope of policy, they argue, should be extended far beyond health care to also include such things as income support, street planning and maintenance, and education influencing images of ageing. They outline some of the particular problems faced by this group, many of which arise from discrimination and lack of understanding. This is an important point to note, for discrimination against older people seems to be endemic to many western societies and provides the basis for many other problems. It can encompass a broad range of social practices, from institutional policies and activities which abuse and harm people to 'ageist' remarks which dismiss, belittle and insult them (Phillipson 1982:xi). And the dominance of medical and psychological explanations of old age which emphasize individual biological and mental changes that take place with ageing undoubtedly contributes to the strong association of old age with decay, senility and reversion to child-like behaviour (Phillipson 1982:xiii).

Discrimination may extend to health promotion programs themselves, which often fail to take into account older people's views. The importance of taking into account these views is emphasized by data presented in this chapter which show that, despite statistics showing a high level of chronic illness, few older people rate themselves as having poor health. A key factor in this self-definition, the authors argue, is independence of action and the ability to maintain social involvements. (On this, also see Chandraratna & Cummins 1988:28.) The authors conclude that the future health of older people will depend upon both the political strength of older people themselves and of the new public health ideologies.

Helen Keleher invites nursing and allied health practitioners such as physiotherapists to take up the challenge of the new public health and actively participate in the development of public policy (Ch. 25). She argues that much of their energies during the 1970s and 1980s have been directed towards professional and intra-professional struggles to the relative neglect of 'more global issues of social justice in health'. Yet of all health practitioner groups, nurses would seem to have articulated policies which are most in line with those of the new public health; for example, the Colleges of Nursing and the Australian Nursing Federation (ANF) have prepared policies spelling out the relationship between nursing and primary health care and pointing to the influence of social and environmental influences on health.

According to Keleher, there has been a conflict between the pursuit of professional status, particularly along the lines achieved by the medical profession, and their involvement in processes and in the development of knowledges that advance the goals of public health. As she puts it, 'the interests of the community are not necessarily served by the elitism inherent in professionalization, with the tendency to moral superiority which is exhibited by some professionals'. In terms of their numbers alone, nurses and allied health workers possess a great potential to effect change. If they are to take a more active role in promoting the public's health, they need to exploit this potential by developing skills in effecting change in a health care system currently oriented towards treatment. And an important part of effecting change is having greater involvement with people in the community and re-orientating professional practice away from its major focus on individual client care towards 'population based health promotion strategies'.

A more sceptical view of the new public health is offered by John Duff in his chapter on nutrition policy and public health (Ch. 26). In contrast to many commentators, Duff sees the new public health as involving not a broadening of perspective, but a *narrowing* of perspective; a change from action at the collective level to action at the individual level. This has been due to the consolidation of the power of medicine which has redefined public health problems as medical problems requiring clinical intervention. Reflecting this broader change in the definition of public health, nutrition policy has been increasingly directed at individual lifestyle change 'and in the process limited food and eating pretty much to a matter of biology...'. Moreover, nutritional campaigns and dietary policy more generally have become matters of scientific understanding and management to the relative neglect of economic, political, and social processes underlying the marketing and production of food. Much of the health science and health promotion effort is directed towards identifying 'at risk' groups and changing their priorities, behaviour and even lifestyles. And it seems that those who are most likely to respond to the health promotion messages are the higher socioeconomic groups.

This last point indicates one of the key problems of the so-called rational choice model of behaviour underlying much of the health promotion endeavour. It is simply assumed that, given the right information, individuals will make 'correct, healthy' choices. However, this denies the constraints on choice; for example, those pertaining to ethnic and class background. Duff contends that, in the case of nutrition policy, 'this model allows all too readily the conclusion that those who do not respond to health promotion are not acting rationally, or have failed to inform themselves properly'. As it happens, it is those who have least resources who are vulnerable to this charge. The difficulty in changing this situation, however, is the privileged position of the scientific view upon which the power of 'experts' depends. As Duff says, there needs to be more encouragement and room for sociological and anthropological research into food and eating and into the underlying economic, political, and social processes.

The final two chapters, by Lynne Hunt (Ch. 27) and by Dorothy Broom (Ch. 28), are on the women's health movement and women's health services. They have been placed together at the end, not because they are less important than the others, but because their critical approaches are the only ones which confront directly the entire edifice of the 'male-stream' health movement and mode of health delivery—its curative *and* preventative aspects.

Lynne Hunt traces the origins of the women's health movement to women's concerns about the inappropriateness of the medically dominated health services which deal with illness rather than health. These services have not only failed to recognize women's different patterns of health risk, but are permeated with sexist values. As Hunt indicates, much of women's contact with health services is a consequence of women's reproductive concerns such as contraception, pregnancy and childbirth. These are not diseases, but tend to be 'medicalized' when dealt with by mainstream health services.

The women's health movement, which is an international movement, begins from the premise that women have not had ultimate control over their own bodies and their own health (Zimmerman 1987:443). It has sought to rectify the injustices women face in caring for their health by creating health centres providing services geared to the specific needs of women, and in working for broader change. The criticism Hunt levels at mainstream health promotion is its male bias, focussing on lifestyle factors which cause today's 'major killers'—heart attacks and cancer—to the relative neglect of women's health issues such as menstruation, post-natal depression, and male violence against women. She argues that health education messages tend to concentrate on single messages (for example, stop smoking, reduce fat intake), but ignore 'the interconnected nature of women's lives and the complexity of individual constructions of health'. The women's movement, says Hunt, works with a 'social action model' of health that moves beyond compliance with professional notions of positive health behaviour to seeking changes of those conditions which adversely affect women's lives. This makes 'health promotion' an essentially political approach which, as Hunt points out, may lead to a conservative backlash.

In fact it was in reflecting upon the result of such a backlash in Australia that led Dorothy Broom to write her chapter. This deals with a legal case brought against women's health services to the Human Rights and Equal Opportunities Commission by a Dr Alex Proudfoot of the Australian Capital Territory. The complaint was made on the basis that such services 'are discriminatory against men under the Sex Discrimination Act because men cannot access them, because men's health is worse than women's, and because the services address problems that are not unique to women'. In the event, the case was lost. But the ruling leaves a number of questions unanswered, which are raised by Broom in the chapter. The health services were found to be discriminatory, despite having being exempted by a section under the Act. This raises a question about the legal definition that permits women's health services to be found discriminatory despite men having suffered no detriment from their activities.

The case also raises a number of interesting questions for the student of sociology of health and illness, a few of which are discussed in the chapter. One is, should judges be able to adjudicate on cases involving resource allocation, which until now have been considered the province of the legislative and administrative branches of government which have taken into account a number of perspectives? Another is, is it appropriate that the very institutions whose dominant male practices and discourses had motivated the establishment of women's health services in the first place be able to adjudicate on whether these same services should be allowed to continue to function?

The chapter ends by welcoming a new interest in 'men's health'. Broom sees this as providing the opportunity to make visible the significance of gender to health 'instead of relegating it to the marginalized status of 'women's issues''. This new interest offers the potential to explore the ways in which gender and health interact so that more effective models of both women's health and men's health can be developed, and the organization and delivery of sick care and health services improved.

REFERENCES

Chandraratna D, Cummins M 1988 Ethnicity and ageing: the Anglo-Asian experience, SWRC reports and proceedings no. 73 June. The Social Welfare Research Centre, The University of New South Wales, Kensington
Palmer G R, Short S D 1989 Health care and public policy: an Australian analysis. Macmillan, South Melbourne
Phillipson, C 1982 Capitalism and the construction of old age. Macmillan. London
Zimmerman M K 1987 The women's health movement: a critique of medical enterprise and the position of women. In: Hess B B, Marx Ferree M (eds) Analyzing gender: a handbook of social science research. Sage, Beverley Hills

22. AIDS and the new public health

Michael W. Ross

The health of the people is the highest law.

Cicero, De Legibus 3,3,8

The Acquired Immune Deficiency Syndrome (AIDS) is a fatal condition caused by the Human Immunodeficiency Virus (HIV), and the clinical syndrome may occur many years (on average 8-10 years) after infection. It is a modern epidemic caused by an agent which was not isolated until 1983 and which did not appear to have occurred outside of Africa until the 1950s. It is thus a new epidemic in both historical and virological terms, and its spread appears in part to reflect the new conditions which have lead to altered patterns of disease since that time: greater mobility through international travel, changes in sexual and drug-using practices, and population movements and their associated dislocations and relocations. The epidemiology of HIV/AIDS thus reflects these social and historical factors.

HIV was first identified in blood samples in central Africa which had been kept in blood registries for research dating from the late 1950s. It was not identified in blood samples kept in North America until the late 1970s. By the time AIDS was first described as an epidemic of opportunistic infections and the cancer Kaposi's sarcoma in homosexually active men in 1981, it had spread to the Caribbean, Europe and North America. In the Caribbean, it appeared to have been carried from central Africa by aid workers and to be heterosexually transmitted as in sub-Saharan Africa. In North America, it was most common in homosexually active men. The virus had thus found its niches in new populations as a function of a number of social factors: frequent air travel which transferred its carriers rapidly across the world (the jumbo jet has begun to replace the mosquito as a major vector of disease), and changes in sexual practices. The growth of transport networks along rivers and roads and the concomitant growth of cities lead to the dislocation of many central African men to cities in search of work. This in turn lead to the growth of sex worker services for these men who were away from traditional family settings. The heterosexual spread of HIV in sub-Saharan Africa (where the World Health Organization estimates that more than 10 million people are infected) was also transferred to the Caribbean and Europe. Transmission to homosexually active men probably occurred in the

323

Caribbean in areas where there was male prostitution and which were popular holiday venues for the gay population of the major North American metropolises.

Once established in homosexually active men, HIV spread was again assisted by a social change arising from the liberalization of sexual mores (both homosexual and heterosexual) in the late 1960s and 1970s, which made it possible for gay communities and facilities servicing them to develop. These conditions made it possible for homosexually active men to have greater numbers and frequency of sexual partners, which lead to an explosion of HIV infection in this population.

In parallel, injecting drug use had also arisen in the 1960s as a function of both the same revolution in morality which occurred in the western world in the 1960s and the concomitant development of the drug trade and opiate (particularly heroin) growth and manufacture. One of its great stimuluses was the Vietnam war, in which the geographical location close to the golden triangle of opium production and the overwhelming conditions of the war led to very high rates of drug use in United States troops. Many returned to the United States with established opiate addictions. HIV became established in injecting drug users and because of its easy spread through blood, and through social policies which made the possession of injecting equipment illegal (and thus it was necessary to share needles and syringes), an epidemic in injecting drug users (IDUs) also occurred.

Because blood donation in the United States is often paid, and because IDUs are frequently unemployed and in need of money for drugs, contaminated blood entered the blood banking system and people who received infected donations also became infected with HIV. In Europe, infection occurred from two sources: through heterosexual contact between people who had contracted HIV in sub-Saharan Africa, and by contact with homosexually active tourists from North America. In other parts of the world, the HIV/AIDS epidemic followed the pattern of the mode of introduction of the virus: in India, it was probably introduced through the strong links of expatriate Indian settlers in east Africa with their culture of origin and the well-developed sex services in Indian cities. In contrast, in Australia and New Zealand, the epidemic arose in homosexually active men who had visited North America, and then spread through the established gay subcultures in the major Australasian cities. Limited contact with IDUs overseas has meant that there is a low prevalence of HIV in Australasian IDUs at the time of writing, and that the majority of infected IDUs in Sydney probably acquired their HIV through sexual contact (Ross et al 1992a). However, the spread of the heterosexual epidemic through south-east Asia and the frequency of sex tourism between Australia and south-east Asia has also raised the possibility of the introduction of a heterosexual focus to the disease.

The epidemiology of HIV is thus dependent on social and historical factors: the growth of national and international transport, the movement of people to cities and the development of sexual and drug-using subcultures, sex tourism, changes in social mores, and social policies relating to prosecution of drug users. The point that must be made clear is that the very epidemiology of HIV is based on historical, social and anthropological factors, and will continue to be. The pattern of the HIV epidemic (in some countries, predominantly heterosexual; in some predominantly homosexual; in some, also associated with injecting drug use; in some, medically acquired through transfusion by the lack of finance for medical equipment, which led to re-use of injecting equipment, as in some parts of eastern Europe) is a social pattern. It thus follows that social policy is central in controlling HIV spread.

Social epidemiology and the inverse care law

In the past, other diseases have also followed social patterns. Examples were epidemics which disproportionately affected those most disadvantaged and in lower socioeconomic levels, who lived in more crowded conditions, which were more conducive to spread of aerosol transmitted diseases such as tuberculosis, parasite transmitted diseases such a bubonic plague (the Black Death), and diseases transmitted through poor sanitation and water supplies such as cholera. In addition, people at lower socioeconomic levels had poorer nutrition, which made them more susceptible to becoming ill, or more seriously ill. Social factors in the transmission and development of disease have always been important, but the more non-random the mode of transmission of a disease, the more social and environmental conditions may affect its distribution.

People in more socially disadvantaged positions have not only a greater burden of disease, but they also have a greater disadvantage in terms of services, which is described as Hart's inverse care law (1972). This law draws attention to the fact that those at lower socioeconomic levels generally have the poorest health and health care, and that conditions detrimental to health occur more frequently in the underprivileged. In the case of HIV/AIDS, Krueger et al (1990) have reported that, when all other factors are controlled for, it is those with lower income in the United States who are most likely to be HIV seropositive. They suggest that poor access to risk-reduction information and less support for implementation of such strategies may explain some of this difference. At a global level, the importance of social factors underlying illness has been emphasized by the World Health Organization (WHO) in both the Declaration of Alma Ata and the Ottawa Charter, which emphasize the importance of community advocacy and mediation and development of personal skills to create environments supportive for health. It is precisely the lack of political and social power which helps to perpetuate the lack of community advocacy and thus the continuation of poorer health and poorer access to health care in disadvantaged communities. It is precisely these disadvantaged communities who are most affected by HIV/AIDS. The 'new public health' has been designed to attempt to respond to this inequitable situation.

The new public health

The new public health grew from the WHO objectives for the development of primary health care. These include the promotion of lifestyles conducive to health, the prevention of preventable conditions, and the development of rehabilitation and health services (Ashton & Seymour 1988). In contrast with the older public health, in which the emphasis was on treatment when people became ill (tertiary prevention), the emphasis is on primary prevention through health promotion. Such health promotion will actively involve the population in the setting of everyday life, will be directed to removing the causes of ill health, and involves community development and organization, health advocacy and legislation, and the encouragement of environments which are supportive for health. Such health promotion sees health in the widest possible context, including enabling people to exercise more control over their health and their environment, and developing skills to make healthy choices. There is thus a close relationship between risk taking and lack of empowerment. The older public health, in contrast, had no commitment to either population coverage or to sharing and demystifying power and there was a potential conflict between the clinical model based on individual transactions and the new public health model based on a social contract with the entire community (Ashton & Seymour 1988). It is thus no coincidence that Bacon's dictum that knowledge equals power has been used as a slogan by AIDS activists who seek greater control over their condition and the policies which surround HIV/AIDS treatments. The tension between the new and the older public health is essentially one of the locus of control, and thus should be seen as a political issue as much as a health one: as Virchow indicated, 'Medicine is a social science and politics is nothing else but medicine on a large scale' (Ashton & Seymour 1988). Since the accent of the new public health is on change (at social as well as at organizational and individual levels), change to the conditions which lead to less physically and mentally healthy environments has been the target for reducing the impact of AIDS. Inevitably, given that HIV/AIDS affects stigmatized (and thus disadvantaged) groups disproportionately, and that HIV infection itself may stigmatize, issues of social justice and health are closely intertwined.

Homosexuality and AIDS

A basic proposition of the new public health is that people who are disadvantaged socially and politically are in a poor position to modify risk behaviours. Homosexually active men are discriminated against both socially and, in some jurisdictions, legally. The effect of legal discrimination may operate at several levels to increase HIV risk behaviours. First, where behaviours are forced underground by legal sanctions, it is difficult if not impossible to target them appropriately and accurately for risk reduction education. Second, legal sanctions are likely to mean that where there are homosexual encounters, they are fleeting and anonymous and probably more likely to be under time constraints or in locales which are not conducive to taking proper precautions, for example condom use. Third, people who are frightened, depressed or anxious are less likely to take appropriate health measures. Each of these propositions will be examined, but as the response of the health system is also important in providing appropriate health education and services, it is important to examine that first.

The political and social aspects of homosexual health care were examined in Ross (1986), where I argued that what distinguishes the health issues of homosexuals compared with heterosexuals is the degree and form of social stigmatization to which they are subject. At a direct health level, this has clearest implications for mental health (particularly self-esteem, depression and anxiety), but also for psychosomatic disorders. However, I also noted that sexually transmissible diseases (STDs) distinguish homosexual from heterosexual people: homosexual men have a higher level of STDs than heterosexual men, while lesbians have a lower level than heterosexual women. This latter point appears to relate not to stigmatization but to the double standards which apply to male and female relationships, and in some cases to political and ideological variables as well.

Lower levels of health care may also (as noted in Hart's (1972) inverse care law) have a major impact on the health care of homosexuals. Pauly and Goldstein (1970) reported that three quarters of a sample of 1000 medical practitioners acknowledged that knowing that a male patient was homosexual would adversely affect their medical management of him. Davison and Friedman (1981) found that when two groups of psychologists were given a case history of a male, and one group were told incidentally that the patient was also homosexual, most of the patient's problems were construed by the latter group in sexual terms, and that area concentrated on. Thus there is not only overt discomfort leading to poorer medical management, but also a narrowing of the field of perception of the patient's health problems and an attribution of them as being associated with sexual orientation.

More indirectly, stigma may also lead to mental health problems. Ross (1990) studied life events and mental health in Australian homosexual men and found that for normal life events such as finances and work, as well as the effects of stigmatization and discrimination, stigmatization amplified the emotional distress reported. His data support the contention that the more socially disadvantaged, the greater the impact of life events. In an earlier study of homosexual men who were married (to women), Ross (1983) found that the worse the anticipated reaction against the individual's homosexuality, the more likely they were to marry and to live a double life (with negative consequences for their psychological adjustment). However, Ross (1990) also found that the greatest negative mental health consequences were associated with HIV/AIDS in his sample: the psychological ramifications of

HIV extended far beyond those in the sample who were infected (less than 9%). These data suggest that the combination of a pre-existing stigmatization and the impact of HIV lead to greater mental health stresses in homosexual men, which will also impact on psychosomatic illness.

In addition to the mental health consequences of being a member of a stigmatized minority group, and the direct effects of this on the thoroughness of the attending medical practitioner, the propositions that legal and social stigmatization will make it more difficult to target homosexual men are born out by two studies. Connell et al (1989) carried out a large study of homosexually active men in Sydney, and found that there was significantly better HIV-preventive behaviour among those men who were associated with, or considered themselves as members of, the gay community. Their data confirm that the existence of a sense of community, and the activities of the gay community, are associated with greater reduction in risk activities. That gay community norms are the variable most closely associated with intention to use a condom was demonstrated by Ross and McLaws (1992), who found that it was the perception of support from significant others for safer sex rather than positive attitudes toward condom use which were the best predictor of intention to use a condom and previous condom use. Thus, the development of community norms (itself dependent on the opportunity to develop a community) is associated with increased preventive behaviour and illustrates the importance of the social and legal climate in reducing the risk of HIV infection.

In an environment in which legal or social sanctions lead to people having to hide their orientation or operate 'underground', the community mobilization and support which has lead to peer education, and the development of gay community norms supportive of safer sex, would be far less successful. An additional factor which must also be considered is that people are less likely to come forward for HIV testing and associated risk reduction education and counselling, in a climate of discrimination and sanction, real or anticipated. In a comparison of the impact of decriminalization of homosexual behaviour between consenting adult males in two Australian states, Sinclair and Ross (1986) found that the consequences of decriminalization did not include any increase in the negative aspects of homosexuality (such as solicitation or STD), and that in fact the data suggested that STD incidence was lower. There was also an increase in both total homosexual friends and close homosexual friends reported by homosexual men in the state which had decriminalized homosexual acts, which supports the contention that decriminalization may have a positive effect on the development of community.

These data suggest that policies which make the development of a community, appropriate community norms, and peer education possible are likely to increase the practice of behaviours which reduce HIV transmission. This is an important objective of the new public health, which seeks to alter health behaviour by changing the environment and context to promote health behaviours. This context will include a consideration of the legal, social and policy factors which discourage health behaviour, and their modification to improve health through improving social and legal equity.

Injecting drug use and AIDS

Similar considerations attend the health and public health aspects of IDUs, although they are in most jurisdictions even more socially stigmatized and more legally disadvantaged. However, the principles of the new public health also apply equally: the parallels between homosexually active men and IDUs are close. However, because of their drug use, many regular IDUs are also unlikely to be employed and therefore resort to illegal activities to obtain drug supplies, thus putting them in a generally more disadvantaged position than homosexually active men.

Adequate medical services for IDUs are likely to be even more difficult to find. IDUs use medical services for as wide a range of health related reasons as the general population (Stowe et al 1992) and not just to obtain drugs as is commonly imagined. Yet Roche, Guray and Saunders (1991) found that most medical practitioners in Australia were antipathetic to IDUs, wanted nothing to do with them, and did not want to become involved in their treatment. The typical response to IDU patients was to refer them quickly to a government clinic, and most practitioners expressed a vehement dislike of them. It is clear that under such circumstances, IDUs could not expect optimum treatment for conditions even other than their drug use.

The social context of injecting drug use is a major determinant of the HIV-related harm that may ensue. In a major and elegant demonstration of this, Grund et al (1992) compared IDUs in Rotterdam, and the Bronx. In the Netherlands, most addicts have regular housing and social welfare, free medical care on demand, and ready access to drug treatment. Drug problems are viewed as one of a number of social problems which cannot be solved by repression, and policy is based on controlling the use of drugs and their damage rather than on their elimination. This has resulted in stable availability, and relatively high purity of drugs (most commonly heroin and cocaine). Most drugs are sold at house addresses where users can buy and sell drugs in a relatively calm atmosphere.

In contrast in the United States, the Bronx is a socially and physically dilapidated area with a large number of permanently homeless and with overcrowded medical facilities which are not receptive to anything but the emergency needs of drug users and then only reluctantly. The majority of drug sales occur in unstable and dangerous settings, through holes in barred up doors or by small groups of people who wander a particular block (Grund et al 1992). Large numbers of young homeless drug users live together in abandoned buildings without access to clean water, and the purity and stability of price of heroin is low because of the difficulty of supply due to the so-called 'war on drugs'. Since, in contrast to the Netherlands, possession of injecting equipment is illegal, renting equipment in 'shooting galleries' where the same equipment is used over and over again by people who have no relationship is common.

The social, physical and legal context of injecting drug use has become associated with obvious differences in HIV risk behaviours. While it has been assumed that IDUs are so socially deviant or disorganized that they are unable or unwilling to change their behaviour, the comparison between Rotterdam and the Bronx illustrates that Dutch addicts share things such as housing, food, money, clothing and child care and help one another with daily problems associated with the addict life (Grund et al 1992). In contrast, the more disintegrating world of the inner city New York addict emphasizes the competition, violence and mistrust of a different social and physical setting. In Rotterdam, the free availability of sterile needles and syringes has made sharing injecting equipment a deviant act in the IDU subculture, with there being no structural scarcity justifying the sharing of injecting equipment. The relative availability of comparatively stable and pure drugs has meant that there is a lower need to supplement use with whatever drug is available and under conditions which are associated with desperation, urgency and a need to inject immediately which are not conducive to prevention of HIV transmission. Grund et al argue that norms, policies and responses to illicit drug use have important consequences on the everyday practice of drug users.

The stereotype of IDUs as being disinterested in their health and living only for their next 'fix' may be as much a function of the milieu in which they exist as of their addiction. In Australia, the Australian National AIDS and Injecting Drug Use Study (1991) found that IDUs in four major cities had extensively modified the injecting practices which put them at risk of HIV infection, to the point where most were using clean equipment, injecting with only one or two close friends, and cleaning contaminated equipment. Since 1986, needles and syringes have been available on an exchange basis and by purchase from pharmacies, and their ready availability and the decriminalization of possession of injecting equipment have been a major step in keeping the HIV seroprevalence level low. Further, knowledge about HIV and its modes of transmission among IDUs is high and accurate (Ross et al 1992b). The 'harm reduction' model has been promoted to reduce HIV transmission in IDUs in Australia; this model uses a multi-step approach which makes it possible for the individual to reduce the risk of infection at the level at which they are capable. Ideally, it is preferable not to use illicit drugs at all. If that is not possible, then people should use drugs by a non-injecting route. If that is not possible, IDUs should use new equipment. If that is not possible, then used equipment should be decontaminated by bleach or methylated spirits. In Australia, where injecting is the most common form of administration of opiates, the median percentage of time that new needles and syringes were used was more than 75% (ANAIDUS 1991). Grund et al (1991) note that in Rotterdam, the harm reduction model has been taken one step further, with less than a quarter of IDUs injecting as a means of drug taking, with the majority smoking their drug. These points illustrate the effect that policies such as provision of readily available needle and syringe exchange, and higher purity of drugs which make it possible to use administration routes other than injecting, have on HIV risk. Both are part of a harm reduction model which, while not condoning illicit drug use, put in place a variety of services ranging from a greater number of treatment places to provision of education, facilities and equipment to minimize risk.

However, as HIV became established in Australia initially in homosexually active men, there is an erroneous and dangerous perception among both IDUs and some health educators that contaminated injecting equipment is the only significant means of transmission of HIV. In Sydney, Ross et al (1992a) have noted that the distribution of HIV infection in IDU men was around 3% for the heterosexually active, 12% for the bisexually active, and 35% for homosexually active, confirming that it is probably the sexual route which has infected most of the HIV seropositive IDUs. This is supported by other evidence (Ross et al 1991) which found that IDUs have a disturbingly high level of STDs. This illustrates the importance of considering the total health, and health risks, of a population rather than a concentration on a single factor, and the reason why the new public health concentrates on the total health environment rather than one or two problems in isolation.

Medically acquired AIDS

Unlike homosexually active men and IDUs, those who have acquired HIV infection through contaminated blood products (primarily haemophiliacs) or through contaminated transfusions in the course of medical procedures do not have a pre-existing stigmatized status. However, by co-categorization (where an infection such as HIV is automatically categorized in the public perception with activities which are perceived as illicit or deviant), those with medically acquired HIV infection are also subject to stigma. The fear of HIV/AIDS is pervasive, and includes unrealistic fears of infection and fears of loss of control, death, and contact with people who are 'different' (Arrindell et al 1989, Ross & Hunter 1991). Hunter and Ross (1991) looked at determinants of health workers' attitudes toward people with HIV/AIDS, and found that patients who were infected by sexual contact or injecting drug use were seen as more culpable and responsible for their condition than those infected by transfusion, and that source of infection also influenced respondent's desire for close personal interaction. They suggested that negative attitudes toward people with HIV were probably associated with negative attitudes toward sexual contacts and through the common association of these two areas.

While the occurrence of medically acquired HIV stopped with the testing of all blood donations for HIV in 1985, people who acquired HIV through blood or blood products are still stigmatized by the association of AIDS with sex, death, drugs and moral outrage, with many people not taking the time to distinguish the source of their discomfort. As Sontag (1989) has noted, the symbolism of HIV/AIDS lies in the fact that it is considered a disease of perversity, and associated with phobias and fears of contamination. She draws a parallel between perceptions of AIDS and of plague: disgracing, disempowering, and disgusting. This association in the public perception has both social and personal penalties, and the avoidance and fear engendered by HIV may also have a psychological and social impact on those who are infected but do not have any other stigmatizing features, including their health care.

AIDS and prevention

In the absence of a cure for HIV infection or AIDS, and the possibility that there will not be any cure in the foreseeable future, prevention of HIV infection is the only way of halting its spread. From a public health point of view, this has been achieved by three areas of action: medical, environmental, and educational. The medical area has involved the judicious application of HIV testing, particularly to protect the blood supply in order to stop medically acquired HIV infection. There is a naive view that testing populations is an answer. This seems implausible: one cannot identify, and test, every member of a population particularly given the large numbers of homeless, visitors and tourists, and illegal immigrants in the population as well as large scale population movement). Even if this were possible, what could be done with those who were HIV positive, since there is no treatment? The 'universal testing' argument also confuses infectious diseases (such as tuberculosis) which are spread by aerosol in both public and private social situations with contagious diseases (such as HIV) which are with rare exceptions only spread by volitional physical contact between two people, such as sex or sharing injection equipment. The rare exceptions may include needlestick injuries in health care settings or sexual assault. The cycle of HIV transmission can easily be broken by modifying behaviour to include safer sex (use of condoms for penetration) and safer injecting (use of uncontaminated equipment). Thus, behaviour is the only vaccine.

There is a perception that HIV testing will lead to positive changes in risky behaviour, and there is certainly evidence to suggest that testing is an effective way of changing behaviour (Ross 1988). However, it is those who test positive who are most likely to change their behaviour, and sometimes a negative test result is seen as a confirmation that previous behaviour is 'safe' or that the individual is somehow immune. Until a cure is available, HIV testing can never be more than an adjunct to health education.

Since health education is the only consistent means of altering risk behaviour, it is important to target it as accurately and as powerfully as possible. It has been shown that knowledge is a necessary, but not sufficient, condition to behaviour change, and that various other conditions must be met: persons must also see themselves as being vulnerable or at risk, and the costs of changing behaviour must not outweigh the benefits. Further, the person must believe that the change will be effective. Health education to prevent HIV transmission has also involved making the message most believable, and this has been achieved by using close consultation, peer education, and empowerment. It is axiomatic that those in the communities most affected will know most about the types and distribution of risk behaviours and the best ways of modifying them. More importantly, however, peer educators are more believable and taken greater notice of than authority figures, particularly where (as in the case of IDUs and to a lesser extent homosexually active men) those same authorities have been involved in the persecution or prosecution of those communities.

The third area where HIV prevention has occurred is also most explicitly related to the new public health. Changing the legislative and social context to improve health involves legal, social and political change. Legal change to reduce the spread of HIV has involved decriminalization of homosexual acts between consenting males in some jurisdictions where this was still illegal, as a way of bringing homosexually active men into the open so that HIV prevention and peer education could be more easily achieved. Decriminalization of possession of injecting equipment made it possible to distribute needles and syringes and to increase the injecting equipment in circulation. Removing the restrictions on the advertisement and sale (and places of sale) of condoms made them more widely and easily available. Social change emphasized that HIV was spread by particular behaviours and that HIV made no distinction between mode of sexual behaviour (and was not associated with 'risk groups' but with risk behaviours), and anti-discrimination campaigns sought to break down the discrimination associated with HIV infection. Indirectly, the public education campaigns surrounding HIV risk reduction have made discussion of sexual behaviour and drug policy public currency and have thus also assisted in making communication about HIV risks more socially acceptable and less likely to produce anxiety or discomfort. This latter consequence has undoubtedly helped to make negotiation of safer sexual or drug taking behaviours easier, and to begin to establish a norm of negotiation between potential sexual or drug sharing partners.

AIDS and the new public health in operation

The new public health approach to reduction of HIV transmission has generally been very successful. Some countries have most consistently utilized this approach with early education, the avoidance of counter-productive repressive measures which simply push the problem underground, and empowerment of those groups most affected by partnering them in peer education and attempts to alter the social context in which the risk behaviour occurs. Examples include the Netherlands and Australia, and there has been a notable reduction in new infections in these areas (although it is impossible to attribute all reduction of HIV to such policies since variables such as epidemiology, history, geography, economics, culture and tradition, and even 'luck' will all play a part in the direction and speed of the HIV pandemic).

There have also been problems associated with the implementation of a new public health approach to reduction of HIV transmission. The transfer of power to previously disempowered and often disorganized groups has seen bureaucrats announce that they represent or speak for groups such as IDUs, thus maintaining their own power and blocking the sometimes erratic but socially critical development of appropriate structures. The redirection of scarce research funds to HIV-related research may lead to an influx of carpetbaggers, with little or no previous interest in minority groups, STDs, drug use and other related areas, eager to build empires and reputations. The political and economic power associated with the direction of funds to community groups may lead to infighting over the control of agendas.

Ultimately, we can conclude that the application of the new public health model to the HIV epidemic has been extremely successful. The focus on the social and political components of health care has placed issues of social equity and justice firmly on the health agenda as well as providing a cogent demonstration of the applicability of the new public health model to primary prevention. The example of HIV/AIDS illustrates clearly that the social context of health and the community is central in any alteration of the conditions which promote health and health behaviour, and as integral to the health of both communities and individuals as specific educational interventions or medical procedures.

REFERENCES

ANAIDUS (Australian National AIDS and Injecting Drug Use Study) 1991 Neither a borrower nor a lender be: first report of the Australian national AIDS and injecting drug use study, 1989 data collection. ANAIDUS, Sydney

Arrindell W A, Ross M W, Bridges K R, van Hout W, Hofman A, Sanderman R 1989 Are there replicable and invariant questionnaire dimensions of fear of AIDS? findings from a pilot study with the fear of AIDS schedule (FAIDSS). Advances in Behaviour Research and Therapy 11:69–115

Ashton J, Seymour H 1988 The new public health. Open University, Milton Keynes

Connell R W, Crawford J, Kippax S, Dowsett G W, Baxter D, Berg R 1989 Facing the epidemic: changes in the sexuality of gay and bisexual men in Australia and their implications for AIDS prevention strategies. Social Problems 36:348–402

Davison G C, Friedman S 1981 Sexual orientation stereotype in the distortion of clinical judgement. Journal of Homosexuality 6:37–44

Grund J P C, Stern L S, Kaplan C D, Adriaans N F P, Drucker E 1992 Drug use contexts and HIV-consequences: the effect of drug policy on patterns of everyday drug use in Rotterdam and the Bronx. British Journal of Addiction 87:381–392

Hart J T 1972 Primary care in the industrial areas of Britain: evolution and current problems. International Journal of Health Services 2:349–365

Hunter C E, Ross M W 1991 Determinants of health-care workers' attitudes toward people with AIDS. Journal of Applied Social Psychology 21:947–956

Krueger L E, Wood R W, Diehr P H, Maxwell L 1990 Poverty and HIV seropositivity: the poor are more likely to be infected. AIDS 4:811–814

Pauly I, Goldstein S 1970 Physicians' attitudes in treating homosexuals. Medical Aspects of Human Sexuality 4:26–45

Roche A M, Guray C, Saunders J B 1991 General practitioners' experiences of patients with drug and alcohol problems. British Journal of Addiction 86:263–275

Ross M W 1983 The married homosexual man: a psychological study. Routledge, London

Ross M W 1986 Psychovenereology: personality and lifestyle factors in sexually transmitted diseases in homosexual men. Praeger, New York

Ross M W 1988 The relationship of combinations of AIDS counselling and testing to safer sex and condom use in homosexual men. Community Health Studies 12:322–327

Ross M W 1990 The relationship between life events and mental health in homosexual men. Journal of Clinical Psychology 46:402–411

Ross M W, Gold J, Wodak A, Miller M E 1991 Sexually transmissible diseases in injecting drug users. Genitourinary Medicine 67:32–36

Ross M W, Hunter C E 1991 Dimensions, content and validation of the Fear of AIDS schedule in health professionals. AIDS Care 3:175–180

Ross M W, McLaws M L 1992 Normative beliefs are better predictors of condom use and intention to use than behavioural beliefs. Health Education Research 7:335–339

Ross M W, Wodak A, Gold J, Miller M E 1992a Differences across sexual orientation on HIV risk behaviours in injecting drug users. AIDS Care 4:139–148

Ross M W, Buzolic A, Wodak A, Stowe A, Gold J, Miller M E 1992b Structure and dimension of risk for HIV transmission in injecting drug users. Drug and Alcohol Review 11:231–237

Sinclair K C P, Ross M W 1986 Consequences of decriminalisation of homosexuality: a study of two Australian states. Journal of Homosexuality 12:119–127

Sontag S 1989 Illness as metaphor and AIDS and its metaphors. Anchor, New York

Stowe A, Ross M W, Wodak A 1992 Contact between injecting drug users and general practitioners and its implications for health education. Journal of the Royal Society of Health 112:122-123

23. The changing face of oral health promotion

Leonie M. Short   Alan F. Patterson

This chapter highlights the inequalities of oral health status in Australia and describes a successful oral health promotion program in the Moree district of New South Wales in order to better understand the changes facing health promotion within the context of the new public health movement.

Oral health status

The World Health Organization (WHO) target for the year 2000 for school children's oral health was reached in Australia in 1983, therefore, oral health should not be a high priority area (Grant & Lapsley 1992:253). However, health inequalities do exist, as 15% of school children have 85% of the dental disease in New South Wales, and there is a shortage of dentists in rural and remote areas (Grant & Lapsley 1992:159). This is also true in New Zealand where a recent WHO study of oral health outcomes concluded that there were dentally advantaged and disadvantaged groups in the population with the latter found mainly within the low occupational group and within the Maori population (Hunter et al 1992).

As part of the National Health Strategy (NHS), *Enough to Make you Sick, How Income and Environment Affect Health* states that good health is strongly influenced by what you earn and where you live (McClelland et al 1992). The Australian Council of Social Service and the Consumers' Health Forum of Australia worked together on issues related to health and inequality in Australia for the NHS and the former federal Minister for Health, Brian Howe. They produced the consultation broadsheet on income, environment and health, *Healthy, Wealthy and Wise*, which expressed concern about the large number of people missing out on dental care. In particular, 'with costly private insurance as the only protection against hefty dental bills, the NHS has found that poorer people and their children seem to go to the dentist only in emergencies' (Australian Council of Social Service and the Consumers' Health Forum 1992:1).

Australian Aborigines find themselves in 'a vicious cycle of poverty and powerlessness from which they feel they can never hope to escape' (Franklin & White 1991:33). This demoralizing helplessness is itself one of the major health problems of Aboriginal and Torres Strait Islander people where oral health status is no exception (Franklin & White 1991:33). 'Although the prevalence of dental health problems such as caries was low under traditional living conditions, there are disturbingly high levels of dental disease in the Aboriginal community today' (Anderson 1988:56). Moreover, when put into perspective, dental caries and periodontal disease are now widespread among Aborigines whilst dental disease in the wider Australian population is declining in the younger age groups (Saggers & Gray 1991:107).

The NHS Background Paper No 9, *Improving Dental Health in Australia,* acknowledges that the 'task of organizing further oral health promotion and evaluating progress in removing social inequalities in oral health and access to services requires a long-term commitment to change' (Dooland 1992:62). Moreover, the backlog of unmet dental care is staggering and will take years to correct (Correll 1992:8). The latest National Health Goals and Targets document seeks to redress this imbalance when oral health strategies will be directed to the priority populations of children of low socioeconomic status, such as Aboriginal and Torres Strait Island children, non English speaking background children and children who live in rural communities (Nutbeam et al 1992).

Oral health promotion programs are relatively new in Australia but have already proved to be beneficial—'It's easier than pulling teeth—changing a dental service' for young and Aboriginal people and 'healthy smiles' for the Vietnamese community in Adelaide (South Australian Health Commission and the South Australian Community Health Association 1992:42, Ryan 1992:32–33). A dental health promotion program has been implemented for Vietnamese children in Central Sydney and has proven to be effective (Community Health Service 1992). 'Dental Care for Arabic Speaking Families', 'Dental Care for Vietnamese Speaking Families' and 'Dental Health in Primary School' in Southern Sydney have been innovative whilst 'The Tooth: The Hole Truth and Nothing but the Truth' in Western Sydney is a step in the right direction (Harrison 1993, Health Promotion Unit 1991, Sinclair & Griffiths 1993). The 'Dental Force Kit' from the north coast of NSW forged new ground when it combined theatre with health promotion and is a good example of the new face of oral health promotion (Lismore School Dental Clinic 1992).

Since 'people who practise health promotion are now being asked to show what they have to offer' (Sindall 1992:289, Hawe et al 1990:3), health promotion practitioners must demonstrate the validity and benefits of their programs to government senior executives so that policy support and funding can continue. Moreover, it must be remembered that it is rather difficult to persuade politicians and bureaucrats of the advantages of health promotion programs which might need up to five years before showing any long-term benefits to the community (Sindall 1992:288).

In 1990 Alan Patterson, the Principal Dental Officer for the New England Health Region in New South Wales, conducted the *Who Cares?* study on the dental status of approximately 900 children in the Moree district. Patterson concluded that children in the Moree district were two and a half times more likely to require dental treatment than children in Tamworth (another major rural centre in the New England Health Region) (1990:1). Moreover, Aboriginal children were five times more likely to require treatment than other children in Tamworth and nearly four times more likely than other children in the New England health region as a whole (Patterson 1990:1).

As the Moree Plains Shire was embroiled in a controversial and divisive water fluoridation debate, other long-term oral health promotion strategies were recommended for implementation (Patterson 1990:1–2). These interventions included school based educational programs, 'brush-ins', 'rinse-ins' and canteen food sales (Patterson 1990:1).

'Teeth for keeps' project

The authors were successful in obtaining a grant from the Commonwealth Department of Health, Housing and Community Services for $40 086 through the National Health Promotion Program for 1991. The 'Teeth for Keeps' Project was jointly co-ordinated by the Regional Dental Service and the University of New England, Armidale, and it aimed at promoting oral health and preventing dental disease in the Moree Plains Shire. The Project implemented and evaluated oral health promotion strategies in infants and primary schools of the target communities.

The Moree Plains Shire covers an area of approximately 18 000 square kilometres in the north-west of rural New South Wales. Moree, the major centre with a population of 17 000, lies some 300 kilometres north west of Tamworth, which is the regional centre of the New England Region. Other population centres include Mungindi, population 1000, Boggabilla and the associated Aboriginal community of Toomelah, with a population of about 1000, and Pallamallawa, population 350.

The health status of rural dwellers is worse than that of the Australian average (Humphreys & Weinand 1989:258). They state that 'in many cases non-Aboriginal people living in small rural settlements have a health status more akin to that of the Aboriginal population', though their perceptions of need and status are vastly different and based on the self-reliant attitude of the 'cocky', compounded by lack of access to, and provision of, services (Hunphreys & Weinand 1989:259). In the Moree Plains Shire, all community members are disadvantaged in terms of accessibility and provision of dental health services as well as with the recruitment and retention of suitable dental personnel compared with their urban counterparts (Huntley 1991). Regional descriptive statistics show a ratio of one dental therapist to 4426 children in New England Region when the World Health Organization guidelines suggest the optimum of one dental therapist to 2000 children for non-fluoridated areas. Prior to commencement of the oral health promotion program, only one fixed dental clinic located in Moree was operational. This service catered only for schoolchildren and was provided by one dental therapist and one dental assistant employed by the local district hospital.

The shire is unique in that it includes the largest Aboriginal population outside the Northern Territory but is well known for non-Aboriginal/ Aboriginal hostility and conflicts. A situation is highlighted in *The Last Report* which asserts that sufficient data and information exist to demonstrate that the health of Aboriginal communities is of 'third world' standards (NSW Task Force on Aboriginal Health 1990:115). In the New England Health Region (which includes the Moree Plains Shire), specific issues of concern raised by Aboriginal communities about health service delivery included the 'attitude' of hospitals and their staff, transportation, and the lack of permanent employment for persons who sought training via the Department of Education, Employment and Training (NSW Task Force on Aboriginal Health 1990:87).

The Moree Plains is also Australia's richest agricultural shire, the main crops being cotton, wheat, oil seeds and pecan nuts. Whilst the Moree Plains Shire is a rich agricultural area, the vast majority of individuals living there do not share in that wealth. As an indicator of this, unemployment rates in the Moree area are much higher than in other parts of Australia, especially in the Aboriginal population which represents 10% of the community (NSW Task Force on Aboriginal Health 1990:18). The P A Consulting Group (1989:16) recognizes that poverty and unemployment are related to health status and this factor plays a significant role in the unacceptable state of oral health in a minority of the people who live in the Moree Plains Shire.

From an ecological point of view, community members have raised serious concerns about the possible side-effects of fertilizer spraying of cotton crops on their children's health. Some 2000 people marched down the main street protesting against Moree being considered as a potential site for NSW's high temperature incinerator and blue-green algae is a problem in the Murray-Darling river system as massive amounts of water are needed for the irrigation of the cotton crops.

In summary, the social ecology of this wealthy rural district is marked by non-Aboriginal/Aboriginal conflicts and by threats to the environment and the health status of the members of the community.

In late 1990, a public meeting was called in Moree to discuss the results and implications of the *Who Caries?* study and the then impending commencement of the 'Teeth for Keeps' Project. From that meeting a Dental Health Liaison Committee was formed. This committee included representatives of the Moree District Community Health Services, private and public dental practitioners, the local Aboriginal health services, school principals, Parents & Citizens Associations and the local Shire Council. Smaller meetings were also held in other centres throughout the Moree Plains Shire so that community members could discuss the 'Teeth for Keeps' Project and gain a better appreciation of oral health promotion strategies. The resulting co-operation and encouragement from the participants of the communities has ensured a more widespread involvement in, and acceptance of, the programs which were implemented.

The research

For six weeks in early 1991, The 'Teeth for Keeps' Project employed an interim co-ordinator and then appointed two research assistants, one of whom was Aboriginal, for the six month research period to co-ordinate and implement the various oral health promotion strategies for the schools in the Moree Plains Shire. Given the positive response by the communities to the oral health promotion project, and the requests for its continuation and expansion, it was decided to continue to employ the two research assistants with regional dental services until June 1992.

Health promotion strategies included a one day seminar on oral health in Moree which attracted representatives from early childhood development nurses, community health nurses, Aboriginal health workers, the Department of Education, the Shire Council and community members. In addition, a community development workshop for dental personnel was held at the Public Health Unit in Tamworth. This workshop dealt with issues such as sensitization to Aboriginal culture, community development strategies and health promotion in the 1990s.

School based programs included:

- four classroom based educational sessions, age specific and related to all aspects of oral health (Fig. 23.1)
- school 'brush-in' programs
- school 'rinse-in' programs
- targeting school canteens to attempt to increase 'healthy' food alternatives available to children and staff
- the use of sugar free chewing gum after lunch (salivary stimulation)
- the 'Molar Patroller' mobile dental clinic
- the 'Turtles' posters.

These interventions involved a variety of personnel including community nurses, Aboriginal health workers, health promotion officers, teachers, dental personnel, parents and school children.

The infants and primary schools were assigned (after consultation with Principals) to either the Control, Experimental 1, Experimental 2 or Experimental 3 groups (Fig. 23.2). An attempt was made to make these groups as comparable as possible in terms of Aboriginal and non-Aboriginal children, private and public schools, fluoridated and unfluoridated water supplies, and in-Moree and out-of-Moree schools.

The quantitative data included dental status of decayed, missing from caries and filled teeth (dmft and DMFT), category of treatment needed (urgent need of treatment, routine need of treatment and no treatment needed) and dental plaque scores. The qualitative data included interviews with Co-ordinators and Principals, teacher evaluations, community seminar evaluations and an Oral Health Education Training Course evaluation.

Kindergarten, Year 1 and Year 2
Why we need teeth
How to take care of your teeth
Nutrition and its link to dental health
Revision
Year 3 and Year 4
Why we need teeth
How to take care of your teeth
Nutrition and its link to dental health
Revision
Year 5 and Year 6
Why we need teeth
How to take care of your teeth
Nutrition and its link to dental health
Revision

Control	Experimental 1	Experimental 2	Experimental 3
Philomena's Moree (excluding 3 classes)	St Josephs Moree East	Toomelah Boggabilla Mungindi Pallamallawa	Moree (3 classes)
	Oral health education and promotion	Oral health education and promotion	Salivary stimulation
	School canteen promotion	School canteen promotion	
		Daily tooth-brushing and weekly fluoride mouthrinse program	

Fig. 23.1 'Teeth for Keeps' dental health education and promotion program.

Fig. 23.2 'Teeth for Keeps' research design.

Evaluation

Health promotion strategies are based on the five factors developed by the World Health Organization for primary health care models, namely, (1) accessibility, (2) relevance, (3) community involvement (4) cost effectiveness and (5) intersectoral collaboration (Ashton 1990:390). This model has been used in order to assess the process, impact and outcome effectiveness of the 'Teeth for Keeps' Project which addressed the inequalities of oral health status. We turn first to accessibility.

Accessibility. Certainly, the use of the 'Molar Patroller' and community based oral health promotion activities ensured accessibility to all those who wished to participate in the clinical and promotional interventions. However, Brown (1991:443) posits that some social environments may reinforce health damaging behaviour. Examples to highlight this point include a number of Aboriginal children who did not possess a toothbrush at home; fund raising at one school included selling chocolates to raise money for much needed school equipment; and the local shop at the Toomelah Aboriginal community did not sell toothpaste. These ongoing barriers to improvements in oral health status needed to be addressed in order to create an environment that promoted oral health.

Relevance. Relevance can be applied to dental personnel, community leaders and individuals. The International Conference on Health Promotion in 1986 (Editor 1987:v) argued for a reorienting of health services to a primary health care focus and changing professional education and training. The community development workshop for dental personnel of the New England Health Region has certainly improved the commitment, and empowerment of dental personnel, to instigate health promotion activities in the area instead of focusing on treating dental and periodontal disease.

Whilst support for the project has been widespread, Muhondwa (1986:1248) warns against the assumption that 'all community leaders are motivated by noble intentions'. Certainly some middle class white power brokers in various influential positions in the community still regard poor oral health in Moree as a 'black' problem. Understandably, there still remains some level of suspicion from some sections of the Aboriginal community with regard to paternalism and medical dominance. Moreover, school canteens have resisted change from 'fast' foods to 'healthy' foods as some canteen managers, teachers and parents fear that the inevitable loss of profits will be financially detrimental to the school as a whole.

Kickbusch (1989:128) sees individual health action in the context of health promotion as being dependent on the 'process of structuralization', that is its meaning, norms and power. The *Who Caries?* study was published in 1990 to provide information, in an understandable form, about the severity of dental disease in Moree and its preventability. However, many individuals and communities, especially Aborigines, perceive that they lack the power to produce a positive change or see the report as irrelevant, either because of the cultural values and beliefs involved, or as in the case of the white middle classes, as a notion that oral health can be purchased when required. In this regard, oral health is socially constructed in different ways by different people in terms of the meanings they form about dentistry, the norms about oral health that exist in their community and the economic power they are able to wield.

Community involvement. Whilst better decision making is seen as flowing from community involvement, Dwyer (1989:59) asserts that community involvement is often actually 'seeking to legitimize decisions already made by the bureaucracy'. Admittedly, the dental surveys carried out by Patterson and his dental team were designed to foster a feeling of local involvement in their community's oral health, with an initial long term view of 'educating' the community towards the benefits of water fluoridation. This was an attempt to lower two of the barriers to effective community participation listed by Dwyer (1989:61), professional guardianship of knowledge and the perpetuation of bureaucratic goals. Just as Epp (1987:423–426) sees the fostering of public participation as central to effective health promotion strategies so too did the project managers of 'Teeth for Keeps'.

Moreover, in allowing schools to choose which research group they wished to participate in, and therefore giving them the ability to decide a level of commitment more appropriate to their wishes, problems with co-operation during the project were minimized. As mentioned above, the research groups consisted of a variety of combinations, from school based project interventions to no intervention at all.

In some communities there was also a preoccupation with the need to provide some clinical services urgently, which initially created a block to the acceptance of the oral health promotion activities. Provision of relevant clinical and preventive services in conjunction with oral health promotion strategies has facilitated the acceptance of both. Therefore, in the Moree district, oral health promotion without access to dental treatment for individuals is seen to be unacceptable and inappropriate.

The takeover and complete ownership of the 'Teeth for Keeps' Project by the Dental Health Liaison Committee at the end of 1991 after further funding was secured is evidence of the ultimate goal of any health promotion program—community involvement and control.

Cost effectiveness. Attwood and Blinkhorn (1989:81) report that the costs of dental treatment in a fluoridated town were approximately 57% lower than in non-fluoridated areas whilst Burt (1989:334) notes that the most cost effective strategy next to water fluoridation, costs of which he estimates at between 75 cents to $6.76 per person per annum, is a fluoride mouth rinse program, with savings to be made of up to $15 per tooth surface saved. However, Mann (1988:198) sees fluoride mouth rinse programs as only moderately practical and effective, though Warner (1989:278) concludes that improved cost effectiveness can be observed in non-fluoridated areas with poor toothbrushing practices. Parviainen and Ainamo (1989:298–299) also found that there may be significant benefits for the DMFT rate in children brushing once per day with a fluoride toothpaste. In the Moree Plains Shire, as water fluoridation was too controversial, a weekly fluoride mouth rinse program was seen as the next most cost-effective strategy with daily toothbrushing being beneficial for those children who did not possess a toothbrush at home and/or needed to develop their personal skills in toothbrushing dexterity.

Butler (1991:1–2) concludes that oral health education in schools has at best 'a short term impact', whilst Russell, Horowitz and Frazier (1989:199) reported students as learning and retaining knowledge formally taught, but lacking an awareness and value of the practical application of such knowledge. In the 'Teeth for Keeps' Project it is hoped that the combination of oral health education, self-care practices, availability to dental services, access to better nutrition and a supportive school environment will ensure a long term impact on oral health status.

In line with the views expressed by Warner (1989:273) the 'Teeth for Keeps' Project will need to be monitored longitudinally to assess any problems dealing with opportunity costs, social, economic and environmental factors, priorities placed on the communities' and dental professionals' time and the effect that existing levels of dental disease and toothache have on resource allocation decisions.

Intersectoral collaboration. Russell, Horowitz and Frazier (1989:198) see health professionals as being indispensable in providing disease specific information to communities. In this respect, the W*ho Caries?* study which was initiated and implemented by the dental health team in the New England Health Region has been extensively cited as the reason that oral health is 'back on the agenda' in Moree. More importantly, it is seen in a positive light and not surrounded in controversy.

At the International Conference on Health Promotion it was pointed out that community health needs cannot be met by health services alone (Editor 1987:iii-iv). The Moree Dental Health Liaison Committee provides a good example of how strategies can be developed on a local level to address oral health issues of concern to a defined population. The Dental Health Liaison Committee (1990:1) includes in its terms of reference the following:

• the development of guidelines for activities families should undertake to ensure dental health;
• to recommend appropriate action by the local hospital and community health services with respect to improving dental health in the Moree district;
• to develop and recommend educational strategies for the community;
• to recommend an appropriate role for the Shire Council.

The role of the 'Teeth for Keeps' project managers and co-ordinators (Lucy Allan, Helen Cahill and Dianne Maunder) was seen as that of consultants to that committee. Moreover, the Project would not have been possible without corporate sponsorship to the value of $130 000.

Finally, the innovative use of the press and public relations activities to inform people may be invaluable' (Gardner 1989:425). In Moree, the role of the Moree *Champion,* the 'Everybody' ABC TV show and the local radio station was crucial as the 'Molar Patroller', 'Turtles' and the 'Teeth for Keeps' logo have certainly captured the imagination of the community and have been instrumental in oral health issues receiving more balanced and positive press. Indeed, the 'Turtles' were featured in the *Health Promotion Journal of Australia* (Patterson 1992:64).

Discussion

Differences in health status measure distribution of power and competence in society. Lifestyle diseases are no longer diseases of affluence but an unnecessary burden on disadvantaged groups (Kickbusch 1987: 437).

Muhondwa (1986:1247-1256) questions whether primary health care is an apolitical, value-free, organizational system or a 'stop gap' measure pending socioeconomic improvement in communities and an alternative health care system for the underprivileged. Clarke, Allen, McBay and Heaney (1990:27) conclude that whilst the 'top down' approach to health planning is encountering increasing resistance from consumers, the problem remains that frequently the voice of the disadvantaged is not heard. Taking this into account, the 'Teeth for Keeps' Project can be seen as an example of the interplay between the plight of disadvantaged groups and the capabilities of organizations which resulted in a combined top down/ bottom up approach.

In analysing the notion of 'empowerment' of people in primary health care settings, Grace argues that 'the problem is that professionals are still required to develop, plan, implement and evaluate most programs' based on their own value systems (1991:331). The dilemma for the project managers is that as 'experts', probably the most beneficial strategy to improve the oral health status of *all* persons in the Moree community dramatically would be to fluoridate the water supplies in the area. However, community opposition to such a move is not to be underestimated or devalued, though it is interesting to note that those who would most benefit from fluoridation have little influence in the community and have had little to say on the matter until now. It is also important to state that the rejection by the project managers of water fluoridation as a strategy in the 'Teeth for Keeps' Project, caused a considerable amount of friction with some members of the dental profession and some individuals within the community, which is still being felt today.

The 'role of public values in developing fairer and more rational allocation rules is largely undefined' (Hadorn 1991:773). To take this proposition further, whilst arguing that devolution of power and decision making in areas such as health are undeniably noble objectives, caution must be exercised in not simply substituting bureaucratic value judgements with the value judgements of a socioeconomically and politically powerful minority in a community, for they may be so individually subjective that they largely ignore the 'collective good' of the community. In this instance, the composition of the Dental Health Liaison Committee has come under criticism as it may not be representative of all communities in the Moree Plains Shire.

The results of the project

The Moree 'Teeth for Keeps' Project is continuing. Dental disease is now seen as a health, and not a fluoridation issue, in the community. Moreover, the vast majority of schoolchildren have access to acute care and toothbrushes, and oral health promotion strategies continue to be implemented.

Early analysis of the quantitative and qualitative data analysis from the 'Teeth for Keeps' Project shows that the percentage of children urgently requiring treatment dropped from 13% to 8.5%, children requiring routine treatment dropped from 28% to 20%, and children requiring no treatment rose from 59% to 71%. Following clinical intervention and an increased community awareness with regard to appropriate dental care, the majority of teachers wanted the project to continue and some requested to be more actively involved. The community seminars were seen to be worthwhile and one Principal said that the people involved in the project were the 'first people to ever do anything'. The Oral Health Education Training Course also proved to be a very successful and beneficial day.

The success of the 'Teeth for Keeps' Project can be seen in the fact that the NSW Department of Health continued funding the project for seven months and both the Aboriginal and the non-Aboriginal co-ordinators gained full-time employment through expansion of the Project. Moreover, the Moree Plains Shire Council and the NSW Department of Health agreed to fund the project for a further three years at a shared cost of approximately $60 000 per year. This is the first preventive oral health promotion project to be funded by a local government association in New South Wales, if not

Australia.

In addition to this, corporate sponsorship from dental companies and other corporations including Oral B, Colgate, Wrigleys and Concept Licences totalled $130 000. Since 1990 the NSW Department of Health has contributed a further $21 000 through the Rural Dental Scheme and has supplied funds for a further motor vehicle. Moreover, an additional Commonwealth research grant totalling $103 000 has been obtained to establish a course of studies leading to a Certificate in Oral Health Promotion at the University of New England, Armidale, in conjunction with the NSW Department of Health.

The *Who Caries?* study and the 'Teeth for Keeps' Project, combined with the costs associated with the three year funding for the additional dental officer and dental assistant, attracted corporate sponsorship and government funds in excess of $922 000.

Finally, the project has stimulated the active involvement of dental professionals in oral health promotion as well as intersectoral collaboration between corporate sponsors and various sectors of local, State and federal governments. It has also aroused the active participation of the local community, which now 'owns' the 'Teeth for Keeps' Project.

Conclusion

The strategies utilized in the 'Teeth for Keeps' Project to reduce inequalities in oral health status also created conditions for empowerment and community-building in line with the new public health movement, a scenario which the alternate strategy of water fluoridation would not have been able to achieve. The primary health care strategies implemented with this project amount to an about face in promoting oral health and preventing dental disease in a sensitive rural area of New South Wales.

REFERENCES

Anderson I 1988 Koori health in Koori hands: an orientation manual in Aboriginal health for health-care providers. Health Department Victoria, Melbourne
Ashton J 1990 Public health and primary care: towards a common agenda. Public Health 104:387–398
Attwood D, Blinkhorn A S 1989 Reassessment of the effect of fluoridation on cost of dental treatment among Scottish schoolchildren. Community Dental Oral Epidemiology 17:79–82
Australian Council of Social Service and the Consumers' Health Forum 1992 Healthy, wealthy and wise: a consultation broadsheet on income, environment and health. Australian Council of Social Service, Sydney
Brown E R 1991 Community action for health promotion: a strategy to empower individuals and communities. International Journal of Health Services 21(3):441–456
Burt B A (ed) 1989 Results of the workshop on cost effectiveness of caries preventive measures. Journal of Public Health Dentistry (Special Issue) 49(5):331–340
Butler R J F 1991 Dental health education for schoolchildren: a strategy for prevention or merely a public relations exercise? Unpublished paper
Clarke R M, Allen G, McBay S, Heaney S 1990 Improving the quality of community health surveys and community health promotion campaigns by feedback from the community:

experience from the Wallsend community health project. Community Health Studies XIV(1):27–33

Community Health Services 1992 Dental health promotion programme for Vietnamese children. Central Sydney Health Service, Camperdown

Correll D 1992 National health strategy and Medicare agreements. Health Forum 24:7–9

Dooland M 1992 Improving dental health in Australia: national health strategy background paper no 9. Department of Health, Housing and Community Services, Canberra

Dwyer J 1989 The politics of participation. Community Health Studies, XIII(1):59–72

Editor 1987 Ottawa charter for health promotion. Health Promotion 1(4):iii–v

Epp J The Hon 1987 Achieving health for all: a framework for health promotion. Health Promotion 1(4):419–428

Franklin M-A, White I 1991 The history and politics of Aboriginal health. In: Reid J, Trompf P (eds) The health of Aboriginal Australia. Harcourt Brace Jovanovich, Sydney

Gardner H 1989 The politics of health: the Australian experience. Churchill Livingstone, Melbourne

Grace V M 1991 The marketing of empowerment and the construction of the health consumer: a critique of health promotion. International Journal of Health Services 21(2):329–343

Grant C, Lapsley H M 1992 The Australian health care system 1991. University of New South Wales, Sydney

Hadorn D C 1991 The role of public values in setting health care priorities. Social Science and Medicine 32(7):773–781

Harrison L 1993 Dental health in primary school, first draft. Southern Sydney Area Health Service, Kogarah

Hawe P, Degeling D, Hall J 1990 Evaluating health promotion. MacLennan & Petty, Sydney

Health Promotion Unit 1991 Dental care for Arabic speaking Families. Southern Sydney Area Health Service, Kogarah

Humphreys J S, Weinand H C 1989 Health status and health care in rural Australia: a case study. Community Health Studies XIII(3):258–272

Hunter P B, Kirk R, de Liefde B 1992 The study of oral health outcomes: the 1988 New Zealand section of the WHO second international collaborative study. Department of Health, Wellington

Huntley B 1991 Problems in recruitment, retention and continuing professional education of health professionals in rural and remote areas. Thesis, University of New England, Armidale

Kickbusch I 1989 Self-care in health promotion. Social Science and Medicine 29(2):125–130

Lismore School Dental Clinic 1992 The dental force kit. Brainstorm Productions, Byron Bay NSW

Mann M L 1988 Planning for community programs. In: Jong A W (ed) Community dental health, 2nd edn. Mosby, St Louis, pp 180–206

McClellan A, Pirkis J, Willcox S 1992 Enough to make you sick: how income and environment effect health. Department of Health, Housing and Community Services, Canberra

Muhondwa E P Y 1986 Rural development and primary health care in less developed countries. Social Science and Medicine 22(11):1247–1256

NSW Task Force on Aboriginal Health 1990 The last report: report to the NSW minister for health. December, Sydney

Nutbeam D, Wise M, Bauman A, Leeder S 1992 Review and revision of the national health goals and targets, progress report. University of Sydney, Sydney

P A Consulting Group 1989 Review of NSW rural health and aged care services. P A Consulting Group, North Sydney

Parviainen K, Ainamo J 1989. Influence of increased toothbrushing frequency on dental health in low, optimal and high fluoride areas in Finland. Community Dental Oral Epidemiology 17:296–299

Patterson A F 1990 Who caries? a report on the dental status of children in the Moree district, New England, NSW. Unpublished

Patterson A F 1992 'Teeth for keeps' oral health promotion program. Health Promotion Journal of Australia 2(2):64

Russell B A, Horowitz A M, Frazier P J 1989 School based preventive regimens and oral health knowledge and practices of sixth graders, Journal of Public Health Dentistry, 49(4):192–200

Ryan P 1992 Cases for change: CHASP in practice. Australian Community Health Association, Sydney

Saggers S, Gray D 1991 Aboriginal health and society: the traditional and contemporary Aboriginal struggle for better health. Allen & Unwin, Sydney

Sinclair D, Griffiths M 1993 The tooth: the hole truth and nothing but the truth. Blacktown and Mt Druitt Community Health Services, Blacktown

Sindall C 1992 An overview of theory and practice. In: Baum F, Fry D, Lennie I (eds) 1992 Community health policy and practice in Australia. Pluto Press, Sydney

South Australian Health Commission and the South Australian Community Health Association 1992 The changing face of health: a primary health care casebook. South Australian Health Commission, Adelaide

Warner K E 1989 Issues in cost effectiveness in health care. Journal of Public Health Dentistry (Special Issue) 49(5):272–278

24. Promoting the health of older people

Colette J. Browning   Hal Kendig   Karen Teshuva

Considerable attention is being given to the growing numbers of older Australians. On the positive side, there is more recognition of the political power of older people and the continuing capacities and contributions of the vast majority of them. Yet stereotypes of older people as frail and dependent remain very powerful and continue to undermine their self respect and life chances. The media frequently portrays population ageing as a 'demographic doomsday' which will impoverish governments (Minichiello et al 1992). These contradictory social images of ageing are reflected in dilemmas and inconsistencies in developing health policies and delivering health care. They underscore the need for developing policies which are based on a careful appreciation of social values concerning older people and the facts concerning their diverse preferences, capacities, and vulnerabilities.

There are a number of reasons for taking age into account when considering the fairness of health outcomes and health systems. Negative attitudes towards older people can limit their chances of having access to resources on the basis of their needs (Sax in press). In the competition for scarce resources, there are strong pressures for health systems to provide better for powerful groups (such as middle aged men) or highly valued groups (such as new born babies) than for groups such as very old and poor women. Fair provision for older people in the mainstream of health services requires advocacy to break down barriers in gaining access to care and ensuring the provision of sensitive and appropriate services (Andrews & Carr 1990, Kendig 1989). A small minority of older people, who have severe and multiple difficulties, may be able to receive appropriate and fair provision only when they have specialized services.

Our knowledge of the ageing process and health is limited but there is encouraging evidence for taking a positive approach to health in old age. It is a major social achievement that people are living longer. As compared to earlier cohorts, Australians now entering old age have more personal and economic resources (Rowland 1991) and overseas studies suggest that health on retirement also is better than in the past (Svanborg 1988). Older people are as likely as any other age group to be satisfied with their life and the vast majority remain substantially independent and socially involved.

Moreover, there is increasing evidence that health in old age can be improved through action throughout the life span with benefits forthcoming in old age (Teshuva et al 1993). For example, moderate exercise can improve well-being as well as mobility for people in their seventies and eighties. For people who have a chronic illness or disability, a small margin of extra fitness can have a critical bearing on maintaining capacity.

Older people of course are concerned about illness and death but they tend to view health primarily as a resource which influences how they feel and what they can do in their daily lives. From this perspective medical 'treatment' is one of many influences on health. Equally if not more important are lifestyles, the supportiveness of family and friends, and 'structural' factors which extend beyond the individual. Structural forces such as social class, prevailing social attitudes, and physical environments have important health consequences over the entire life course and have particularly strong effects in old age. The various individual and structural factors can interrelate in complex ways. For example, an older woman may be frail and have osteoporosis. A fall, broken hip, and then entry to a nursing home may reflect a chain of events which could also include an unsafe footpath, side effects of medication, delays in resetting the fracture, insufficient rehabilitation, and not having anyone (or enough money) to have help to return home.

The complex relationships between ageing and health make it imperative to adopt a broad view of health promotion for older people. As the above example suggests, the scope of relevant policy can extend far beyond health care to include also income support, street planning and maintenance, and even education influencing images of ageing. It requires a balance in meeting diverse needs which vary greatly within as well as between age groups. Further, it involves developing actions which are acceptable to all parties involved including older people themselves, providers of services, funding bodies, and the general public.

The health status of older people

In order to promote good health in old age it is necessary to understand how health is conceptualized by both the research community and older people themselves. Older people's own health goals have often been neglected in health promotion programs and improving quality of life and independence are relatively recent goals of interventions (Teshuva et al 1993).

The traditional way of measuring the health of populations is to determine mortality (deaths), morbidity (illness and disability) and risk factors associated with various illnesses. An alternative way to conceptualize health is to seek older people's views using qualitative methodologies. This approach is discussed later in the chapter.

Table 24.1 Life expectancy for Australian males and females, 1901–1910 and 1990

| Year | Life expectancy (years) | |
	Males	Females
1901–1910	55.2	58.8
1990	73.9	80.0

Source: Australian Bureau of Statistics 1992 Social Indicators. AGPS, Commonwealth of Australia copyright, reproduced with permission.

Mortality

During this century Australia and other western countries have experienced a steady decline in mortality rates. Table 24.1 shows that over this century the life expectancy at birth has increased by approximately 19 years for men and 22 years for women; women are even more likely now to live longer than men. Among those who have already reached 60 years of age, men can expect to live another 18 years and women can expect another 23 years. As a result of declining death and birth rates, the proportion and numbers of people over 65 years of age have increased over this period. There will be especially large rises in the number of people aged 75 years and over during the 1990s and the numbers aged 60 years and over will rise rapidly next century when the large 'baby boom' cohort reaches old age (Minichiello et al 1992).

The leading causes of death for both males and females 65 years and over

Table 24.2 Causes of death, 1990

| Cause of death | Males | Females |
	% of deaths	
65–74 years		
Cancer	39	41
Cardiovascular disease	36	33
Obstructive airways disease	9	7
Cerebrovascular disease	8	11
75–84 years		
Cardiovascular disease	38	47
Cancer	31	24
Cerebrovascular disease	13	20
Obstructive airways disease	10	–
85 years and over		
Cardiovascular disease	47	54
Cancer	22	14
Cerebrovascular disease	17	27

Source: Australian Bureau of Statistics 1992 Social Indicators. AGPS, Commonwealth of Australia copyright, reproduced with permission.

Table 24.3 Hospital admission rates in New South Wales and South Australia, 1988

Age group (years)	Admission rate (per 1000 population)		
	Males	Females	Persons
65–74	471.0	351.2	405.9
75 and over	649.0	498.0	552.7
All ages	197.4	237.9	216.0

Source: Australia's Health 1992: the 3rd biennial report of the Australian Institute of Health and Welfare 1992. AGPS, Commonwealth of Australia copyright, reproduced with permission.

are cancer, cardiovascular disease, cerebrovascular disease and obstructive airways disease. These patterns vary, however, across age group and sex (see Table 24.2). For males, cancer and cardiovascular disease remain the main causes of death in all older age groups. For women this relationship holds until 85 years and over where cardiovascular disease and cerebrovascular disease are the two main causes of death.

Morbidity

Morbidity of a population has typically been measured by hospital admissions. This type of data focuses on serious episodes of illness and does not necessarily indicate the types of illnesses and disabilities present in the community (Australian Institute of Health and Welfare 1992). The figures in Table 24.3 indicate that people 65 years and over have about twice the rate of admissions to hospital than the general population and men show higher rates of admission than women. Overall, older people use approximately half of the bed days in acute hospitals. The relatively high use of hospitals is a major reason why the health care costs to government are much higher for older people than for younger people (Goss 1992).

The National Health Survey (Australian Bureau of Statistics 1991a) collected information on Australia's health status, health-related actions and

Table 24.4 Proportion of recent illnesses per 1000 of population, 1989-1990

Age group (years)	Proportion (per 1000 population)	
	Males	Females
65–74		
Hypertension	304.5	382.9
Arthritis	171.9	237.6
75 and over		
Hypertension	242.4	393.7
Arthritis	194.3	289.5

Source: Australia's Health 1992: the 3rd biennial report of the Australian Institute of Health and Welfare 1992. AGPS, Commonwealth of Australia copyright, reproduced with permission.

Table 24.5 Handicap, percentages by age and sex, 1988

Age	Sex	% with disability
60–74	Males	37.6
	Females	29.7
75 and over	Males	53.0
	Females	61.1

Source: Australian Bureau of Statistics 1990 Disability
and Handicap Survey 1990. AGPS, Commonwealth of
Australia copyright, reproduced with permission.

health risk factors. Table 24.4 shows the proportions of older men and
women who have experienced recently two of the most common and serious
illnesses in people over 65 years of age: arthritis and hypertension. It should
be noted that hypertension is a risk factor for cardiovascular disease and
cerebrovascular disease, two of the major causes of mortality and morbidity
in older people. Arthritis is a disabling condition which can lead to a
reduction in mobility, independence and quality of life.

To understand the effects of health on people's lives it is important to
move beyond the statistics on hospital admissions and recent illnesses. The
World Health Organization (WHO) defines disability as '...any restriction or
lack of ability to perform any activity...considered normal...' (1980:28). The
Australian Bureau of Statistics (ABS) has conducted surveys which measure
disability and handicaps. Their definition of a handicap is a limitation in
capacity to perform functional tasks related to self-care, mobility, verbal
communication, schooling or employment. Table 24.5 shows that, in the
group 75 years and over, more than half report having a 'handicap'.

Another way of looking at health in old age is the idea of active life
expectancy (i.e. 'disability free' years). Studies in the United States (Manton
1988) and Australia (Mathers 1991) suggest that increasing longevity is
resulting in more years of disability than years of relatively good health.

The health perceptions and practices of older people

The statistics on illness and disability paint a grim picture of old age.
However, a different picture emerges when older people are asked to assess
their own health. The paradox is that 70% of older people have one or more
chronic illness, but studies consistently show that only 10 to 20% would rate
themselves as having poor health. The explanation is that older people
generally rate their health as good when they can cope with stress or pain and
can maintain their daily activities and social contacts (Blaxter 1990). A
qualitative study in Sydney found that older people associated the 'feeling of
health' with social involvement with family, friends and young people,
regular engagement in activities, independence and a healthy mental state
(Saltman et al 1989).

A study of frail older Australians found that many who would be classified as disabled by ABS criteria did not regard themselves in this way and still tried to maintain a high level of independence (Davison et al 1992). A 95-year-old informant, who had several chronic illnesses and difficulty walking, says:

I have managed here all these years. It's only just lately that I haven't been able to do quite so much. I haven't been able to do all the things, but I practically do everything. I have only had a helper once a month that—well, they don't do anything anyway, not very much, but that doesn't matter. They just call in and I find them a little job, a bit of shopping if necessary. I've just carried on ever since. I've done everything myself, cleaned the place and shopped, cooked and every-thing. I had Meals on Wheels once for three weeks; I thought I would try them and I had three weeks and I couldn't eat it...So I used to always like cooking, so that was no trouble...so I still cook.

It is also interesting to note that older people's rating of their own health has been found to be a good predictor of mortality (Mossey & Shapiro 1982).

Behavioural factors in the health of older people

The relationship between personal health behaviours and health outcomes has been well established through epidemiological studies. For example, cardiovascular disease is linked to sedentary lifestyles, smoking and a high fat diet; and cancer is linked to poor diet and smoking (Svanborg 1988). This knowledge has given rise to health promotion programs which have attempted to target these behaviours for change. Health promotion has traditionally aimed to prevent premature illness and death by targeting risk behaviours early in the life span. There is increasing interest in health promotion for older people including guides for action by older people themselves (Gingold 1992).

Controversy exists over the benefits of protective health practices in older persons. Branch and Jette (1984) examined the effects on mortality of five health behaviours: physical activity, sleep patterns, smoking patterns, alcohol use and regularity of meals. Smoking by women (but not men) was the only health behaviour associated with higher risk of mortality. The authors concluded that these results do not support the findings with younger groups that health-protective behaviours reduce mortality. However, Guralnik and Kaplan (1989) report prospective evidence relating lifestyle and health behaviours to functional ability and emotional well-being. Similarly, Green and Gottlieb (1989) concluded that health related behaviours over the entire life span are key influences on quality of life and the self-reported health status in old age. These findings are important because promoting health in old age involves more emphasis on independence and quality of life than on illness prevention. Examining the health behaviours and beliefs of older people can help us design appropriate interventions.

A number of studies show that older people are more likely to practise good health habits than younger people. Bausell (1986), for example, reported compliance with various health behaviours among younger and

Table 24.6   Health behaviour indicators by age and sex, 1989-1990

	Consumes alcohol (%)	Current smoker (%)	Does not exercise (%)	Overweight or obese (%)
Males				
18 to 65	75.4	34.4	35.1	44.5
65 to 74	64.6	19.7	34.8	50.6
75 and over	52.8	11.1	41.4	33.7
Females				
18 to 64	73.9	27.6	34.1	29.7
65 to 74	39.3	13.8	38.8	41.2
75 and over	31.2	6.3	57.1	31.9

Source: Australian Bureau of Statistics 1992 National Health Survey 1989-90: Summary of Results, Australia. AGPS, Commonwealth of Australia copyright, reproduced with permission.

older people. Although there was great variability in compliance between behaviours, the older group were more compliant for nine of the 20 behaviours (including blood pressure checks, the avoidance of foods with high salt and fat content). The older group placed more importance on health behaviours that are thought to help people live longer and healthier. The younger group were more optimistic about the control they had over their future health.

In Australia, the National Health Survey (Australian Bureau of Statistics 1992b) asked people about their health practices and behavioural risk factors (Table 24.6) In terms of alcohol consumption in the week preceding interview, both men and women 65 and over are less likely to consume alcohol than those aged 18 to 64. Older people also consume less volume of alcohol than those aged less than 65. Similarly, for both males and females the rates of smoking for people 65 and over are considerably less than for those less than 65 years. Older people also tend to smoke fewer cigarettes per day than those aged under 65 (Australian Bureau of Statistics 1992b).

Older people are less likely than younger people to exercise. Exercise refers to physical exercise (recreational, sport or health and fitness) undertaken in the two weeks prior to interview. The largest proportion of non-exercisers are women 75 years and over. Walking was very important to the older age groups and it was the only form of exercise for 68% of people aged 75 years and over. Although this level of activity may not improve aerobic fitness, it may be sufficient to reduce some mobility problems and improve quality of life (Teshuva et al 1993).

At all age levels males are more likely than females to be overweight or obese. Between the ages of mid-fifties to mid-seventies there was a decline in the proportion of people overweight or obese (Teshuva et al 1993). In the age group 75 and over about one third of people are overweight or obese. In the two years prior to interview, the group least likely to have changed their diet were those 65 and over. The main reasons that older people had changed their diet were ageing or physical changes and to improve their health.

In summary, although older people are likely to engage in some healthy lifestyle practices, there is still a significant proportion of people over 65 years who could reduce their weight, give up smoking and exercise more. McPherson (1986) states that more than 50% of older adults have no health restrictions on physical activity, suggesting that psychosocial factors are important contributors to a sedentary lifestyle. The potential benefit of lifestyle changes (Horwath 1991) are considerable. For most older people, probably the single most important health message is to achieve or maintain at least moderate levels of physical activity. The health benefits of exercise include cardiovascular, musculoskeletal, psychosocial benefits, and improvement in fat and carbohydrate metabolism (Evans & Meredith 1989).

Studies like the National Health Survey provide information about the types of behaviours that need to be targeted for promoting health in older people. However, we need to know much more about 'modifiable' influences on health-related outcomes in old age (Ory 1991). Loss of control, excessive stress, the absence of social supports, life events, life strain, and loneliness have all been linked to decreased longevity and a decline in well-being (Revicki & Mitchell 1990). Ory (1991) suggests that health knowledge and beliefs are important predictors of health-protective behaviour. A major literature review of the field (Teshuva et al 1993) suggests that broader efforts to improve the social status and living conditions of older people would yield substantial returns in improved health and better quality of life.

Priority health conditions for older people

A working party on the Health Status of Older People, convened by the Victorian Health Promotion Foundation, identified priority health issues for older adults in Australia. The researchers, program planners, and clinicians on the working party determined that priority should be directed to health conditions which are potentially preventable or postponable; have a significant bearing on the independence and well-being of older people; and have important consequences for the health system. The six priority health conditions, as reviewed below, have a broader focus than the prevention of specific diseases. Similar priorities in health promotion for older people are found in other countries, for example, the United States (US Department of Health and Human Services Surgeon General's Workshop 1988). An extensive review of each of these conditions is available in Teshuva et al (1993).

Physical capacities

Physical limitations are the main causes of the high rates of disability among older people. These include musculoskeletal problems, visual and hearing impairments, foot problems and loss of balance (Imms & Edholm 1979, Manchester et al 1989). These conditions can be painful and reduce functional ability, leading to isolation, loss of independence, psychological reactions and reliance on support services. Losses in physical capacities are also related to other health conditions such as the likelihood of falling and fluctuations in appetite (Grieg et al 1986). Good foot, vision and hearing care, movement and exercise play an important role in preventing disability (Robinson 1989, Ayalon et al 1987, Hopkins et al 1990). Helme et al (1991) present Australian findings on ways to control pain, and consequent distress and debilitation, by combining medication, physiotherapy and psychological interventions.

Inappropriate use of medication

Older people are reported to have a high use of prescribed drugs, especially psychotropic drugs, and they are likely to use several drugs simultaneously (Australian Bureau of Statistics 1991b). While medication is of course central to the treatment of many illnesses, inappropriate use of drugs can cause confusion, agitation, depression, postural hypotension and dyskinesias (McMillan et al 1986). Older people are reported to experience approximately 25% of adverse drug reactions in Australia leading to hospitalization. Australian and overseas research shows that drugs are prescribed for social and personal problems such as anxiety, sleeplessness or a family crisis, and that this is often done without attempting non-medication strategies (Mant et al 1988). Environmental and behavioural interventions have been proposed as preferable to psychotropic drugs in addressing problems such as anxiety and insomnia (Chapman 1976). The risks of medication and the benefits of alternatives are receiving increasing attention in health education for older people, medical practitioners, and pharmacists.

Falls and injuries

Community studies in Australasia and abroad (Campbell et al 1981, Tinetti et al 1988) estimate that a third of persons aged 65 years or more have fallen once or more per year. Among older people falls are the major cause of injury and a significant cause of death, hospitalization, and loss of independence (Fildes et al 1990). Overseas studies show that falls can seriously increase anxiety, loss of confidence, and social withdrawal (Romer & Macfadyen 1987). Strategies for preventing falls by older people include thorough education and assessment of at risk individuals, monitoring medication use, and elimination of environmental hazards (Fildes 1993, Walker et al 1991).

Cardiovascular health

The results of the ABS National Health Survey (1991c) suggest that declining mortality from cardiovascular disease is resulting in more people living with consequent disabilities. Unfortunately, most current assumptions about exercise, diet, and other influences on cardiovascular disease in older people are based on data extrapolated from studies of people in middle age. However, a recent review of hypertension in people over 65 years concludes that hypertension remains a risk factor for cardiovascular morbidity and mortality in those aged up to 80 years (Leaverton et al 1990). Australian cardiovascular disease prevention programs, such as the Australian National Blood Pressure Study, have focused on a wide age range with little attention to possible differences between the middle and older age populations. Increasing exercise among older people has been shown to significantly improve the cardiovascular health of older people.

Psychological well-being and depression

Of the various psychological difficulties which can be faced at any age, depression is especially widespread with an estimated 15 to 20% of older people. Diagnosis of depression is problematical and the condition in older people is often confused with dementia resulting in incorrect treatment (Kiloh 1981). Depression has a direct and obvious effect on quality of life and also elevates mortality rates (Murphy et al 1988) and it is by far the most common psychiatric illness leading older people to attempt suicide (Pierce 1987). On present knowledge there is ample scope for prevention and treatment of depression (Livingstone et al 1990). General practitioners have a significant role to play in diagnosing and treating late-life depression (Yeatman 1991). The emotional well-being and mental health of older people also can be expected to benefit considerably from broad based social strategies which increase the incomes, social status, and social involvement of older people.

Urinary incontinence

Urinary incontinence is a distressing condition estimated to affect about 800 000 adults in Australia, including up to 15% of older people in the community (Fonda et al 1988). Women are especially at risk. Urinary incontinence can have profound psychosocial effects such as shame, isolation, and depression (Ory et al 1986). It also is estimated to cost hundreds of millions of dollars each year for care in hospitals and nursing homes and is a major factor for the institutionalization of older people. Difficulties with urinary incontinence among older people can be limited, however, by behavioural therapies and exercise of pelvic muscles and bladder control. Appropriate use of medication is another important influence in reducing the prevalence of urinary continence.

Health promotion policies and programs

Governments in Australia have begun to promote the health of older people actively. The *Health for All* report (Health Targets and Implementation

Committee 1988) established the health of older people as a priority area and set increasing independence as a goal. Subsequently the Older People Project Planning Team, on the basis of extensive consultations, recommended initiatives to promote social participation, integrate health and welfare services, and develop more informed interventions (Lin 1989). The National Better Health Program also placed special emphasis on older people (Department of Health, Housing and Community Services 1993). The National Goals and Targets for Australia's Health (Nutbeam et al 1993) identify many areas where older people are mentioned as a priority target for improving health status.

Health services

The older person's interaction with health care services and professionals provides a very significant avenue for promoting health. Andrews and Carr (1990) and Sax (in press) outline how general practitioners can have a crucial role in leading a holistic response to the health of older individuals. Preliminary studies (Saltman et al 1989) suggest that general practitioners (along with spouses, adult children, and friends) are an important influence on older people's knowledge, attitudes and health behaviours. Nonetheless, prevention is only recently gaining attention in the literature on Australian general practitioners (Macklin 1992) and other health professionals.

A recent study of people who used general practitioners showed that people over 60 years of age can articulate their requirements of doctors (Dickens et al 1993). A major theme in this study was that older people wanted their doctor to not just provide technical care but to provide reassurance and empathy. For example one informant expressed his needs as follows:

Young people...would obviously regard doctors as a kind of technical person... to get information and...treatment...but as you get older you depend on a doctor not only just simply for advice and treatment and medication but you are looking for a kind of understanding a kind of sympathy, a kind of relationship which makes much more demands on the doctor himself to give you total satisfaction...

These views are probably related to the type of problem that older people present to doctors. Many informants expressed the view that they went to the doctor for a check-up. For example, another informant, in referring to his father (aged 88) who visits the doctor once a month states:

...my father goes to the doctor every month and that keeps him going because he is reassured that everything is working, his pacemaker...the doctor becomes a reassuring factor...

The National Health Strategy recently released an issue paper on the future of general practice in which it was argued that one of the roles of general practitioners is to engage in prevention such as cancer detection and encouraging preventive health and also to manage '...chronic illness to improve people's quality of life...' (Macklin 1992:29). The National Health

Strategy's 'Pathways to Better Health' (Macklin 1993) and the Evaluation of the National Better Health Program (Department of Health, Housing and Community Services 1993) argue that the entire health care system, including acute hospitals, have important responsibilities to promote health and prevent illness as well as treat disease. Health promotion objectives (Nutbeam et al 1993) are being incorporated into the Medicare Agreements which form the basis for Commonwealth funding of State services. However, the spate of recent policy documents all recognize that a reorientation of health systems towards more health promotion is a difficult and long term process which will require major changes in the cultures and perceived interests of providers of health care as well as the public.

Health promotion programs

The National Better Health Program set the health of older people as its only population based target group and 31 projects (8% of the total budget) were funded. The Victorian Better Health Committee (1991) and the Victorian Health Promotion Foundation have argued for combining a life span perspective in health promotion while maintaining a focus specifically on older people for particular projects. In New South Wales the Healthy Older People Project (NSW Department of Health 1989) recommended a comprehensive strategy that emphasized increasing the information, skills, and resources of older people.

The National Better Health program and State Health Promotion Foundations have funded a number of interventions which aim to increase opportunities for exercise, self care, social involvement, and appropriate medication use (Department of Health, Housing and Community Services 1993). Approaches range from social marketing and community education through to community development and advocacy. The national evaluation of the program noted that the health promotion projects for older people generally had been small scale, community based efforts. It was noted that the programs were hampered by short time frames and were considered to be at an early stage of development. Only a few examples can be found for projects that are being thoroughly evaluated; for example, the Self Help for Older People Project (National Better Health Program 1991). Overseas evidence is also scanty on ways to implement effective health interventions for older people (Hickey & Stillwell 1991). Sax (in press) argues that the major impact of the National Better Health programs may be to facilitate the emergence of a strong lobby of older people who will take more control of actions to improve their health.

Towards structural change

McKinlay (1989) among other writers has emphasized that race, class, and gender inequalities in health status are heavily influenced by exposures to social and physical environments. The National Health Targets and Goals report (Nutbeam et al 1993), after a good deal of discussion and lobbying on earlier drafts, eventually produced a strong statement arguing for creating healthy environments through concerted public and private reform in transport, housing, community services, and the workplace. Governments are recognizing the complementarity among preventive strategies, aged care and health care (Commonwealth Department of Health, Housing, and Community Services 1991, Victorian Better Health Committee 1991).

Marshall (1989) articulates the Canadian experience with multi-sectoral action as part of Healthy Public Policy initiatives for older people. These policies have emphasised a life span approach rather than separate treatment of particular life cycle groups. They have had a strong emphasis on making social structures more conducive to health rather than to change the behaviour of individuals (Marshall 1989, 1992). The government in Ontario has pursued healthy policies in a wide variety of areas with leadership coming from the top political levels rather than from within health organizations. There is no doubt of the desirability and potential effectiveness of these policies particularly for older people.

In Australia as well as other countries, the main issues for the future of health depend on the political strength of older people and the 'new public health' ideologies. Both of these social movements will need to be very strong to bring about significant change across the full range of sectors which influence the capacities of older people to live healthy, independent, and enjoyable lives.

REFERENCES

Andrews G, Carr S 1990 Health care for the aged. In: Kendig H, McCallum J (eds) Grey policy: Australian policies for an ageing society. Allen & Unwin, Sydney

Australian Bureau of Statistics 1990 Disability and handicap survey 1988. Australian Government Publishing Service, Canberra

Australian Bureau of Statistics 1991a National health survey 1989–1990. Australian Government Publishing Service, Canberra

Australian Bureau of Statistics 1991b National health survey 1989–1990: summary of results, Australia. Australian Government Publishing Service, Canberra

Australian Bureau of Statistics 1991c National health survey 1989–1990: cardiovascular conditions, Australia. Australian Government Publishing Service, Canberra

Australian Bureau of Statistics 1992a Social indicators. Australian Government Publishing Service, Canberra

Australian Bureau of Statistics 1992b National health survey 1989–1990: health risk factors. Australian Government Publishing Service, Canberra

Australian Institute of Health and Welfare 1992 Australia's health 1992: the third biennial report of the Australian Institute of Health and Welfare. Australian Government Publishing Service, Canberra

Ayalon J, Simkin A, Leichter I, Raifmann S 1987 Dynamic bone exercises for postmenopausal women: effect on the density on the distal radius. Archives of Physical Medicine and Rehabilitation 68:280–283

Bausell R 1986 Health-seeking behavior among the elderly. The Gerontologist 26(5):556–559

Blaxter M 1990 Health and lifestyles. Tavistock/Routledge, London

Branch L, Jette A 1984 Personal health practices and mortality among the elderly. American Journal of Public Health 74:1126–1129

Browning C 1992 Psychological aspects of ageing. In: Minichiello V, Jones D, Alexander L (eds) Gerontology: a multidisciplinary approach. Prentice Hall, Sydney

Campbell A J, Reinken J M, Allan B C 1981 Falls in old age: a study of frequency and related clinical factors. Age and Ageing 10:264–270

Chapman S 1976 Psychotropic drug use in the elderly. Connexions 7(5):10–14

Commonwealth Department of Health, Housing and Community Services 1991 Aged care reform strategy mid-term review 1990–1991: progress and directions. Australian Government Publishing Service, Canberra

Davison B, Kendig H, Stephens F, Merrill V 1993 It's my place: older people talk about their housing. Australian Government Publishing Service, Canberra

Department of Health, Housing and Community Services 1993 Towards health for all and health promotion: the evaluation of the National Better Health Program. Australian Government Publishing Service, Canberra

Dickens E, Browning C, Jellie C, Thomas S 1993 Older people's satisfaction with the services provided by general medical practitioners, Lincoln Papers in Gerontology no 18. Lincoln Gerontology Centre La Trobe University, Melbourne

Evans W J, Meredith C N 1989 Exercise and nutrition in the elderly. In: Munro H N, Danford D E (eds) Human nutrition: a comprehensive treatise of nutrition, aging and the elderly. Plenum Press, New York

Fildes B, Ozanne-Smith J, Hodge K, Dunt D 1990 Injury prevention amongst the elderly: interim report to the health department Victoria on a research project. Accident Research Centre, Monash University

Fildes B (ed) 1993 Injury prevention among the elderly: falls at home and pedestrian accidents. Victorian Health Promotion Foundation, Melbourne

Fonda D, Nickless R, Roth R A 1988 A prospective study of the incidence of urinary incontinence in an acute care teaching hospital. Australian Clinical Review 8:102–116

Gingold R 1992 Successful ageing. Oxford University Press, Melbourne

Goss J 1992 Health care for the elderly: costs and some institutional issues: EPAC background paper no 23, economic and social consequences of Australia's ageing population—preparing for the 21st century. Australian Government Publishing Service, Canberra

Green L, Gottlieb N 1989 Health promotion for the aging population: approaches to extending life expectancy. In: Andreopoulos S, Hogness J (eds) Health care for an aging society. Churchill Livingstone, New York

Greig D E, West M L, Overbury O 1986 Successful use of low vision aids: visual and psychological factors. Journal of Visual Impairment and Blindness 80:985–988

Gurlanik J M, Kaplan G A 1989 Predictors of healthy aging: prospective evidence from the Alameda County Study. American Journal of Public Health 9 (6):703–708

Health Targets and Implementation (Health for All) Committee 1988 Report to the Australian health ministers' advisory council and the Australian health ministers conference: health for all Australians. Australian Government Publishing Service, Canberra

Helme R D, Katz B, Neufeld S 1989 The establishment of a geriatric pain clinic: a preliminary report of the first 100 patients. Australian Journal on Ageing 8:27–30

Hickey T, Stilwell D L 1991 Health promotion for older people: all is not well. The Gerontologist 31(6):822–829

Hopkins D R, Murrah B, Werner W K et al 1990 Effect of low-impact aerobic dance on the functional fitness of elderly women. The Gerontologist 30(2):189–192

Horwath C C 1991 Nutrition goals for older adults: a review. The Gerontologist 31(6):811–820

Imms F J, Edholm O G 1979 The assessment of gait and mobility in the elderly. Age and Ageing 8:261–267

Kendig H 1989 Direction on ageing in New South Wales. Office on Ageing, New South Wales Premier's Department

Kiloh L G 1981 Depressive illness. Medical Journal of Australia 2:550–553

Leaverton P E, Havlik R J, Ingster-Moore L M et al 1990 Coronary heart disease and hypertension. In: Cornoni-Huntley J C, Huntley R R, Feldman J J (eds) Health status and well-being of the elderly: national health and nutrition examination survey—1 epidemiologic follow up study. Oxford University Press, New York

Lin V 1989 Healthy older people: a national strategy. NSW Health Promotion Conference.,7th August, Westmead

Livingston G, Hawkins A, Nori G, Blizzard B 1990 The Gospel Oak study: prevalence rates of dementia, depression and activity limitation among elderly residents in inner London. Psychological Medicine 20(1):137–146

Macklin J 1992 The future of general practice: the national health strategy issue paper no 3. Australian Government Publishing Service, Canberra

Macklin J 1993 Pathways to better health. National health strategy issues paper no 7. Australian Government Publishing Service, Canberra

Manchester D, Woollacott M, Dederbauer-Hylton N, Marin O 1989 Visual, vestibular and somata-sensory contributions to balance control in the older adult. Journal of Gerontology 44(4):M118–M127

Mant A, Duncan-Jones P, Saltman D et al 1988 Development of long-term use of psychotropic drugs by general practice patients. British Medical Journal 296:251–254

Manton K G 1988 A longitudinal study of functional change and mortality in the United States. Journal of Gerontology: Social Sciences 43(5):S153–S161

Marshall V W 1989 Lessons for gerontology from healthy public policy initiatives. In: Lewis S J (ed) Aging and health: linking research and public policy. Lewis Publishers, Michigan

Marshall V W 1992 Workshop on health promotion and aging: working together for a state of better health, May 25–26. New South Wales Department of Health, Sydney

Mathers C 1991 Health expectancies in Australia 1981 and 1988. Australian Government Publishing service, Canberra

McKinley J B 1989 Bringing the system back in: the social production of inequalities in health. The Public Health Association of Australia, Annual Conference, 24–27th September. University of Melbourne

McMillan D A, Harrison P M, Rogers L J et al 1986 Polypharmacy in an Australian teaching hospital: preliminary analysis of prevalence, types of drugs and associations. Medical Journal of Australia 145:339–342

McPherson B D 1986 Sport, health, well-being and aging: some conceptual and methodological issues and questions for sport scientists. In: McPherson B (ed) Sport and aging. Human Kinetics Books, Champaign, Ill

Minichiello V, Browning C, Aroni R 1992 The challenge of studying ageing. In: Minichiello V, Jones D, Alexander L (eds) Gerontology: a multidisciplinary approach. Prentice Hall, Sydney

Mossey J, Shapiro E 1982 Self-rated health: a predictor of mortality among the elderly. American Journal of Public Health 72:800–808

Murphy E, Smith R, Lindesay J 1988 Increased mortality rates in late-life depression. British Journal of Psychiatry 152:347–353

National Better Health Program 1991 Victorian projects. Victorian Government Publishing Service, Melbourne

NSW Department of Health 1989 Healthy older people project—report. Health Promotion Unit, NSW Department of Health, Sydney

Nutbeam D, Wise M, Bauman A, Leeder S, et al 1993 Review and revision of the national health goals and targets. Department of Health, Housing and Community Services, Canberra

Ory M G, Wyman J, Yu L 1986 Psychosocial factors in urinary incontinence. In: Ouslander J (ed) Urinary incontinence. Clinics in Geriatric Medicine pp 657–672

Ory M G (ed) 1991 Ageing, health and behaviour. Sage Publications, Newbury Park

Pierce D 1987 Deliberate self-harm in the elderly. International Journal of Geriatric Psychiatry 2:105–116

Revicki D A, Mitchell J P 1990 Strain, social support and mental health in rural elderly individuals. Journal of Gerontology: Social Sciences 45(6)S267–S274

Robinson J 1989 The Aldersgate Study. Flinders Medical Centre, Adelaide

Romer C J, Macfadyen D M 1987 The prevention of falls in later life. Danish Medical Bulletin, special supplement series no 4 (Foreword)

Rowland D T 1991 Pioneers again: immigrants and ageing in Australia. Bureau of Immigration Research, Melbourne

Saltman D, Webster I, Therin G 1989 Older persons' definitions of good health: implications for general practitioners. Medical Journal of Australia 150:426–428

Sax S in press Ageing and public policy. Allen & Unwin, Sydney

Svanborg A 1988 Health and vitality. Swedish Medical Research Council, Sweden

Teshuva K, Stanislavsky Y, Kendig H 1993 Health status of older people: literature review: a small grant study for the Victorian health promotion foundation. Collins Dove Publishing, Melbourne

Tinetti M, Speechley M, Ginter S 1988 Risk factors for falls among elderly people living in the community. New England Journal of Medicine 319(26)1701–1707

US Department of Health and Human Services 1988 Health promotion and aging proceedings. Surgeon General's Workshop, Mayflower Hotel, March 20–23, Washington DC

Victorian Better Health Committee 1991 Promoting health and preventing illness in Victoria: a framework. Health Department Victoria, Melbourne

Walker C, Boldy D, Spickett J, Stevenson M 1991 Preventing falls at home in old age: a broad approach. Australian Journal on Ageing 10(1):3–9

World Health Organization 1980 International classification of impairments, disabilities and handicaps. WHO, Geneva

Yeatman R 1991 Carers of depressed elderly patients. Royal ANZ College of Psychiatrists

25. Public health: challenges for nursing and allied health

Helen Keleher

During the 1980s and early 1990s, the principles of access and equity in health care appeared to have gained wide acceptance by policy makers. However, the 'new public health' extends that moral ground in health, by challenging health practitioners not just to practise the science and art of healing, but to participate actively in the development of public policy, and to ensure that the conditions of living on which health status depends are safe and sustainable. The principles of social justice in health, then, are most strongly espoused in the new public health movement.

The Ottawa Charter for Health Promotion unequivocally states the case in these terms:

> The fundamental conditions and resources for health are peace, shelter, education, food, income, a stable ecosystem, sustainable resources, social justice and equity. Improvement in health requires a secure foundation in these basic prerequisites...people in all walks of life are involved as individuals, families and communities. Professional and social groups and health personnel have a major responsibility to mediate between differing interests in society for the pursuit of health (Terris 1990:42).

Since Ottawa, public health has indeed become fashionable. As with all health trends, the published literature on public health has abounded. This chapter will begin with an examination of the definitions of health that purport to underpin sound public health practice. It is argued that the definitions of health on which disciplines base their educational programs are a critical factor to their potential for involvement in public health. The orientation of practitioner groups to public health practice is ameliorated by their intra-organizational unity or conflict, and in particular, their striving towards professionalism. Challenges then arise for greater support and participation in public health policy making and activities by nurses and allied health practitioner groups. The theme of this chapter will be that Health for All has a much greater chance of success if nurses and allied health personnel can become effectively oriented towards the principles and practices of the new public health. In doing so, these groups will be politically strengthened and philosophically enriched, whilst the general public stands to benefit from the unity of action from such an orientation.

Ownership of public health

Three basic areas of public health policy are set out by Terris (1990), and can be used as a yardstick of involvement in public health by all health practitioners, including medicine, nursing and allied health. They are in order of importance (a) health promotion, in its broadest sense of improving standards of living, (b) disease prevention and (c) medical care, or treatment services.

The politics of public health are at one level, about advocacy for the achievement of healthy outcomes on particular issues. However, at the level of practitioner groups, a somewhat paradoxical debate has arisen over who 'owns' public health.

Analysis of the various philosophical approaches suggests that public health is a highly political movement in health, where different paradigms compete for ownership, rather than complement each other. Their claims to legitimacy are in terms of their priorities, as well as their orientation towards, and definitions of the health problems experienced by people and how those problems can be ameliorated or treated.

Inglis (1958), in his seminal work on the history of the Royal Melbourne Hospital, refers to the medical profession's hostility to the early public health movement. In recent years however, an observable shift has occurred, with medicine actively increasing its stake in public health issues. Yet, the individualistic focus of the medical treatment model combined with the professional ideology of doctors' ownership of 'expert' knowledge, seems incompatible with public health philosophies that respect lay knowledge and self-help (Ashton & Seymour 1988).

In paradigmatic terms, the biomedical model is based on logical positivism, whilst the humanist paradigm underpins the social/community model. Their differences become evident if the 'new public health' is conceptualized. For example, one of the fundamental differences between the two models derives from their understanding of the determinants of ill health; who or what is responsible for ill health and perhaps more contentiously, what should be done about it. In the following definitions, key words in public health practice have been italicized.

Lawson (1991:3) articulates a biomedical approach to public health, defining it as 'essentially concerned with the prevention of *disease and injury* among *populations* as distinct from individuals', further suggesting that *epidemiology* is the primary science on which public health practice should be based. This definition can be politicized by pointing out what it omits, rather than what it includes. For example, it does not make the links between health, social factors and inequalities in society, nor to the relationship between public health practitioners and consumers.

Compare this definition with those based on the Health for All edict which take as their frame of reference, the WHO declarations and initiatives, first conceptualized at Alma Ata in 1978, and further advanced at the Ottawa (1986) and Adelaide (1988) conferences. For example, Kickbusch (in

McPherson 1992:125) describes public health as '*ecological* in perspective, *multi-sectoral* in scope and *collaborative* in strategy'. He postulates that improvements to the health of communities will best occur through organized efforts that '*enable communities* and individuals to achieve their full health potential' and specifically refers to the responsibilities for health practitioners to *mediate* between interest groups in society for the pursuit of population based health goals.

Ashton & Seymour (1988) see the *elimination of inequalities* in health as a key strategy for public health, a strategy which is firmly built on the concepts of *primary health care* and *health promotion*. They incorporate the social dimensions and determinants of ill health and the influence of lifestyle on well-being, expanding their explanatory model to incorporate the development of healthy public policy as fundamental to healthy people. The two latter definitions make those links apparent, revealing the potential for public health and its impact on society. Thus, the World Health Organization (WHO) is uncompromising in its belief that the humanistic approach has the greater potential for improving the health status of people. Through their history making International Conferences, the WHO have set the agenda for change in health practice.

A public health care system

The image of our present health care system is one of hierarchies of power and sophisticated treatment modalities. At the top are the professionals, who claim special expertise and knowledge about people's health. Hierarchical arrangements have historically been based on disciplinary regimes and the sexual and technical divisions of labour that have served to control the rights of practitioners to practise certain healing and treatment tasks (Gamarnikow 1978, Willis 1989). The dominance of the medical model based on the logical positivist paradigm, has produced a health system that is actually a monolithic treatment service, although there is evidence of change. For example, progress to incorporate health promotion and illness prevention programs has allowed them to claim a more central place among the range of services the health system offers. However, the dominance of the biomedical paradigm over other forms of knowledge about health and caring has contributed to the lower status of nurses and allied health practitioners and thus to a devaluation of their skills (Short et al 1993). In turn, the strategies of professionalism employed by these groups to achieve power and control over the labour process have led them to emulate the activities of the medical profession. The interests of the community are not necessarily served by the elitism inherent in professionalization, with the tendency to moral superiority which is exhibited by some professionals.

Today, the medical treatment model, the basis of medical power, remains influential. This can be deduced from health expenditure figures, which show the medical treatment model as attracting an overwhelming proportion of available health dollars (Duckett 1992). Consumers however, once powerless in the hierarchies of health, have shifted the balance of power through interest group activities participating in policy development to give voice to their experience of the health care system and to demands that service delivery become more user friendly (Howe 1992).

The public health and community movements have long argued for a shift in resources away from the technologically hungry, acute, hospital sector. Such moves would be towards a system that ensures a basic level of care for all, where 'a sound and widespread system of primary health care' is the most fundamental strategy for improving the health of all people to enable them to lead fulfilling, productive lives (Sax 1990:167).

It is within this environment that nurses and allied health practitioners have pursued their own strategies of professionalization—in their desire to become self-regulating or at the very least, to be equal with, yet remain separate from, medicine (Coburn 1988). In doing so, they have sought to secure their share of the patient care market with both professional and union activities. Whilst these activities have been beneficial to the pay, conditions, and status of these groups, they have contributed to a shift in focus, turning the politics of care inwards towards intraprofessional or organizational conflicts. Thus the politics of care becomes directed more at protecting territories or perhaps, seeking alignment with more powerful groups, as with nursing and physiotherapy in recent years. Another consuming activity of these groups has been concerned with defining their product, which has particularly been a preoccupation with nursing theorists within the context of professionalism. In the process, nurses and allied health practitioners have actually become isolated from the politics of care as it is played out in health care arenas, somewhat 'sidetracked into providing illness-oriented services', rather than playing an active role in the development of public health policy (Gibson in Clay 1992:16).

Voices in the policy process

Nurses account for nearly 70% of all people in health occupations, compared with 5.5% for allied health workers (Palmer & Short 1989:124). The treatment and hospital system remains the major focus of these groups, although significant numbers of physiotherapists are engaged in private practice. These groups are characterized by their femaleness, a historical orientation of handmaiden status to the medical profession, and also by the medicalization of their work content (Palmer & Short 1989).

My own research into policy development and implementation in health organizations, has demonstrated that health organizations are not passive, but active and highly political, with the policy process operating through both formal and informal mechanisms. The informal channels of discussion and information dissemination are directly reflective of the social relationships between the participants. Women health workers experience a dual socialization into disciplined patterns of subservience, deferring or demurring to the voices of authority and dogmatism. Individual nurses or allied health personnel demonstrate a timidity or reluctance to put forward their views, and rarely make public statements on professional issues.

Moreover, health organizations give restricted opportunities for nurses and allied health to participate actively in the policy process. For example, the formal committee structure of hospitals is arguably more powerful than the informal channels described above, with the most powerful people in the organization securing committee membership. Those who have accessed this level of power understand the communication necessary to control the policy process. It is a level of privileged communication that supports and reinforces a class distinction between health professionals. Degeling and Anderson (1992) argue that the policy process within health organizations is contingent on relationships of power, conflict and control. Thus, membership of a committee does not guarantee a voice. The voices of nursing and allied health are not generally heard above the voices of more powerful and more politicized groups in health, specifically the medical profession and health administrators. Despite the rhetoric about gender equality over the last 20 years, female dominated health professions still suffer from powerful sexist ideologies about femininity and masculinity, and the inherent power relations and prejudices involved (Short 1986). Values about medical science and its practitioners have remained powerful (Ehrenreich & Ehrenreich 1975, Ashley 1980), effectively limiting or suppressing other forms of health knowledge (Willis 1989). These factors have underpinned the desire by nurses and allied health practitioners to pursue strategies of professionalism, articulated since the 1970s.

The struggles of nurses to gain a voice in the decision making processes of the hospital system have been well illustrated by the process in Victoria from 1987–1992 to implement the recommendations of the Studies of Professional Issues in Nursing (SPIN) (Keleher 1992). During the SPIN process, nurses attempted to challenge the traditional barriers to their participation in policy and decision making. The degree of participation of practitioner groups with minority status in decision making processes may perhaps be due to their socialization into support roles to medicine, or because of the prevalence of beliefs held in the organization about their place in the politics of care. Socialization is a covert barrier to participation that must be overcome by education to provide a sense of identity, which can be described as being about one's own consciousness and sense of personal autonomy.

Nurses demonstrably became more politicized than allied health practitioners during the 1970s and 1980s. Activities in nursing during this time demonstrate the preoccupation with internal struggles. The dual strategies of professionalism and unionism have been earnestly pursued, with the active construction of agendas that have attempted to resolve conflict between rival interest groups in the politics of care, i.e. between nurses and others with a greater degree of apparent power. In response to the widespread corporatization of hospitals, nurses and allied health professionals have become somewhat insular in their activities, attempting to introduce collegial models of modus operandi within the treatment model, rather than focussing on more global issues of social justice in health.

Creating opportunities for greater participation

Yet, of all health practitioner groups, nursing has articulated the most socially progressive orientation towards public health. Officially, nursing bodies have developed policies concerning primary health care that articulate social justice principles. The Colleges of Nursing and the Australian Nursing Federation (ANF) have prepared a comprehensive and committed policy about the relationship between nursing and primary health care, demonstrating an awareness of social and environmental factors and their relationship to health (Australian Nursing Federation 1990). However, despite the existence of this policy, nursing has found it difficult to overcome the colonization of nurses into the illness sector, and to re-orient its practices away from the medical model towards more community based interventions. Structural barriers that have determined the employment of nurses are slowly being challenged, but the resistance to independent practising nurses remains strong, 'even within the nursing profession there will be conflicting views' (Percival 1989). Restructuring of employment to broaden the scope of services available to the community is only one mechanism available. The establishment of Area Health Boards in NSW for example, has facilitated change in the status of independent practising nurses, but only for a small minority. The majority of nurses still service the hospital sector.

Physiotherapy as a group, though much smaller than nursing, has similarly pursued professionalism. The 'Goals, Objectives & Strategies: 1990–1995', of the Australian Physiotherapy Association, (Victorian branch) summarize the professional and industrial goals of the Association. They are essentially an intra-organizational statement of purpose and make no reference to the wider or more global field of health concerns. The strong alignment of physiotherapy and other allied health groups with the medical model, and its concern, shared with nursing, to pursue professionalism actively, demonstrate central concerns in these groups with status, power and authority (Cosh 1971, Palmer & Short 1989). The acquisition of such attributes associated with professional boundaries, may well be setting up contradictory value systems to those necessary for the participative and collaborative style of public health practice. In other words, the traditional professionalization model does not fit comfortably with the new health care politics.

If the energies of health practitioner groups are consumed by intra-professional conflict, they are less likely to find the energy for the level of advocacy required of public health practitioners, and even less likely to be confident in contributing to the development of primary health care in the community, or to the development of healthy public policy. Since the move of nursing education to the tertiary sector, nurses have begun to articulate a different politics of care to other practitioner groups. For example, the philosophy of many nursing schools of education revolves around the model of the interaction between nursing, the client, the environment and health, re-interpreting the historical orientation of nursing that dates back to Nightingale. Thus, nursing education is actually oriented towards health in context, even though its educational philosophy was sidetracked for many decades by the imperialism of the medical treatment model.

But as a profession, nurses are yet to realize their potential for influence in the arenas where healthy public policies are articulated. As with any instrumental model, the methods for reform or change need to be built into any policy, setting directions and articulating the barriers to implementation and achievement of necessary reforms (Franzway et al 1989, Degeling & Anderson 1992). Undergraduate programs for nurses must therefore realize the challenge to incorporate social theory, political science and studies in health policy to lay the foundations for activism to realize the goals of public health practice.

The challenge

The challenge for health practitioners has a number of components. A recurring theme is about the reorienting of educational programs for health practitioners (Percival 1989) towards enabling them 'to provide leadership in public health service, education and research' (Chambers 1989). As explained, such calls have a sound philosophical basis, but must also be politicized, to recognize the structural barriers that impede the involvement of independent practitioners. Whilst nurses and allied health practitioners rely almost entirely on a health system oriented towards treatment, colonizing their services into treatment programs, such goals will not be met. Thus, the education of allied health and nurses must be broadly based, encompassing the politics of the health system. Understanding *how to effect change* is critical to the articulation of common goals between allied health, nursing and public health.

To be articulate about the principles of health promotion and primary health care, is only one level of change, that goes hand-in-hand with political action. It is an important strategy to gain access to decision making processes, but quite another to operate effectively at that level. Last (1987:382) believes that multidisciplinary teams have been a trend. However, he goes on to say that 'the increasing numbers of physicians and their political power make it unlikely that primary care will become a task for non-medically qualified health workers in the industrial nations in the foreseeable future'. This is a salient reminder of significant barriers to the development of practitioners other than doctors, in primary care.

Nursing and allied health must believe in their ability to work within participative and collaborative models with people in the community. It becomes a matter of orientation towards concerted efforts of practitioners, working towards common goals. That orientation should also recognize the value of consumer groups in articulating community needs, providing the bottom-up balance to our sometimes top-down, professional imposition of values. If the Health for All goals are to be met, then all practitioner groups need to develop an awareness of the necessity to become actively involved in primary health care and health promotion, in occupational health and rehabilitation, not just at the individual client level, but at the population based level and where appropriate, at the cutting edge of public health policy. Thus, these groups have the opportunity to become an influential lobby for the development of healthy public policy, but there are a number of barriers to be overcome. The call by the Ottawa Charter for health personnel to mediate between differing interests draws attention to the structures which restrict the successful co-ordination of public health programs because of interdisciplinary tensions, or perceptions of ownership of particular public health issues.

One major barrier is the orientation of professional practice towards individual client care, at the expense of education for active participation in 'population based health promotion strategies' (Chambers 1989). Another barrier is the professionalization model that inherently assumes a power relationship between patient/client and the health professional, based on assumptions of expertise and greater health knowledge and literacy. If nurses and allied health practitioners are to become effective players in the politics of care of the future, then it is imperative that they understand these barriers themselves and work towards overcoming them. The public health model clearly offers nursing and allied health practitioners exciting opportunities for active participation in the sustainable health of our society and its people.

REFERENCES

Ashley J 1980 Power in structured misogyny: implications for the politics of care: advances in nursing science. Aspen Systems Corporation

Ashton J, Seymour H 1988 The new public health. Open University Press, Milton Keynes

Australian Nursing Federation 1990 Primary health care in Australia: strategies for nursing action. Melbourne

Australian Physiotherapy Association Victorian Branch 1990 Goals, objectives and strategies 1990–1995. Supplement to the APA Victorian Branch Newsletter (VGB 1014) March

Chambers L 1989 Individual client care and public health policy: the dual challenges for public health nurses. Canadian Journal of Public Health 80:315–316

Clay T 1992 Education and empowerment: securing nursing's future. International Nursing Review 39(1):15–18

Coburn D 1988 The development of Canadian nursing: professionalisation and proletarianization. International Journal of Health Services 18(3):437–456

Cosh P 1971 The challenge of physiotherapy education in Australia. The Australian Journal of Physiotherapy XVII(4):113–118

Degeling P, Anderson J 1992 Organisational and administrative dimensions. In: Gardner H (ed) Health policy: development, implementation and evaluation in Australia. Churchill Livingstone, Melbourne

Duckett S 1992 Financing of health care. In: Gardner H (ed) Health policy: development, implementation and evaluation in Australia. Churchill Livingstone, Melbourne

Ehrenreich B, Ehrenreich J 1975 Hospital workers: class conflicts in the making. International Journal of Health Services vol 5(1):43–51

Franzway S, Court D, Connell R 1987 Staking a claim: feminism, bureaucracy and the state. Allen & Unwin, Sydney

Gamarnikow E 1978 Sexual division of labour: the case of nursing. In: Kuhn A,Wolpe A (eds) Feminism and materialism. Routledge Kegan Paul, London

Gray G, Pratt R 1989 Issues in Australian nursing 2. Churchill Livingstone, Melbourne

Howe A 1992 Participation in policy making: the case of aged care. In: Gardner H (ed) Health policy: development, implementation and evaluation in Australia. Churchill Livingstone, Melbourne

Keleher H 1992 The potential power of nursing: why is it unrealised? Paper presented to TASA Annual Conference, Adelaide, December

Inglis K 1958 Hospital and community: a history of the Royal Melbourne Hospital. Melbourne University Press, Melbourne

Last J 1987 Public health and human ecology. Appleton & Lange, Ottawa

Lawson J 1991 Public health Australia: an introduction. McGraw-Hill, Sydney

McPherson P 1992 Health for all Australians. In: Gardner H (ed) Health policy: development, implementation and evaluation in Australia. Churchill Livingstone, Melbourne

Ottawa Charter for Health Promotion. 1986 Canadian Public Health Association, Ottawa

Palmer G, Short S 1989 Health care and public policy. Macmillan, Melbourne

Percival E 1989 Nursing in primary health care. In: Gray G, Pratt R (eds) Issues in Australian nursing 2. Churchill Livingstone, Melbourne

Sax S 1990 Health care choices and the public purse. Allen & Unwin, Sydney

Short S 1986 Physiotherapy—a feminine profession. The Australian Journal of Physiotherapy. 32(4):241–243

Terris M. 1990 Public health policy for the 1990s. In: Breslow L, Fielding J, Lave L (eds) 1990 Annual review of public health, vol 11. Annual Reviews, California

Willis E 1989 Medical dominance:the division of labour in Australian health care. Allen & Unwin, Sydney

26. Eating away at the public health: a political economy of nutrition

John Duff

The recent history of nutrition presents us with this paradox: although improved health has generally followed in the wake of economic development, nutrition seems to be an exception. Among the most affluent nations, nutrition is in fact identified as the primary cause of worsening health. Nutrition appears in many health statistics as the single largest cause of death, mainly nutrition related heart disease and various cancers (Commonwealth Department of Health 1987). But it is not, as one might expect, the most affluent in the developed countries who suffer the most. The figures instead point to the least affluent. This chapter will place this paradox in the context of public health more generally.

The pursuit of health is closely bound up with equal and just access to social resources. Although some groups continue to have worse health and health care than others, recent political initiatives have been taken to close the gap by ensuring a minimum level of health and health care to which all can aspire. The Alma Ata declaration, Medicare's insurance system and community health programs are all signs that the right of all to good health and health care is broadly accepted.

Health promotion and health education have become central elements of modern public health policy. Health workers are aware from their research that people of higher socioeconomic status (SES) respond more readily to health promotion messages—to stop smoking, breast-feed babies (Williams & Carmichael 1983) or avoid being overweight (English & Bennett 1985)—than people of lower SES. As social scientists, we need to question health research which tells us who responds to health promotion but fails to deal with the question of why the different responses occur.

Explaining responses to nutrition promotion requires consideration, among other things, of the way food is produced, marketed, advertised and priced. The conventions of scientific reporting, however, make if difficult for health scientists to deal with those broader issues arising from the political economy of food production and marketing. To the extent that these issues are neglected, researchers by default work from a model of health behaviour in which approved behaviour follows from rational choice based on scientific information. This model allows all too readily the conclusion that those who do not respond to health promotion are not acting rationally, or have failed to inform themselves properly (Crotty et al 1992). From this we can surmise that in the past ill health was more readily accepted as a consequence of too few resources, while now, as Crotty et al (1992) has pointed out, it is more likely to be seen as a consequence of poorly chosen lifestyle or poor education.

But, is this the full story?

Health promotion and individualism

Health promotion plays a major part in Australia's public health program, especially in the area of food and nutrition. The levies raised from tobacco sales in some states are being directed into health promotion research and projects on a large scale, many of them relating to diet (Healthway 1991). At first, this seems like a welcome return to the old public health of the late 19th century which was characterized by action at a community rather than an individual level. The late 19th century saw major initiatives in public health directed towards building regulations ensuring ventilation, and the development of water and sewerage systems. As Davis and George (1993) point out, such action was precipitated largely by the more affluent, who could be kept safe from infectious diseases only through improvement of conditions of housing and hygiene by public works in less affluent areas. The significant point is that action was taken at a political level and enacted on a collective rather than individual basis.

With the development of medical and pharmaceutical control of infection in individuals over the first half of the 20th century, there was a marked change in public health ideology which began favouring clinical intervention at the individual level. The change in focus is evident in the words of the founding Director-General of the Commonwealth Department of Health:

...the concept of preventive medicine, that is the prevention of disease, the preservation of health as a government activity, and the relation of the medical profession to that activity, have passed away from being mainly concerned with the physical environment of man—the external influences which might adversely affect health—to the physical condition of the human individual, and to the use of medicinal agents which can be directly applied to the individual (Cumpston 1978:47).

The change signalled a consolidation of medical expertise, with public health problems being presented primarily as medical problems to which medical solutions were appropriate. It is just this ideology of medical intervention that McKeown (1979) questioned so effectively with the claim that the great reduction in infectious diseases in the 19th and well into the 20th century was achieved more by better food and improved physical environment than by individualized medical means.

McKeown identifies the very paradox referred to earlier. He uses improvements in nutrition to explain improvement in health over the 100 years from 1830 to 1930. McKeown accepts that inadequacies of food followed from circumstances beyond the control of the individual, and could be remedied only by structural intervention at the level of food supply or prices or incomes. 'Overconsumption', on the other hand, the basis of much current nutrition related illness and early death, is taken to reflect personal choice as well as other constraints (McKeown 1979). The acceptance of freely chosen 'lifestyle' as the cause of ill health both explains and justifies the increased reliance on health promotion as an instrument of public health. But it sidesteps the question of constraints on the kinds of choices people are effectively able to make (Crotty et al 1992).

Nineteenth century public health began at a community rather than an individual level. Later, developments which made possible direct clinical contact between public health agencies and individuals (e.g. immunization) were seen as advances. Although public health continues to deal with social goals, many programs are now targeted at individuals and the way they 'choose' to live. Reiger (1985) has argued consistently for looking beyond individual choices and making visible the sociopolitical context in which these choices are made.

The public health of nutrition has increasingly directed its efforts to individual lifestyle change, and in the process limited food and eating pretty much to a matter of biology: in this way of thinking, we need to know about the physiology of food so that we can stoke our furnaces with most benefit and least harm. Armed with this knowledge, and assuming we are committed to good health as a matter of personal interest, we are in a position to lead rational lives. Failure to do so represents the non-rational—lack of knowledge, lack of discipline or both. Others, (e.g. Murcott 1988a) have noted the differences, even contradictions, between people's beliefs about good health or nutrition, and the judgements of health professionals. So long as those judgements come from a highly individualistic and biological framework, there is some question about whether health promotion campaigns incorporating them will serve the interests of those at whom they are directed.

Individualized health promotion has two great advantages: it promises to be more effective and less costly than clinical intervention which is delayed until illness occurs, and it is politically much easier to implement than public health policy which has an impact on structured social interests. It has proved much easier to have information aimed at individual choice printed on tobacco products, than to alter sponsorship arrangements with some sporting bodies, to say nothing of the tobacco producers. With the increase in affluence in wealthy economies, risk is most comfortably represented, from the producers' point of view at least, as a consequence of lifestyles, rather than of commercial initiatives over which individuals have little control.

The strengthening trend towards preventive approaches involving lifestyle has come in the footsteps of McKeown's critique of clinical intervention. While preventive approaches are regarded by health promotion workers as more broadly effective than clinical intervention, there is concern that they may overemphasize individual lifestyles at the expense of politico-economic forces such as food production itself (Davis & George 1993, Griggs 1988)

The new public health

Politico-economic aspects of public health are well recognized by some groups within the new public health movement. There are two important features of the approach taken by one of these groups, the Health Issues Centre (1988). The first is that public health policy cannot be made in isolation from other areas of public policy, especially those relating to housing, income security, and education. Public health, in other words, is not merely a matter for health experts. The second feature involves participation at the level of local communities in health and welfare initiatives. This recognizes the underlying issue reflected in the term 'empowerment' which accepts that choice in lifestyle is related to questions of social justice and economic well-being.

Behind the distinction between a public health which makes prescriptions for individual behaviour and one which acknowledges structured social forces, lies the question of value free science. An approach to public health, and to nutrition in particular, which is committed to the scientific method as accepted by the medical sciences, is characterized by two blind spots. Research methods which are neither quantitative nor directed towards hypothesis testing are seen to be outside the realm of science, and best left to be dealt with elsewhere. Techniques found in sociology or anthropology find little acceptance in the scientific journals in which most health research is reported. The other blind spot is that analyses of social and political forces, such as the use of children's television advertising to promote eating between meals, are thought to threaten the neutrality of science. The campaign against tobacco related illnesses, as a counter example, shows how powerful the consideration of such forces can be (Palmer & Short 1989). It has come to be accepted by public health policy makers that the organization of the tobacco industry had to be taken into consideration when setting goals of minimizing tobacco use. There is little evidence yet that the impact of the organization of the food industry on public health goals has been recognized in nutrition policy. We can now turn to the question of what kind of nutrition research has been available to the makers of nutrition policy.

The foundations of a nutrition policy

Nutrition education campaigns, and dietary policy more generally, have signalled a re-orientation of the way we think of food and eating, from a cultural practice which we carry out routinely to a technical health matter in which we maintain a monitoring role. This transformation has been associated with the rise of health experts (clinical dietitians, nutrition educators, epidemiologists) who study and evaluate food and nutrition as a public health issue. The very different approaches to food practices as part of culture or as a health matter increase the complexity of the study of diet. Competing interpretations stemming from differences between the health sciences and the social sciences have been few only because the social sciences have had so little to contribute (Murcott 1988b). Much of the social analysis of nutrition has been carried out by health scientists, and has sought to identify 'unhealthy' groups by mapping correlations between social indicators such as class, gender and age, and dietary practices. The purpose of these studies is to identify groups 'at risk' so that nutrition education programs can be directed towards 'modifying the food choices' individuals make.

In 1986 the Commonwealth Department of Health issued dietary guidelines for Australians as a way of implementing national dietary goals. The reasons for these goals seemed fairly straightforward: nutrition related disorders had come, according to the statisticians' categories, to account for more deaths in Australia than any other cause. The purpose of the dietary guidelines is to improve the health of the nation and lessen the financial and social costs of ill health (Commonwealth Department of Health 1987).

This is generally interpreted as requiring change of behaviour, and the whole business of health promotion and health education is directed towards changing individuals' priorities, behaviour and even lifestyles. What is important to note in the emphasis on lifestyle to which much health promotion is directed, is the move away from the great tradition of public health: the public good which needs to be achieved by collective action. Little allowance is made for the shaping of choices by cultural tradition, by rhythms and routines imposed by work or place of residence, or the force of interests concerning the production and marketing of food. The assumption that public health is to be pursued on the basis of individual decisions in such a framework has two important repercussions: it throws responsibility for risk of illness more firmly onto the individual whose 'chosen' lifestyle is held responsible for the risk, and it draws the attention of researchers to individuals and their actions, rather than to structured environments.

The remainder of this chapter will look at the nutrition survey, the main instrument for determining what food habits are to be targeted in health promotion, and point to some of the broader structural factors that should be taken into account when creating nutrition policy from this research.

Social nutrition

The nutrition survey, as the principal tool for studying food choices, can have two purposes. The first, typically requiring a large scale survey, is to provide a population profile on nutrition as a guide to food policies. The first major national survey of this kind in Australia took place in 1936. Organized by the Nutrition Section of Commonwealth Department of Health which served the National Health and Medical Research Council (NH&MRC) Nutrition

Committee, it concentrated on health deficiencies. It was a notable survey, combining clinical assessment of part of the sample within the larger survey of reported diet (Clements 1986). The survey found only limited evidence of health problems related to diet, mainly pertaining to localized iodine deficiencies (Australia-Advisory Council on Nutrition 1939). The Commonwealth Department of Health organized a second major survey in 1944, again concluding that there was little evidence of malnutrition in Australia. Individual choice and sufficient purchasing power, it appeared, combined to provide good health.

This situation was to change. There was evidence by the 1970s that individual food choices, combined with perhaps too much purchasing power, were resulting in an increase in deaths related to diet (Walker & Roberts 1988). In 1983, another national survey was conducted, this time by the Commonwealth Department of Health in association with the National Heart Foundation (Commonwealth Department of Health 1986). This survey confirmed the influence of the affluent diet on death rates, and was influential in the development of national dietary goals by the Commonwealth Department of Health (1987) and a major campaign of health promotion by the National Heart Foundation.

The second purpose of the nutrition survey is to correlate social variables such as gender, age, class and ethnicity with food habits. This helps health education and promotion, which, it is argued, can be more effective when targeted at specific groups with specific messages. Complex studies of this kind are difficult to mount and require substantial resources, and consequently are more limited in scale. The Nutrition Section of the Australian Department of Health took an active role in promoting these social correlate studies in the 1940s, which were first known as 'social nutrition' (Duff 1990). Later, following the opening of schools of nutrition at Australia's newer universities, the term 'food habits' research has come to be more widely accepted (Trusswell & Wahlqvist 1988).

Food habits research has been carried out principally by people trained in the sciences, and reported in scientific journals and forums, following the conventions of scientific publishing. This has considerable influence over the way research questions are approached. The positivism of normal science favours a study design built around hypothesis testing using quantifiable variables. Indeed, some onlookers from the laboratory sciences are concerned to see that only 'rigorous' pieces of scientific research are published in the journals (Woodward 1988); the imprecise and interpretive methods of sociology are treated with suspicion. Quantitative studies can, with increasing precision, identify the food consumption patterns of different groups within different parts of Australia, and confirm, for example, that lower socioeconomic status mothers are more likely to bottle feed their babies (Williams & Carmichael 1983, Bailey & Sherriff 1992). The question of how such patterns might be explained in terms of social power, access to resources, continuity of culture or the nature of community is systematically excluded from consideration by the conventions of scientific reporting.

A question now presents itself: does the 'scientific' approach to the study of individual action increase the chances of individuals being blamed for their own ill health? The implication of some aspects of health promotion, i.e. that individuals have to be persuaded to change their lifestyles, is that those with the worst health chances have 'chosen' bad lifestyles. This question of choice deserves further consideration.

The increasing affluence in the years after the second world war seemed to extend the range of choices people could make. Nutrition problems seemed to be no longer those of limited choice imposed by poverty, but related to extended choice imposed by affluence. How then should we explain the finding (Commonwealth Department of Health 1987) that death rates are higher for lower socioeconomic groups? Health education works on the assumption of ill informed food habits, with education being the key to improvement. The Nutrition Task Force, set up by the Australian Government to help meet the Health for All by the Year 2000 target of the World Health Organization produced national dietary guidelines (Commonwealth Department of Health 1987); these guidelines have formed the basis of substantial programs of health education and health promotion. (See Navarro 1984 on the unwillingness of WHO agencies to acknowledge the politico-economic impediments to achieving this target.)

The focus of food habits research on the choices individual people make about their food creates a highly privatized orientation to public health. The national dietary guidelines present the problem as one of individual knowledge, and the willingness to act on it rationally. The 'technical rationality' of the health sciences, in other words, appears to assume that the individual is freely and rationally making choices based on better or worse technical knowledge. The role of the health professional is taken to be one of improving the availability of knowledge about food, and persuading individuals to act rationally on it.

Even a cursory application of sociological principles to food and eating would suggest there is much more to 'food habits' than this, but sociology has yet to offer much in the study of food and eating (Beardsworth & Keil 1990). Many studies of the cultural meanings of food and eating have come out of the anthropological and social historical traditions. The place of food in the culture of different groups in contemporary society remains an important but relatively neglected area. Douglas (1984) has long pointed to the rules governing the use and sharing of food in traditional cultures. Mennell (1985) has studied the long friction between the British and the French over food and its meaning for 'civilized' culture. Symons (1982) describes the shaping of the Australian diet as if we had gone, well provendered, on an extremely long picnic from the British Isles. Despite these small beginnings, there is no doubt that this is an area of research which has yet to cast much light on what is otherwise regarded as 'ill informed' choices made by people about their food.

Anne Murcott (1983, 1988a, 1988b) is one of the few sociologists to have carried out community studies into the changing cultural meanings of food in modern industrial societies. She has focused on changes in what women in different British cultural groups understand by providing a 'good meal' for their family, and emphasized the way cultural traditions shape choice.

While culture remains important to an understanding of food and its uses, regional or ethnic traditions have undergone rapid change in modern economies. High rates of internal and external migration are obvious contenders for explaining this change, but two other forces need to be taken into account: one is the inclusion of popular science into modern culture, and the application of 'science' to diet. The second force for change is the manipulation of meanings attached to food through commodification, i.e. the manufacture of culture as part of product advertising and promotion.

Producers have long recognized that the economic rewards of large scale production can be enjoyed only so long as there is matching large scale consumption. The advertising and marketing industry is the means by which this consumption is ensured, with constant efforts to replace foods produced in the household with 'value added' foods from the commercial sector (Ewen 1976). Jelliffe and Jelliffe (1977) have campaigned with a similar argument against multinational companies who manufacture and market infant formula. The Jelliffes emphasize the force of marketing to explain changing infant feeding patterns, especially in the Third World. Douglas and Isherwood (1979), without taking on the politico-economic perspectives of Ewen or the Jelliffes, attempt to deal with the difficult question of why people consume goods at all, pointing out that it is a central question which has been almost totally neglected.

Studies in the political economy of agriculture have also pointed to the shaping of national food habits by the politico-economic development of agriculture. Mintz (1986) explains the introduction of sugar, cocoa, coffee and tea into the English diet in these terms. For Mintz, the creation and control of markets for the agricultural produce of colonial territories was required to secure their incorporation into the Empire. Lawrence (1987) analyses for Australia the enormous force for shaping food production, and thus consumption, brought about by production strategies which have as their goal domination over markets. In this analysis, as that of Mintz, production drives consumption rather than the other way around. The consequences for the sugar-cane and beef cattle industries of the tropical north of Australia would need to be taken very seriously if sugar and red meat consumption were to be reduced significantly.

Conclusion

People of higher SES appear to respond to health promotion and health education programs in the way their architects intended, and it is they who benefit most from gains in health. The contradiction revealed by much of the work in nutrition research is that private choice is the centre of attention, and those who are the least affluent, the least powerful, and with the fewest resources, are the ones who show up as 'failing' to make choices in their own interest. Rather than blaming such people for yet another disadvantage, nutrition research needs to return to the political, economic and social circumstances which shape the choices people can plausibly make.

The health sciences, particularly in scholarly publishing, allow little scope for dealing with political processes, political economy, or cultural practices which can be studied only interpretively. Of course in their work health practitioners deal with all these, but paradoxically their claim to expert status depends on their scientific research which they present in scientific journals. Crotty (1987) points out how important this privileging of science is, since it means the difference between experts directing social groups 'from the top' using the limited assumptions which have shaped nutrition and dietetics studies, and encouraging community groups to set their own goals in the terms of their own cultural practices and meaning systems.

The challenge is to provide encouragement and room for sociological and anthropological research into food and eating. This should reflect more of the complexity of the social, political and economic processes involved than most current forums for research in the health sciences allow. And, as with tobacco smoking, it may well become clear that the organization of production, the marketing of the products, and the linkages to the broader economy, deserve as much attention as the imputation of individual choice.

REFERENCES

Australia-Advisory Council on Nutrition. Final Report 1939. In: Parliament of the Commonwealth of Australia, Parliamentary papers, Session 1937–38–39–40 vol IV. Commonwealth of Australia, Canberra, pp 253–426
Bailey V, Sherriff J 1992 Reasons for the early cessation of breast-feeding in women from lower socioeconomic groups in Perth, Western Australia. Australian Journal of Nutrition and Dietetics. 49:(2)40–45
Beardsworth A, Keil T 1990 Putting the menu on the agenda. Sociology 24(1):139–151
Clements F 1986 A history of human nutrition in Australia. Longman Cheshire, Melbourne
Commonwealth Department of Health 1986 National dietary survey of adults, 1983, no 1, foods consumed. Australian Government Publishing Service, Canberra
Commonwealth Department of Health 1987 Towards better nutrition for Australians: report of the nutrition taskforce of the better health commission. Australian Government Publishing Service, Canberra
Crotty P 1987 Rose's prevention paradox = the nutrition educator's dilemma: an issues paper prepared for the NHMRC workshop on research priorities in public health aspects of nutrition, (Mimeo)
Crotty P, Rutishauser I, Cahill, M 1992 Food in low income families. Australian Journal of Public Health 16(2):168–174
Cumpston J 1978 The health of the people: a study in federalism. Roebuck Society, Canberra
Davis A, George J, 1993 States of health: health and illness in Australia. Harper & Row, Sydney
Douglas M, Isherwood B 1979 The world of goods: towards an anthropology of consumption. Allen Lane, London

Douglas M, (ed) 1984 Food in the social order: studies of food and festivities in three American communities. Russell Sage Foundation, New York

Duff J, 1990 Nutrition and public health: division of labour in the study of nutrition. Community Health Studies 14(2):162–170

English R, Bennett S 1985 Overweight and obesity in the Australian community. Journal of Food and Nutrition 42(1):2–7

Ewen S 1976 Captains of consciousness: advertising and the social roots of consumer culture. McGraw Hill, New York

Griggs B 1988 The food factor: an account of the food revolution. London, Penguin, Ch 25

Health Issues Centre 1988 Getting it together for the year 2000: a social health strategy for South Australia. Health Issues 13:26–28

Healthway 1991 Healthway: newsletter of the Western Australian health promotion foundation, Issue 1

Jelliffe D, Jelliffe E 1977 The infant food industry and international child health. International Journal of Health Services 7(2):249–254

Lawrence G 1987 Capitalism and the countryside: the rural crisis in Australia. Pluto Press, Sydney

McKeown T 1979 The role of medicine: dream, mirage or nemesis? Princeton University Press, Princeton

Mennell S 1985 All manners of food: eating and taste in England and France from the middle ages to the present. Basil Blackwell, Oxford

Mintz S 1986 Sweetness and power: the place of sugar in modern history. Penguin, New York

Murcott A (ed) 1983 The sociology of food and eating. Gower, Aldershot

Murcott A 1988a A finger in every pie: the variety of approaches to the study of food habits. In: Truswell A, Wahlqvist M (eds) Food habits in Australia. Rene Gordon, North Balwyn, pp 15–39

Murcott A 1988b Sociological and social anthropological approaches to food and eating. World Review of Nutrition and Dietetics 55:1–40

Navarro V 1984 A critique of the ideological and political position of the Brandt report and the Alma Ata declaration. International Journal of Health Services 14(2):159–172

Palmer G, Short S 1989 Health care and public policy: an Australian analysis. Macmillan, South Melbourne

Reiger K 1985 The disenchantment of the home: modernising the Australian family 1880–1940. Oxford University Press, Melbourne

Symons M 1982 One continuous picnic: a history of eating in Australia. Duck Press, Adelaide

Truswell A, Wahlqvist M (eds) 1988 Food habits in Australia. Rene Gordon, North Balwyn

Walker R, Roberts D 1988 From scarcity to surfeit: a history of food and nutrition in New South Wales. University of New South Wales Press, Kensington

Williams H, Carmichael H 1983 Nutrition in the first year of life in a multi-ethnic poor socioeconomic municipality in Melbourne. Australian Pediatric Journal 19:73–77

Woodward D 1988 Some methodological issues in research on food habits. In: Truswell A, Wahlqvist M (eds) Food habits in Australia. Rene Gordon, North Balwyn, pp 252–258

27. The women's health movement: one solution

Lynne Hunt

The women's health movement has emerged over the last 25 years as a solution to problems experienced by women with mainstream, medical model, health care. This account of how and why the movement developed, draws on the writer's international study of 71 women's health agencies in nine western countries (Hunt 1991). The analysis illustrates the relationship between ideology and praxis in the introduction of an alternative model of health care designed to provide appropriate, just and equitable access to health.

At first sight the concepts of justice and health may seem incompatible because justice concerns social issues while health, on the face of it, is a function of capricious biological disposition. Yet analyses of health data (Kane 1991) do reveal social patterns in health, illness and mortality which suggest that both social and biological factors affect health and well-being. In other words, who we are, biologically and socially, affects our prospects for good health. Gender, in particular, has been shown (Kane 1991) to be a significant factor influencing morbidity and mortality. For example, women in Australia live seven years longer than men. This apparent advantage, however, brings little joy because, as Kane (1991:57) indicated, a large proportion of women's longer life span is 'actually spent in pain or ill health'.

Biological factors offer an obvious explanation for the differences between female and male mortality and morbidity rates. However, Kane (1991) showed that most biological accounts of male-female differences in health opportunities are at worst sexist and at best equivocal. She took the analysis further to show that the very statistics which have given rise to biological accounts of gender differences are themselves suspect. Women, for example, are commonly cast in the role of the greatest users of health services, yet she found that women had higher rates of hospitalization in only about one third of the diagnostic categories, and that much of their apparent excess use of health services was related to the female reproductive system. In fact, women's higher use of medication, Kane (1991) found, can be largely accounted for by the use of the oral contraceptive pill. What emerged from Kane's overview of women's health statistics from around the world was a picture of genuinely different patterns of health risk for women which requires the development of appropriate health services, such as those developed through the women's health movement during the last quarter of the twentieth century.

The women's health movement emerged as a response to women's complaints about the inappropriateness of mainstream, medical model, health services which, in reality, deal with illness rather than health. The medical model of health care was described by Russell and Schofield (1986) in terms of three key characteristics: it is cure focused; individualistic in orientation; and interventionist in nature. However, much of women's contact with health services arises from reproductive concerns such as contraception, pregnancy and childbirth. These are not diseases and do not, necessarily, require interventionist treatment.

A particular problem for women has been the uncritical adoption by mainstream health services of patriarchal social values. Dally (1991) showed how, from its very inception, the medical profession confirmed prejudices about women and raised sexist judgements to the status of scientific propositions.

An example of prejudice masquerading as medical science may be found in the 'conservation of energy' theory. During the nineteenth century the quantity of energy in the human body was held to be constant. Consequently 'because reproduction was the sole purpose of women's existence...women ought to concentrate their physical energy internally, toward the womb' (Dally 1991:39). Reflecting this theory, the medical advice offered to women was to refrain from physical activity particularly at puberty and during menstruation. The result was that many middle and upper class women were effectively inhibited from participation in public life. Working class women meanwhile worked in factories and mines.

So powerful was the influence of sexist values on the development of medicine that Virchow, recognized as one of the greatest pathologists of the nineteenth century, wrote: 'woman is a pair of ovaries with a human being attached; whereas man is a human being furnished with a pair of testes' (Dally 1991:84). This embodiment of women in terms of their reproductive function continued into the present century, influencing medical research in a manner which had appalling consequences for the women involved in the 'unfortunate experiment' at the National Women's Hospital, Auckland, New Zealand.

The 'unfortunate experiment', conducted over a twenty year period to the mid 1980s, was motivated by the desire of the doctor in charge of the research to reduce the number of hysterectomies performed on women with positive Pap smears indicating carcinoma in situ. In his view it was a woman's 'heritage' (Coney 1988:50) to keep her uterus intact. He hypothesized that carcinoma in situ was a non-invasive cell abnormality. To prove his theory, women with positive Pap smears were denied correct treatment over a period of some 20 years in spite of local and international evidence that carcinoma in situ is invasive. As a consequence many women died and many others were left physically and emotionally scarred. In one poignant case study of 'Mrs

M', Coney (1988:85) showed that in the doctor's attempts to preserve her uterus she had visited the hospital 65 times and had at least 50 vaginal examinations and 12 general anaesthetics. All this for a woman in her forties who had already been sterilized. She died 'with her uterus intact, though with no bowel, and no function in her bladder and her vagina scarred beyond recognition' (Coney 1988:85).

Some doctors at the Auckland hospital tried unsuccessfully to stop the experiment, but the principal researcher held a powerful position and was able to squash opposition. Where doctors failed, consumers had little hope. In any case the women involved in the experiment had not been informed of the true nature of their condition nor had they been asked for their consent to participate in the experiment. Two central points emerge from this case study of the 'unfortunate experiment'. The first is the continuing embodiment of women in terms of their reproductive function by a patriarchal medical profession. The second concerns the power relationships, on the one hand between doctors in hierarchical medical organizations and, on the other, between doctors and their patients. The problem for women, therefore, is not only the medical model of health care but also patriarchy and power as these operate in medical practice.

The link between medicine and patriarchy, Ehrenreich and English (1979) suggested, has not been coincidental, passive or benign. Rather, the medical profession has been actively involved in the suppression of women and their traditional knowledge of health and healing. This understanding places the women's health movement's objective of asserting women's rights in health care at the 'cutting edge of sexual politics' (Coney 1988:16).

In concrete terms the problems which women have faced in their contact with mainstream health services have included the medicalization of the natural processes of pregnancy and childbirth; the trivialization of their health problems; the treatment of social and emotional problems with medical solutions such as tranquillizers; patronizing attitudes of doctors; and the mismanagement of women's mental health problems.

The point, however, is not just to document the injustices which women face in caring for their health. The point is to rectify them. This has been an objective of the women's health movement born of the resurgence of feminism at the end of the 1960s. Faced with the enormity of the problems and the complexity of the issues, the women's health movement had to seek innovative ways of promoting women's health. How this was done was described in a recent international study (Hunt 1991) which revealed that, although the work of women's health activists in a range of developed countries varied with local circumstances, their work was informed by three fundamental ideologies: feminism; empowerment; and the social model of health. In order to comprehend their work it is important not only to understand something of these ideologies but also the importance of ideology in shaping any social change.

Contemporary feminism is not a unitary ideology. Indeed, Tong (1992) documented seven major strands of feminist thought with many shades of opinion in each. More commonly, feminist thought is typified as comprising three major bodies of opinion: liberal, radical and socialist feminism. The difference between the three perspectives lies in the identified source of women's oppression and the consequent political agenda for change.

On the whole, liberal feminists tend to be more supportive of the status quo and seek equality within it. Socialist feminists focus on the inequalities for women which are inherent in the capitalist system. By contrast, radical feminists lay bare the structures of patriarchy which are everywhere apparent regardless of the economic structure of society. In spite of these different perspectives, what all feminists have in common is the goal of empowering women.

Empowerment is about the creation of a just society in which people may become self-directed through the creation of opportunities to choose between realistic alternatives. A clear account of what people need in order to be empowered was developed by the Youth Affairs Council of Australia (1983). It called for: new forms of organization; new knowledge; skills development; access to resources (including funding); and social and political action to create equitable social systems. In the case of the women's health movement the goal is a just system of health for women.

The issue of justice in women's health care extends the vision beyond biological health because many of women's health concerns have been identified as being social in origin. As a consequence, feminist health workers, along with those working with disadvantaged groups such as Aborigines, have developed a social as distinct from a medical model of health. The social model of health recognizes the interconnected nature of people's complex lives and contextualizes biological health in its social, economic, cultural and psychological dimensions. The social model of health incorporates wellness, a philosophy which moves beyond freedom from illness to models of human fulfilment and self-discovery. The solutions go beyond cure, illness prevention and health promotion to social action for a healthier society.

If social action is to succeed, observed Kaplan (1992), the oppressors must be dealt with. There are, she noted (Kaplan 1992:273), only three ways of doing this: 'kill them, force them to leave, or force them to undergo ideological re-education'. As none of these presents a realistic alternative, feminist health workers sought a different solution. They side-stepped mainstream health services, moved around the medical profession and set up an alternative system of women's health centres. From this base they have continued to lobby for change in mainstream health services and in society.

Women's health centres in the western world vary from small organizations, which act as information and referral centres, to larger establishments which offer a full complement of medical, counselling and health promotion services. Women's health centres are distinguished from mainstream health services by process. When challenged to identify the difference, feminist health workers most commonly reply 'we listen' (Hunt forthcoming).

Of itself, the willingness to listen seems to offer little of a distinctive nature by which to identify process in the women's health movement. However, in the context of women's evidence that doctors do not listen (Broom Darroch 1978, Miles 1991), it remains a significant achievement. Further, women's health centres are deliberately designed to be homely, fostering an environment in which women are actively encouraged to talk. This contrasts with the clinical and hurried atmosphere of medical centres. Finally, feminist health workers identified empowerment as a process of providing women with the necessary information and resources to make their own decisions (Hunt 1991). By so doing they seek to avoid creating in women's health centres the dependency which has been characteristic of women's role in patriarchal society in general and in their relationship with health professionals in particular.

It would be contradictory for feminist health workers to empower women by facilitating personal decision making if the workers themselves were subject to hierarchical controls. Women's health centres have, therefore, tried to establish new forms of organization—usually a collective or at least a flattened managerial structure. McShane and Oliver (1987) identified some of the main characteristics of feminist organization. These included consensus or collegiate decision making; the representation of women's rather than experts' viewpoints; personalized interaction rather than the impersonal nature of relationships in bureaucracies; and an accountability to consumers and the collective rather than external or government agencies.

At times, experiments with new forms of organization have created difficulties and contradictions. In the Australian context, Broom (1991) documented the achievements and problems of Australian women's health centres and analysed the difficulty of trying to be different in a funding context which constrains the organizational form of health centres to conventional models and government requirements. Hunt (1991) found that the centres which best preserved their feminist organization were those which maintained independent funding sources. These centres, though, faced the dilemma of being poorly funded and, therefore, potentially less effective in promoting women's health.

It is part of the empowerment philosophy that, wherever possible, client and provider groups should be matched in terms of social characteristics because: 'our own race, class and background must influence our familiarity with different client groups and our skill in maintaining contact and dealing effectively with them' (Helean & Huygens 1986:194). Consequently, women's health centres are invariably run by women. This practice is developed further in multicultural women's health centres which are staffed by women drawn from local ethnic groups.

The extent to which separate centres should develop catering for distinct needs is viewed as problematic by some women's health workers (Hunt 1991). Some lesbian women, for example, felt that their needs should be met within women's health centres—to do otherwise would be to bow to the homophobic tendencies of society and to marginalize lesbian health care. In Amsterdam, by contrast, a lesbian doctor found that her clientele largely comprised lesbian women, suggesting a need for a lesbian-centred service (Hunt 1991). One of the difficulties in developing services for special groups of women is that they may incorporate an essentialist approach which suggests that all women in a particular group are the same. One women's health worker, interested in lesbian health care, raised this concern: 'I don't know if you need a separate place...I mean it is a really diffuse group of people anyway' (Hunt forthcoming).

Without exception, women's health centres seek to empower women through information sharing. However, given the patriarchal construction of medical knowledge about women (Dally 1991), it has been necessary for women to develop their own health information. In this sense knowledge is not an unchanging set of facts and figures, rather it is socially structured. It can, therefore, be restructured. A significant landmark in the development of women's knowledge about their own health was the publication of the book *Our Bodies Our Selves* (Boston Women's Health Book Collective 1971). It was revolutionary not only in the intention to empower women with health information, but also in the manner in which women's own experiences were incorporated as a legitimate form of knowledge alongside scientific evidence. The publication highlighted a number of features in the creation of women's health information: the women worked collectively; fact and feeling were mingled; lay women showed that they could handle technical/medical information and relay that knowledge in understandable language; and, finally, the book included an acceptance of self-help and alternative health care strategies.

Women's health workers have developed unique processes for the sharing of health information which differ from mainstream health promotion strategies (Hunt 1992). In general, government sponsored, mainstream, health promotion has emphasized personal health skills and concentrated on changing lifestyle factors which cause diseases. In particular, attention has been focused on today's major killers: heart attacks and cancer. These health education priorities have been criticized by feminists for their male bias and neglect of women's health issues such as menstruation, post-natal depression, and male violence against women.

More significantly, in focusing on single aspects of negative health behaviour, health education messages have ignored the interconnected nature of women's lives and the complexity of individual constructions of health. This point may be illustrated by reference to the work of feminist Ann Oakley (1989), who spoke at length with pregnant, working-class women who had continued to smoke even though they understood health education information about the harmful effects of smoking on the fetus. Some women had, in fact, incorporated the health promotion information into their own constructions of health and were deliberately smoking in order to keep their babies small so as to facilitate childbirth. Others continued to smoke to create some personal space for themselves in a life rendered unpredictable by poverty and unsuccessful marriage.

The parameters of an alternative, feminist model of health promotion have been sketched by Whatley (1988) and fleshed out by Shaw and Tilden (1990). In essence they moved health promotion beyond compliance with professional notions of positive health behaviour into a social action model which starts with women's stated needs.

Directed by the social model of health and their own experience, feminist health workers have focused on changing the alienating circumstances of women's lives rather than altering negative health behaviours. The reason for this was made clear by a counsellor working at an Australian women's health centre: 'I've been here [for a number of] years and in that time I've only seen one woman whose problem was not explained by her context or her life history' (Hunt 1992). Persuaded by the view that it is better to deal with the source of the problem rather than to 'band-aid' the symptom, feminist health promotion workers have challenged women's role in society and revealed in sharp profile the essentially political nature of health promotion. In Dublin, this approach has resulted in a government backlash. There, women's health workers have, for several years, been placed under legal injunction not to give women information about abortion, or even information about where to get information.

The issues of abortion and freedom of choice for women in their own reproductive concerns are central to any feminist agenda for change. Without adequate birth control techniques, including abortion, women will be forever condemned either to celibacy or the unpredictable processes of conception, child bearing and child rearing. Motivated by the desire to create choice for pregnant women, feminist health workers lobby in support of abortion services. Their stance is best characterized as pro-choice rather than pro-abortion. To illustrate this point, Rowland (1984) referred to China where the one child per family policy has resulted in enforced abortions in the eighth month of pregnancy.

Neither in Ireland nor China do women themselves have a free choice. Indeed Chattoo (1990:333) referred to a range of studies (Reed 1987, Mies 1987) to substantiate the view that 'ever since the advent of agriculture, no society has ever left the choice to reproduce totally to the individual'. To oppose state control of reproductive issues and assert women's right to freedom of choice, by definition thus transforms health promotion into a political activity.

Networking has been the basis of feminist political activity. By working together and sharing information, coalitions of small women's health groups, such as the Amsterdam based Women's Global Network on Reproductive Rights, have provided a broad basis for social action. On some issues, such as the defective intrauterine device, the Dalkon Shield, and the misuse of the drug, diethylstilbestrol (DES), women's health groups have lobbied with considerable success. The Dalkon Shield, which damaged women's health and fertility, has now been withdrawn from the market and compensation, won through class action in the United States, paid to victims.

DES was used in North America and Europe from the 1950s to the 1970s, being prescribed to prevent miscarriage. This was so even though its efficacy was in doubt. Some daughters of the mothers who used the drug are now presenting with rare forms of vaginal cancer. Tudiver (1986) recounted the success of DES action groups around the world which researched this problem and disseminated information with the result that people at risk are now being monitored rather than ignored.

In the critical stand which it has adopted, the women's health movement may be understood as part of the wider analysis (Illich 1976) of the limits of medicine as it has come to be practised in the western world. Yet, it is more than this because it has moved on to establish its own alternative vision of health care for women. This vision changes in accordance with local circumstances. As Shaw and Tilden (1990:7) so aptly pointed out, what actually happens is a combination of what feminist health workers would like to do and the constraints placed on their activities by the immediate context. This kaleidoscope of images makes it difficult to encapsulate the essence of the movement. In any case, defining the women's health movement is almost impossible because social movements of this kind exist in and through the perspective of others. The women's health movement has, therefore, been hailed as visionary by some and reviled by others. Kaplan (1992:3) did offer some opportunity for a more substantive, less relativistic, definition in her observation that the 'outstanding feature of postwar movements lies in their self-definition'. This being so it has been possible in this chapter to draw on Hunt's (1991) analysis of the international women's health movement as seen through the eyes of feminist health workers. From this study emerged a picture of the women's health movement as a revolutionary response to the problems presented to women by patriarchal, medical model health care. That response has been guided by a unique combination of feminist and health theory and has resulted in a range of innovative women's health centres which care for women's immediate health needs while continuing to challenge the social circumstances which circumscribe women's opportunities for well-being, justice and health.

REFERENCES

Boston Women's Health Book Collective 1971 Our bodies our selves. Simon Schuster, New York
Broom Darroch D 1978 Power and participation: the dynamics of medical encounters. Unpublished PhD thesis, Australian National University, Canberra
Broom D 1991 Damned if we do: contradictions in women's health care. Allen & Unwin, Sydney
Chattoo S 1990 A sociological study of certain aspects of disease and death: a case study of Muslims in Kashmir. Unpublished PhD thesis, University of Delhi

Coney S 1988 The unfortunate experiment. Penguin, Auckland

Dally A 1991 Women under the knife: a history of surgery. Hutchinson Radius, London

Ehrenreich B, English D 1979 For her own good, 150 years of the experts' advice to women. Anchor/Doubleday, New York

Helean J, Huygens I 1986 Empowerment in alcohol services: a model for developing human resources. Proceedings of the 8th conference of the international federation of non-governmental organizations for the prevention of drug and substance abuse, Alcohol and Drug Foundation, Canberra

Hunt L 1991 Women's health promotion, an international perspective. Centre for the Development of Human Resources, Edith Cowan University, Perth

Hunt L 1992 A feminist critique of health education. Paper presented to the Sociological Association of Australia conference, Adelaide

Hunt L (forthcoming) An institutional ethnography of the women's health movement: the study of a solution. PhD thesis, University of Western Australia, Perth

Illich I 1976 Limits to medicine: medical nemesis: the expropriation of health. Marion Boyars, London

Kane P 1991 Women's health: from womb to tomb. Macmillan, London

Kaplan G 1992 Contemporary western European feminism. Allen & Unwin, Sydney

McShane C, Oliver J 1987 Women's groups as alternative human service agencies. Journal of Sociology and Social Welfare 5(5):615–626

Mies M 1987 Sexist and racist implications of new reproductive technologies. Alternatives XII:323–342

Miles A 1991 Women, health and medicine. Open University Press, Buckingham

Oakley A 1989 Smoking in pregnancy: smokescreen or risk factor? toward a materialist analysis. Sociology of Health and Illness 11(4):311–335

Reed J 1987 History of contraceptive practices. In: Spicker S F, Bondeson W B, Engelhardt H T (eds) The contraceptive ethos. Reidel, Dordrecht, pp 15–38

Rowland R 1984 Reproductive technology. Deakin Media Production, Geelong

Russell C, Schofield T 1986 Where it hurts, an introduction to sociology for health workers. Allen & Unwin, Sydney

Shaw L, Tilden J 1990 Creating health for women: a community health promotion handbook. Brisbane Women's Community Health Centre, Wooloongabba

Tong R 1992 Feminist thought. Routledge, London

Tudiver S 1986 The strengths of links: international women's health networks in the eighties. In: McDonnell K (ed) Adverse effects, women and the pharmaceutical industry. Women's Educational Press, Toronto

Whatley M H 1988 Beyond compliance: towards a feminist health education. In: Worcester N, Whatley M H (eds) Women's health: readings on social, economic and political issues. Kendall/Hunt, Dubuque, pp 131–143

Youth Affairs Council of Australia 1983 Creating tomorrow today. Youth Affairs Council of Australia, St Kilda

28. Taken down and used against us: women's health services

Dorothy H. Broom

Reflecting on some recent cases before the Human Rights and Equal Opportunities Commission (HREOC), one might wonder about the original purpose of the Sex Discrimination Act (1984)(SDA). A major objective of the Act is to give effect to Australia's ratification of the UN Convention on the Elimination of All Forms of Discrimination Against Women. Although many women have been able to use it effectively, weaknesses in the Act have given a tool to men seeking to constrain women's claims and inhibit affirmative action. The 'Proudfoot' complaint against women's health centres (described below) is a cautionary case in point. Indeed, when the House of Representatives Standing Committee on Legal and Constitutional Affairs published its 'Report on the Inquiry into Equal Opportunity and Equal Status for Women', it called the case a 'challenge to the effectiveness of the SDA' (p265). This chapter presents a brief summary of what transpired, followed by a few comments about problems and questions that emerge from the case and the decision.

The case

This case had its inception in July 1990 when Dr Alex Proudfoot (principal adviser to the Therapeutic Goods Division of the Commonwealth Department of Health, Housing and Community Services) filed a complaint with the Human Rights and Equal Opportunities Commission. The complaint claimed to act on behalf of all men in the Australian Capital Territory (ACT), and asserted that they were 'persons aggrieved' by the ACT government's efforts to identify women's special health needs, by its provision of services specifically to women, and by funding such services. The complaint alleged that special women's health services are discriminatory under the Sex Discrimination Act because men cannot access them, because men's health is worse than women's, and because the services address problems that are not unique to women. Gynaecological and reproductive health services were explicitly excluded from the complaint, as indeed they would have to be since the Act permits services that can, by their nature, only be delivered to members of one sex. Consequently, the case concerned only services and information concerning conditions that, at least theoretically, occur in both sexes.

Proudfoot named the ACT Government, the ACT Board of Health (the ACT's name for its health department), and the Canberra Women's Health Centre as respondents. At the time the complaint was lodged, the Canberra Women's Health Centre had not yet begun operations. It had an interim management committee and was in the early planning stages, but there were no premises or staff or services available from the Centre. The ACT Board of Health had been running a women's health service for several years, and this service—which had not previously provoked a complaint—was also threatened. Subsequent to the original complaint, two other men filed related complaints. They named the Commonwealth and complained about its consultative activities leading to the formulation of the National Women's Health Policy as well as the allocation of funding under the National Women's Health Program and the services provided. The three complaints were considered jointly. Unlike the majority of complaints before HREOC, conciliation was considered to be inappropriate, and the complaints went to a hearing at which two of the three complainants were present.

When all the complaints are taken into account, the respondents in the case were the Commonwealth of Australia, the ACT Government, the ACT Board of Health, and the Canberra Women's Health Centre (an independently incorporated community based women's health centre jointly funded under the National Women's Health Program by the Commonwealth and ACT governments). The Commonwealth sought to have itself joined to the original complaint because it recognized the relevance of the complaint to its National Women's Health Program, but in any event it was named by the second and third complaints.

Clearly, much was at stake in this complex case, with its obscure legal points, concrete community based health services, government policies and programs and numerous (and various) participants. To my knowledge, women's services had never before been subjected to legal attack in Australia. The matter was regarded by everyone involved as a test case for women's health services all over the country, and potentially for other women's services. Several of the legal arguments had not been tested previously, so the case is legally significant as well as substantially significant to women's services. It would clearly be an important landmark in interpretation of the Sex Discrimination Act. Although race and age discrimination are prohibited by other Commonwealth and State acts, there was concern in some quarters that the decision might influence thinking about other forms of discrimination.

At law, the case turned on three basic questions, elaborated below: standing; discrimination (as defined by the Sex Discrimination Act); and exemptions.

Standing. This concerns who is entitled to bring complaints before the Commission. It is not enough to have an emotional or intellectual interest; one must be a 'person aggrieved' in order to have the Commission investigate or hear a complaint. Quoting an English legal precedent from Lord Denning, Chris Ronalds, acting for the ACT, argued that a person aggrieved does not include 'a mere busybody interfering in things that do not concern him'. None of the complainants had sought services from a women's health facility, nor have they been affected by the services they sought to close. Ronalds argued that the complainants do not qualify as persons aggrieved and hence that the action should not proceed. Proudfoot claimed being a doctor gave him standing. He also claimed that, because he is a man, the very existence of the services complained of gave him standing. This is a circular argument which would have required a prior determination that the services were discriminatory, when the submission on standing questioned his right to have his complaint heard in the first place. The third complainant based his claim to standing simply on his masculinity, again a tautological argument.

Discrimination. This is closely related to the matter of standing. Traditionally, two criteria must be met to sustain the definition of 'discrimination' under the Sex Discrimination Act. First, the person complaining must have suffered a *detriment* from the differential treatment. Second, the *circumstances* of the aggrieved party and the other sex must be 'the same or not materially different'. Complainants argued that men's higher age specific mortality (and certain kinds of morbidity) show that health needs of men are greater, and by implication signal detriment. The respondents argued that no discrimination had occurred because neither criterion for discrimination could be fulfilled: the complainants had not suffered any harm from the acts complained of; and in any event, the circumstances of women and men seeking health services are materially different.

Exemptions. Even if an act is found to be discriminatory, it may be lawful if it is exempted under one of several sections of the Sex Discrimination Act providing a defence for discrimination. Advocates for the respondents argued that women's health services were protected by at least two exemptions which I will discuss in a moment.

To the legally uninitiated, it was not always easy to tell which of these elements was at issue. The arguments were often remarkably similar as Ronald Wilson dealt with each of them in turn. The hearing and associated preparation absorbed months of time. ACT women's health workers were deflected from delivering services to fighting for the survival of the services, and for the survival of women's health centres all over the country. There were four days of hearings, hundreds of pages of evidence, exhibits, submissions and transcripts. Distinguished witnesses gave evidence defending women's health initiatives. None of the complainants' witnesses were called, so they pursued their argument by presenting their own submissions and cross examining witnesses for the respondents. Three barristers, four solicitors and numerous public servants from the ACT and the Commonwealth applied their expertise to the matter. The complainants represented themselves, and used this fact frequently to highlight their alleged underdog status. Because most of those involved participated as part of their normal work duties (or perhaps, more accurately, in addition to or instead of their usual tasks), it is not possible to determine how much the battle cost, but it was surely expensive.

The decision

Finally, in March 1992, the President of the Human Rights Commission handed down his judgment. The bottom line—quite literally—of Justice Wilson's decision is that he finds 'all the complaints unsubstantiated. They are therefore dismissed.' The decision results simply in legal legitimation for women's health services to continue doing what they were doing before they were interrupted by the complaint.

Wilson did not, in the end, discuss the question of standing, despite having received submissions on the matter. However, he found that the services are discriminatory under the definition of discrimination in Sex Discrimination Act, but he ruled that they are exempted, in one case (the ACT Women's Health Service) by Section 32 (which permits 'services the nature of which is such that they can only be provided to members of one sex') or Section 33 (the so-called 'affirmative action' or special measures section which was considered to apply to both the Service and the Canberra Women's Health Centre). Thus, women's health services in the ACT are lawful, and so, presumably, are similar services around the country. None of the complainants appealed against the decision.

To the services, the important result is that they are now free to get on with the job. The judgment acknowledges that women are disadvantaged in obtaining adequate and appropriate health services, and that some of their health needs (not only reproductive and gynaecological) are best addressed through special, targeted services. Furthermore, it confirms that it is lawful for governments to consult about, fund and deliver such services. These findings will come as no surprise to people involved in public health policy and programs in Australia, and one can only be relieved that Sir Ronald Wilson was able to write a judgment that leaves these activities unconstrained by the operation of the Sex Discrimination Act. However, the conduct of the case, and certain aspects of the decision, reveal a number of unanswered questions.

First, one might well wonder about a legal definition of discrimination that would permit women's health services to be found discriminatory despite the fact that—as Wilson acknowledges—men suffer no detriment from their activities. The legalistic comparison based definition of discrimination is a product of the political compromises of the mid 1980s, compromises which are often hazardous to women and ought to be reconsidered in the 1990s. To establish discrimination, the Act relies on statistical comparisons between groups rather than disadvantage to women, as the UN Convention on the Elimination of All Forms of Discrimination Against Women might have suggested. The spuriously 'balanced' or neuter definition made it possible for this costly complaint to proceed. The question of whether discrimination had occurred was reduced by the complainants to a simple question of supposedly statistical 'fact': which sex is 'sicker'? On this reasoning, if a group can establish *any* deficit compared to another group, that deficit might be argued as 'evidence' of discrimination. Oddly, a similar line of reasoning—and clear demonstration of material deficit—has not been outstandingly successful in women's efforts to establish indirect or structural discrimination in claims for equal pay, for example. One is left to wonder why it is simply good business to pay child care workers less than plumbers, but it is 'discrimination' to provide health services specifically to women.

Elements of the decision also show both strengths and weaknesses in the Act. The application of Section 32 to the activities of the ACT Women's Health Service is regarded in some circles as a 'courageous' decision which 'makes law', and certainly that part of the judgment shows real insight into a social view of health and well-being, and a willingness to use the law to protect targeted services. However, there are complications. Wilson has exempted the respondents using two sections of the Act, but he does not make clear why only Section 33 was applied only to the Canberra Women's Health Centre, while both Section 32 and Section 33 were applied to the ACT Women's Health Service. The absence of clinical services from the Centre may be relevant, but the decision does not say so. (Perhaps it was simply an oversight in the submissions for the Centre.) Nor is it apparent to the lay reader why the argument about women's distinctive health needs (which forms the basis of Wilson's decision to accept Section 32 for the Service) was not relevant to the original question of discrimination. If this matter had been decided against the complaints, resort to the exemptions would have been preempted. The apparent inconsistency reinforces the impression that the Act's definition of discrimination is flawed.

Finally, reliance on Section 33 to protect women's services, although effective at the moment, must leave one with a sense of unease. The recent report of the House of Representatives Standing Committee on Legal and Constitutional Affairs acknowledges that women's needs should be defined by women themselves (p248) which would have made a stark contrast to the definition of needs deployed in the discrimination hearing, but more of that in a moment. However, Lavarche's recommendations merely suggest that the Attorney-General's Department consult with HREOC to 'determine if an amendment is necessary to Section 33' (p265). One would think, after this hearing, that an additional inquiry had become superfluous! Given that 'special measures' are, by vague definition, temporary, one is prompted to wonder how durable a Section 33 exemption will be, and on what basis it might be terminated. Of course, governments do not need to rely on the Sex Discrimination Act to close women's services: they can do that through the simple economic or political expedient of withdrawing funds. But for the lawfulness of women's services to hang on such a slender thread is a cause for some disquiet to anyone who believes in the value and usefulness (let alone the cost effectiveness) of the services that were put on the line. This appears to be a defect not in the decision but in the legislation being interpreted. To this lay observer, Wilson has done the best he could with a cumbersome and defective Act.

The questions

To the student of the sociology of health and illnesses, a number of interesting questions are raised by this case. I will discuss only a few of them.

The location of this debate in the setting of a hearing before the Human Rights and Equal Opportunities Commission creates a disturbing precedent for the involvement of the law in health. Previously, the law has been mobilized in two broad medical domains:

1. Professional questions such as licensing, regulation of the right to practice, and adjudication of malpractice; and
2. Contested clinical matters such as the right to die, establishing who may give permission for procedures for patients who may not be capable of giving informed consent, and when death has occurred.

That this case effectively concerned resource allocation rather than professional or clinical questions makes it a novel involvement of the law in health, and potentially attributes to judges a capacity to interpret and rule on public health matters. Of course judges are often required to rule on issues containing technical questions with which they have no expertise, and one could say that health should be no exception. Matters of resource allocation, however, have until now been considered the province of the legislative and administrative branches of government where a number of perspectives are taken into account, and where decisions are the responsibility of groups of experts, not one individual.

Quite apart from the implications arising from that precedent, having this *particular* case decided on the basis of a quasi-judicial hearing creates a poignant dilemma. Most readers will be aware that Australian women's health centres have been created by women who mobilized action from their analysis of the political nature of women's individual, personal experiences (Broom 1991: Ch. 2). In brief, that analysis identified deficiencies in mainstream medicine, deficiencies that arose out of the patriarchal foundations of medical institutions and medical training (Ayanian & Epstein 1991, Broverman et al 1970, 1972, Ehrenreich & English 1973, McRae 1981, Martin 1987, Miles 1991, Nathanson 1975, Prather & Minkow 1991, Standing 1980, Steingart et al 1991, Waitzkin 1991, Wallen et al 1979). The Women's Movement was constantly confronted with women's accounts: accounts of being ignored, trivialized, over-medicated and mutilated by doctors. Academics were often of little help because many of them accepted the medical view of health, including women's health, and anyway, academic research into women's health was limited in scope, quantity and quality (Council on Ethical and Judicial Affairs, American Medical Association

1991, Dresser 1992, Kane 1991a, 1991b, O'Connor et al 1990, Sibbison 1990). Consequently, the women's health movement sought to establish women centred/women run services that would provide an alternative to mainstream facilities, a site where health development might occur, a base for advocacy, a place to gather and disseminate information, a research focus, and a model from which the mainstream might learn. Central to the motivation was (and is) the explicit conviction that the personal is political, that women's lives and feelings and experiences count.

By mounting the case in a quasi-legal setting, the issue of what would be accepted as evidence was heavily weighted against such convictions. There was considerable emphasis on epidemiological, medically based statistics, and medical authority in the form of published reports of clinical research. Academic authority was also at a premium, although the complainants sought to discredit all witnesses except those in active medical practice. In other words, the very institutions whose hegemonic male practices and discourses had motivated the establishment of women's health services in the first place were now to adjudicate on whether these same services would be allowed to continue to function. Women's services were forced to engage the debate on a terrain and in a language that were systematically hostile to their fundamental raison d'etre. The same body of medical research that had been unable to envisage women's health as anything more than breasts and uteri was now the only legitimate source of statements to defend women's health services that were under attack precisely *because* they extended beyond reproductive matters. Evidence about women's unhappiness, the inadequacies of mainstream/'malestream' services, the absences in research and the slurs and silences in training might have seemed 'soft' and diffuse alongside age-specific death rates and incidence of high blood pressure. The Human Rights Commission is not bound by strict rules of evidence, but the ambiguity of the decision—finding discrimination but ultimately dismissing the complaints—suggests that the academic and statistical may have been persuasive, and the respondents were only partially successful at introducing alternative ways of formulating the issues.

Another issue is the formulation of a health resources allocation debate in terms of a 'zero-sum game'. The basic argument of the complainants, and one which a hearing of this kind is utterly unable to render problematic, is that if women benefit, men must suffer. If women are better off, then men must, by definition, be worse off. If any resources are being invested in women's health, it must be at the expense of men's health resources. Therefore, the only way to improve men's health is to stop activities designed to benefit women. Of course, at the simplest level such an argument is true: money spent on X (or XX) cannot be spent on Y (or XY). But this is not the model of health resources allocation by which governments (let alone the private sector) currently operate. If it were, all Australia's medical resources would be invested in Aboriginal health services instead of being concentrated as it is overwhelmingly on the non-Aboriginal population. However, from the public health perspective, the issue is far more complex and interactive than that, and the zero-sum model obscures more than it reveals as an approach to allocating health resources where they will be effective. It assumes a simple comparability of any given health need or service for women with a direct cognate need or service for men, a confusion that may appeal intuitively but does not withstand thoughtful analysis.

The new interest in 'men's health' can become a welcome development. It encourages service providers, policy makers and the general population to take seriously the relevance of gender to health instead of relegating it to the marginalized status of a 'women's issue'. Often, the activities of the women's health movement have been seen in some quarters as making a 'special case' of women, asking for privileges and resources to be allocated to women that are not accorded to the population at large. This mentality informed the complainants in the HREOC case. But fortunately, the complainants do not hold a monopoly on models for men's health. Indeed, when pursued constructively, attention to men's health will help us to understand that gender is potentially relevant to everyone's health, not just women. By exploring when and in what ways gender and health interact, we may develop more useful and effective models of women's health as well as men's, and improve the ways various sick care and health services are organized and delivered. The women's health movement has cleared significant theoretical and policy terrain. Now, like the women's health movement, a positive men's health movement has the potential to contribute to the health of the whole community.

REFERENCES

Ayanian J Z, Epstein A M 1991 Differences in the use of procedures between women and men hospitalized for coronary heart disease. New England Journal of Medicine 325:221–225

Broom D H 1991 Damned if we do: contradictions in women's health care. Allen & Unwin, Sydney

Broverman I K et al 1970 Sex role stereotypes and clinical judgments of mental health. Journal of Consulting and Clinical Psychology 34:1–7

Broverman I K et al 1972 Sex role stereotypes: a current appraisal. Journal of Social Issues 28:59–78

Council on Ethical and Judicial Affairs, American Medical Association 1991 Gender disparities in clinical decision making. Journal of the American Medical Association 226:559–562

Dresser R 1992 Wanted: single, white male for medical research. Hastings Center Report (Jan-Feb):24–29

Ehrenreich B, English D 1973 Complaints and disorders: the sexual politics of sickness. Feminist Press, Old Westbury NY

House of Representatives Standing Committee on Legal and Constitutional Affairs 1992 Half way to equal: report of the inquiry into equal opportunity and equal status for women in Australia. AGPS, Canberra

Kane P 1991a Women's health: from womb to tomb. Macmillan, Melbourne

Kane P 1991b Researching women's health: an issues paper. AGPS, Canberra

Martin E 1987 The women in the body. Beacon Press, Boston

McRae F B 1980 The politics of menopause: the discovery of a deficiency disease. Social

Problems 31:111–123

Miles A 1991 Women, health and medicine. Open University Press, Milton Keynes

Nathanson C 1975 Illness and the feminine role. Social Science and Medicine 9:57–62

O'Connor D et al 1990 A sliver—not even a slice: a report of a study on expenditure on women and health research. Melbourne District Health Council, Melbourne

Prather J E, Minkow N V 1991 Prescription for despair: women and psychotropic drugs. In: Van Den Bergh N (ed) Feminist perspectives on addictions. Springer, New York, ch 6

Sibbison J B 1990 Women's health, women's rights. The Lancet July 21:166

Standing H 1980 Sickness is a women's business? In: Birke L et al (eds) Alice through the microscope: the power of science over women's lives. Virago, London, pp 124–138

Steingart R M et al 1991 Sex differences in the management of coronary artery disease. New England Journal of Medicine 325:226–230

Waitzkin H 1991 The politics of medical encounters. Yale University Press, New Haven

Wallen J, Waitzkin H, Stoeckle J D 1979 Physician stereotypes about female health and illness. Women and Health 4 (2):135–146

Epilogue

The genesis of this book was the Australian Sociological Association's (TASA) annual meetings at Murdoch University, Perth. Half of its chapters are revised versions of papers presented there. The other half were solicited from scholars also doing research in what may be called, 'health anthrosociology'. Together, the chapters provide a comprehensive coverage of the field for undergraduates and a firm basis for postgraduates and colleagues to undertake future research. But the chapters do more: being research in handson settings, they offer the practical for health practitioners and promoters.

The book began with the letter below (somewhat abridged) sent to each contributor:

Dear

Alan Petersen and I have just contracted to put a book together and we want your work to be part of it. The book is entitled *Just Health:...* (any ideas for a subtitle are welcomed) and is being published by Churchill Livingstone. Some details about the book are:

1. Its general theme is social justice in the broadest sense of that term;
2. Its focus is on health, illness, health care and policy in Australia and New Zealand;
3. It includes anthropological and sociological researchers since we think that at least in this area they have more in common than difference (e.g. eschewing reductionism and explaining social behaviour by locating it in its socio-cultural context);
4. It is primarily oriented to second and third year students but should also serve as a basis for future postgraduate and other professional research;
5. Each chapter is to be research based so that students see anthropology and sociology as activities and not merely as entities that live on a shelf.

Your chapter should be approximately 5000 to 6000 words. It should be directed to students not colleagues and therefore is not so much an article as scholarly work that you know students will read.

With all the above in mind, Alan and I want you to feel free, flexible and bold in your writing so that students can appreciate the anthropology and sociology of health, illness, health care and policy in Australia and New Zealand.

Alan and I are very keen about *Just Health* and think it will build upon the good works already being used in our courses.

Thank you.

Kind regards,

Charles Waddell

We present this letter here not so much so that you can see how we put this book together but because the letter raises several fundamental points about anthro-sociology that we want to hammer home to you. The first is the theme: just health. Just health is the most common theme running through health anthro-sociological research and so, it seemed the obvious theme and title for this book.

It also says something about anthropologists and sociologists; our work is committed to social justice issues.

The second point is that anthropology and sociology have more in common than difference: both eschew reductionism—trying to explain human behaviour by reducing it to its smallest possible part (e.g. bio-psychological pathology) in much the same way that we explain algebraic equations by reducing them to their smallest components, or explaining chemical solutions by their molecular structure or principles of matter by their atomic properties. Anthro-sociology, instead, tries to see patterns of shared human behaviour rather than the more common idiosyncratic view of behaviour; and it tries to explain these patterns of behaviour by locating them in the sociocultural context within which they occur (some leaning more to structural explanations such as political economy and others leaning more to cultural explanations such as shared logic and perceptions of reality).

For example, the great efforts already in train to halt the spread of AIDS have generally taken two forms: (1) laboratory work searching for a cure and finding a vaccine to immunize people against contracting HIV (the AIDS virus); and (2) public health promotion of safer sex and intravenous drug use techniques, presumably based upon the current knowledge of laboratory scientists. As laudable as these efforts are, biochemical wizardry and safer sex and drug techniques are both a reductionist approach to the AIDS epidemic. These are common and useful approaches, but hardly anthro-sociological, for they interpret AIDS and AIDS prevention by reducing them to the smallest common denominator—molecular structures in the view of laboratory workers and, to a great extent, the exchange of bodily fluids in the field of health promotion people.

But, the AIDS epidemic is more than biochemicals and the lack of safety techniques; like so many aspects of illness, its care, and prevention discussed in this book, it is tied into the very social fabric within which we live. How we relate to each other sexually and how we alter our 'states of mind' are not randomly distributed nor can they be explained solely by biological reductionism. The structures and cultures which we create, maintain and change and which largely create, maintain and change us effect our sex and drug using behaviours.

The third and final point is that health anthro-sociology is an activity not an entity. It is a research enterprise of trying to capture human reality and explain it conceptually; to talk in the tongue of concepts but with the voice of our respondents and informants; to ask what do the people being researched see themselves as doing while simultaneously asking what are these people doing in terms of their illness, its care and prevention? A goal of this activity is just health and, as you have seen through the chapters in this book, we have a long way to go before achieving this goal. And so we invite you to engage in this activity.

Index

Note: bold page numbers refer to
major discussions of a topic.